MW01141614

# The New Middle Ages

Series Editor

Bonnie Wheeler
English & Medieval Studies
Southern Methodist University
Dallas, Texas, USA

The New Middle Ages is a series dedicated to pluridisciplinary studies of medieval cultures, with particular emphasis on recuperating women's history and on feminist and gender analyses. This peer-reviewed series includes both scholarly monographs and essay collections.

More information about this series at
http://www.springer.com/series/14239

Patricia Skinner

# Living with Disfigurement in Early Medieval Europe

palgrave
macmillan

Patricia Skinner
College of Arts and Humanities
Swansea University
Singleton Park, Swansea, SA2 8PP, United Kingdom

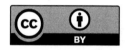

The New Middle Ages
ISBN 978-1-349-95073-7      ISBN 978-1-137-54439-1   (eBook)
DOI 10.1057/978-1-137-54439-1

Library of Congress Control Number: 2016959489

Cover illustration: © Malcolm Freeman / Alamy Stock Photo; released under a Creative
Commons Attribution 4.0 International License (CC BY 4.0)

Printed on acid-free paper

This Palgrave Macmillan imprint is published by Springer Nature
The registered company is Nature America Inc.
The registered company address is: 1 New York Plaza, New York, NY 10004, U.S.A.

*For LHM and JP, and all campaigners for equality*

# Acknowledgements

The academic profession, particularly in the UK, does not easily accommodate the non-traditional career pattern. Institutions are wary of appointing people whose age profile, or career history, do not meet certain, unwritten, criteria relating to a smooth and preferably continuous progress from doctoral study to first post and uninterrupted employment. It is a pleasure, therefore, to record my gratitude to the Wellcome Trust for the three-year fellowship (Grant number 097469) that enabled me to return to the profession after a five-year gap, and to the College of Arts and Humanities at Swansea University where I held most of it. So many people have supported the writing of this book in different ways: at Swansea, Liz Herbert McAvoy, Roberta Magnani and other colleagues within the Centre for Medieval and Early Modern Research, and Elaine Canning, Nathan Roger and the staff of the Research Institute for Arts and Humanities. I should also like to thank Peter Biller, John Henderson and Peregrine Horden, whose challenging questions helped me shape a better project; David H. Jones and colleagues at Exeter for welcoming a pre-modern specialist into their discussions on facial disfigurement in the past two centuries; James Partridge and Henrietta Spalding at Changing Faces, for their inspiration and guidance as the project progressed well beyond its original, medieval parameters; Suzannah Biernoff, Mark Bradley, Emily Cock, Luke Demaitre, Guy Geltner, Chris Mounsey, Kat Tracy, David Turner, Wendy Turner, Garthine Walker, Michelle Webb and Edward Wheatley for their insightful comments and interventions along the way; Elisabeth van Houts for her continuing friendship and support (and advice on the Normans); colleagues participating in the IMEMS seminar of Welsh universities;

Elma Brenner and Ross MacFarlane at the Wellcome Library in London; Bonnie Wheeler for her generous comments and inclusion of the book in the wonderful New Middle Ages series; the anonymous reviewer of the manuscript for their careful and engaging comments; Ryan Jenkins and Paloma Yannakakis at Palgrave US for their handling of the manuscript into an Open Access book (the first in the series, I understand!); and finally, my family, who have lent support in so many ways.

# CONTENTS

# CHAPTER 1

# Introduction: Writing and Reading About Medieval Disfigurement

"Probably from a social point of view, a simple facial disfigurement is the worst disability of all—the quickly-suppressed flicker of revulsion is, I am certain, quite shattering."[1] This statement, made by a person reflecting on his own social challenges living as a muscular dystrophy sufferer in in the 1960s, expresses succinctly the horror that facial disfigurement holds for modern observers, and its perceived place in the spectrum of social disability. Whilst modern medicine has in the intervening five decades largely perfected the process of "improving" the appearance of the disfigured face through prosthetics, surgery, skin grafts and sophisticated cosmetics, the aesthetic and technical genius of some modern medical prosthetics units is often up against deep-rooted psychological damage in the subject, which finds its expression in dissatisfaction with the "new" facial features, and may even lead to outright rejection.[2] The ingrained sense of disgust that facial damage is said to provoke in its victims and observers alike is even the subject of psychological studies, where the assumption that an impaired face *will* evoke such a response is taken as a given fact.[3] William Ian Miller puts it succinctly: "There are few things that are more unnerving and disgust evoking than our partibility... severed hands, ears, heads, gouged eyes...Severability is unnerving no matter what part is being detached."[4] The high-profile, modern cases of individuals who have "fought back" from severe facial damage, whether through burns, acid attacks or mutilation, have gone some way toward challenging such attitudes; and as historians reflect on the centenary of the destruction and loss of life inflicted in World War I, the facial disfigurement of returning soldiers from two World

© The Author(s) 2017
P. Skinner, *Living with Disfigurement in Early Medieval Europe*,
DOI 10.1057/978-1-137-54439-1_1

Wars has featured in a number of research projects, interested not only in the human story of such men, but in the early attempts at surgical and prosthetic intervention.[5] As Suzannah Biernoff comments, "being human is an aesthetic matter as well as a biological one."[6]

All of this work, however, and the very few studies that have sought to trace the history of aesthetic or cosmetic surgery, start from the assumption that acquired facial disfigurement is and was, universally, a stigmatizing—worse, a *disgusting*—condition.[7] Reading early accounts such as Ward Muir's *The Happy Hospital*, published in 1917, it is hard to avoid the sense of horror that accompanies the loss of facial features.[8] The explosion of work in the 1960s on stigma, social identity theory and deviance in the social sciences, including the influential studies of Erving Goffman and Henry Tajfel but echoing the earlier work of Durkheim on *anomie*[9] contributed toward reinforcing the apparent marginalization of *the* impaired or disfigured. Earlier generations of historians, whilst stimulated in their research questions by sociological and anthropological models, were rather too accepting of the assumptions underlying such studies, assumptions that they themselves might share. Thus physical difference, in all of its manifestations, was implicitly labeled as abnormal almost before the study began. The "impairment"—disfiguring injury—led to the "disability"—society's response to the injured face.[10] This owes much to the modern discourse within the history of medicine and surgery of the "progress" made in those fields, the ever-increasing ability of the profession to "fix" faces and bodies, and restore the individual to some kind of "normal" life. Thus both those with congenital conditions, such as cleft lip or palate, as well as those whose disfigurement is acquired during their life course, are subject (or subjected) to surgical repair, and even [physically] non-threatening conditions such as birthmarks are lasered out of existence. Yet surgery can itself also disfigure a person, particularly in the case of excision of cancerous tumors. This in turn leads to further intervention to repair the damage, introducing prosthetic replacements for the absent flesh.[11]

The early Middle Ages have not fared well within this teleological framework of surgical and medical progress: it is telling that studies of later medieval medical and surgical texts have highlighted their "rational" nature, and through such apologetic the authors of these studies have revealed their own attachment to post-Enlightenment, scientific approaches to medicine.[12] In terms of surgical treatments for the damaged face, recent attention has lighted upon texts from the early modern period, proposing ways to replace lost or damaged noses.[13] One result of this has been the under-representation of the earlier Middle Ages in histories of medicine, and an over-emphasis on the power of the written medical theory at the expense of work on the social history of medicine and practice in this period.[14]

This book seeks to address such omissions through examining social and medical responses to the disfigured face in early medieval Europe, arguing that head and facial injuries can offer a new contribution to the history of early medieval medicine, as well as offering a new route into exploring the language of violence and social interactions. In its early stages, the research underpinning the book was, it is fair to say, very much shaped by some of the assumptions outlined above—that medieval people would view disfigurement with at best ambivalence and at worst disgust. Yet this assumption has never been effectively tested within previous historiography. Despite the prevalence of warfare and violence in early medieval society, and a veritable industry studying it (largely, if not exclusively, focusing on the later Middle Ages),[15] there has in fact been very little attention paid to the subject of head wounds and facial damage in the course of war and/or punitive justice.[16] The impact of acquired disfigurement, for the individual, and for her or his family and community, is barely registered, and only recently has there been any attempt to explore the question of how damaged tissue and bone might be treated medically or surgically before the thirteenth century.[17] Moreover, whilst the body as a site of physical and metaphorical meaning has attracted the attention of literary scholars and historians of gender since the 1980s, to the extent that it is now a relatively mature field of study and even features work on the *head*, the specific, and to my mind obvious, role of the *face* in medieval social interactions has barely been addressed.[18] Yet one of the pioneers of that field, Miri Rubin, long ago pointed out that examining parts of the body could give an insight into how the whole body functioned or was understood, especially if those parts were in pain.[19] The somewhat marginal field of physiognomy, the practice of determining character traits though the scrutiny of facial features, is largely overlooked in studies of the early Middle Ages, not least because it was not heavily represented in Christian European texts or discourse in the period under review. It was nevertheless recognized as a practice in the early medieval Muslim regions of Europe, and would enjoy more prominence from the thirteenth century as physiognomic texts were circulated with medical works, and new treatises were compiled with royal patronage. Some work, therefore, is now being done on the transmission of such texts between antiquity and the Middle Ages.[20]

In terms of a social history of facial disfigurement, however, newer fields of medieval studies are highlighting the lives of hitherto unnoticed groups, and offering potential approaches to the topic. A growing body of work exploring medieval impairment and disability touches upon the sensory impairments resulting from political and judicial mutilations of the head and face, and studies of specific groups of people with physical impairments in the medieval past are increasingly being published.[21] The now well-established field of research into the medieval emotions, utilizing both medieval descriptions and modern psychoanalysis, and owing much to the work of Norbert Elias, has to some extent legitimized the desire on the part of historians to speculate on the psychological impact of life events on medieval people, as well as to analyze the role of specific emotional states within ritual behaviors.[22] The use of non-medical texts from the centuries before 1200 is beginning to reveal how medical practitioners may have been identified and valued in early medieval society.[23] The field of osteoarchaeology, and increasing samples of material being analyzed from early medieval contexts, is demonstrating that some surgical procedures known in the texts were actually being carried out, and that the recipients of such treatment (and even some who did not get such care) might well survive quite serious head trauma.[24] And visual representations of medieval faces are increasingly coming under scrutiny not just by art historians, but also cultural historians intrigued by representations that were not quite portraits, but whose elements (in particular facial and other hair) were clearly imbued with almost supernatural meanings.[25]

Yet facial disfigurement remains a poorly-understood topic in medieval history, partly because it relates to all of these sub-fields of historical enquiry, and yet belongs wholly in none of them. Combining the insights of historians of disability, forensic archaeologists, scholars of literary and visual culture and the histories of premodern medical practice with a renewed interrogation of early medieval primary sources, it is possible to explore several key questions:

- How prevalent was acquired cranio-facial disfigurement in early medieval Europe (including the Byzantine empire and Mediterranean littoral)?
- How did it occur and why?
- In what contexts, and with what kinds of language, did it come to be recorded?
- How did contemporaries treat the disfigured face (medically and socially)?

The aims of this book are to document how acquired disfigurement is recorded across different geographical and chronological contexts; to examine how the genre of text affects the record of injury and responses to it; to determine the specific medical and health implications that such punishments had for the individual and her/his community; to compare the practical knowledge available in different locations across time to deal with the aftercare of such injury, and ask whether it was applied.

Geographically, the range of the study is wide: sources from Ireland, the Byzantine Empire and most (but regrettably not all) regions in between are mined for examples of disfigured men and women (whether actual, or imagined), and account is taken of regional and linguistic difference, the possibilities of transmission of disfiguring practices, and the potential medical care available at the point of injury. Chronologically, the study ranges from late antiquity (often as reported in early medieval sources) to the pivotal twelfth century. The latter functions as both end point for logistical reasons (the study had to stop somewhere) but also as a point when, besides the legal and intellectual revolution known to older scholarship as the twelfth-century Renaissance, the political landscape of Europe was becoming increasingly defined, and claims to authority (in particular the right to define social outsiders and inflict mutilating punishment) were being negotiated in light of western Europe's increasing interactions with both Byzantine and Muslim neighbors. The impact on the physically impaired of the formation of the "persecuting society" has not yet been fully worked out, except in economic terms,[26] but it seems that there was a heightened awareness, at the end of the period under discussion, of the messages encoded in damaged facial features. Insofar as the source itself was interested in such matters, an attempt is made, therefore, to explore the "before" and "after" of selected cases of acquired disfigurement, and to situate them in the broader social norms of early medieval societies.

## Congenital vs. Acquired Conditions

It is important at the outset to define the parameters of the study, and in particular to explain its focus on acquired, as opposed to congenital, disfigurement. Within medieval society, the birth of a child with a congenital impairment might provoke a series of responses: it might not be cared for as well, in the hope of a swift and early death; its birth might be interpreted as a punishment from God for a perceived misdemeanor by the mother, or both parents; it might be abandoned, or made a "gift" to the church; or it might be nurtured, and allowed its place in the family (it is possible to imagine that a couple who had already had healthy children might respond more positively, whilst an impaired firstborn might be viewed rather differently).[27] Burdened by Philippe Ariès' controversial theory that parents could not afford to invest emotionally in their children due to the high child mortality rate in the Middle Ages, subsequent studies challenging his thesis have rather overlooked the lot of the physically impaired child in their championing of children as a group.[28] The exception to this statement has been the work of archaeologists such as Sally Crawford, who argue that impaired children could be nurtured, and that isolated examples of adaptive technology—such as a specially-shaped drinking cup for a child with a cleft lip or palate—are proof of this.[29] Of course, it is dangerous to generalize on single examples, but the survival of such children, and their integration into their community, might ultimately depend not on attitudes to impairment, but on the relative social status of their parents and wider family (one thinks of the numerous impairments encoded in the epithets accorded to the Carolingian royal dynasty, for instance). Either way, as they grew up their impairment was a constant feature, something that God had shaped, and their presence in the community would have become commonplace, something people were used to, and threatened only by outsiders or a change in their own circumstances (one wonders how far an extended family would step in on the death of parents, for instance). They may, of course, never have grown up, and so their difference did not impact upon their acquisition (or not) of social adulthood. This at least is the conclusion reached in a recent archaeological report, which sought reasons for the undifferentiated burial of an Anglo-Saxon child with a severely deformed jawbone, the result of fibrous dysplasia.[30]

By contrast, the vast majority of references to acquired disfigurement in early medieval sources present it as a sudden transformation resulting from interpersonal or group violence among human beings rather than the result of a supernatural intervention, with the exception of hagiographic texts where a saint suddenly punishes a transgressor for perceived or actual sins.[31] The disfigurement was inflicted on one person (or group) by another, whether or not such actions were legal or moral. Disfigurement often took its place alongside other types of physical mutilation, and could be combined with them, although it is difficult to trace any consistent continuum from one disfiguring act to another.[32] Moreover, these episodes occurred entirely during adulthood,[33] and thus had the potential to destroy or severely damage a pre-existing, and established, social identity. It is this sudden change, and its impact both on the person and her/his community, that is of particular interest, since in the words of Valentin Groebner, the facially-mutilated in later medieval Europe (especially those whose noses were cut off) became Ungestalt—hideous, faceless, non-persons.[34] The term functions as a noun and an adjective, so hideousness, non-person-ness, exist as medieval concepts in the mainly later medieval, German, urban cases he studies.[35] Groebner was chiefly concerned with the visual impact of such violence, and his work largely reinforces long-held stereotypes about the cruelty and violence of the later Middle Ages, but to a great extent it ignores the earlier period, not least because the judicial world in which his subjects lived had been profoundly altered by the resurgence of Roman legal studies in the twelfth and thirteenth centuries, with their emphasis on punitive, rather than compensatory, justice. Groebner's work, however, pointed up the need for more work to be done on the face as a specific site of identity and violence, a need that the present study tries to address.

Lying between the two fields of congenital disfigurement and its sudden acquisition during adulthood is the progressive disfigurement brought about by disease, in particular leprosy.[36] Certainly lepromatous leprosy, the most serious form of the disease, was a disfiguring condition, and an anecdote in the life of the twelfth-century holy woman Oda of Brabant suggests how quickly the signs of leprosy could be identified (in this case, wrongly) and lead to social exclusion.[37] But the disfigurement caused by leprosy, and indeed other skin and fleshly conditions, was not inflicted by others, but interpreted as both a curse as well as a gift from God.[38] Some saints' lives even have the saint praying to be *afflicted* with the disease as part of their journey toward true humility.[39] Lepers were a special case in that they were increasingly excluded and housed in separate spaces from the medieval community, but it was their contagious disease, rather than its visible results, that was the reason. Their condition was one to be pitied, and offered the opportunity for the well to provide charity to this special group. Whilst it is entirely possible that some people with disfigurements were mistaken for lepers, the analytical categories of lepers and disfigured people have far more differences than analogies.

## What is "Disfigurement"?

What, though, does that word "disfigurement" actually mean? The root of the English word is the Latin *figura*, meaning shape or form, so a literal translation from English into Latin would give us the sense of losing shape: *deformatus* in Latin, παραμορφωμένος in Greek. Yet an electronic search for the Latin term in a major source collection such as the *Monumenta Germaniae Historica* reveals only 21 occurrences of this root, most of which refer to abstract deformation of morals or institutions such as the Church. A few refer to deformed body parts, but none refer to the face.[40] "Misshapen," therefore, does not quite seem to capture the sense of "disfigurement" we're looking for here, and it is difficult to find, in the many cases I have gathered, any real equivalent to the English term. "Disfigurare" in the seventh-century Lombard laws refers to unspecified damage caused to a stolen horse, whilst "defigurare" seems to indicate disguise, as applied to the treacherous Eustace the monk, in the chronicles of Matthew Paris recounting the battle of Sandwich in 1217.[41] The same difficulty is true of the few Greek examples: what Freshfield translates as "disfigured" in his presentation of a later Byzantine law on injuring the beard is in fact rendered as αποσφαλτιώσας in Von Lingenthal's edition, and translated by the latter as "interemerit" or "destroyed."[42]

The Latin "mutilatio" and variants occur far more frequently (featuring multiply, for example, in over eighty MGH volumes), but only a small minority of these references deal with injury to the face, and the term far more frequently indicates loss of hands or limbs or, again, injury to institutions such as the Church, the kingdom, or a person's moral wellbeing. Searching on a specific term, of course, inevitably misses out all the facial injuries that are not referred to as "mutilation," including the lengthy tariff lists in early medieval law codes, explored later.

If language constitutes reality, does this lack of a stable term for disfigurement (in the MGH sample at least) mean that medieval society did not conceptualize facial appearance in this way? Does searching for disfigurement ill-advisedly project a modern idea onto a random selection of damaged medieval faces? To answer the first question: there is plenty of evidence for damaged faces being "read" by contemporaries, and appearance being associated with honor or a lack of it. Early medieval legal compilations spoke of the shame of being injured (although "injury" here takes on a wider range of meanings than simply the physical, as we shall see). That the tenth-century compilation of Bald's Leechbooks in England took the trouble to include a surgical procedure for hare lip, and featured remedies for blotchy faces, suggests that (in theory at least) faces mattered.[43] To tackle the second point, the application of modern questions and concepts is an everyday part of medieval history, whether conscious or not, and several scholars have explicitly tried to connect medieval and modern manifestations of social behaviors in order to better understand both.[44] A strong proponent of continuity is William Ian Miller, who argues that "our disgust maintains features of its medieval and early modern avatars," a contention that this book explicitly explores, and that historians are more confident in identifying difference in the past than sameness.[45] A recent criticism of medical history as "moribund" also challenges scholars of more distant pasts to engage critically with modern discourses on their subject, and to recognize that reconstructing the past of minority and marginalized groups is a political act, forcing us to face our own prejudices and examine their possible origins.[46]

Returning to the word "figura," it is useful in this context to use the modern Italian usage, which refers not only to physical shape, but also, in the phrase "fare una bella/brutta figura," to the image of self (good or ugly) that is projected to the world. The potential for a facial or head injury to shame or stigmatize the individual was, it seems, entirely dependent on the circumstances surrounding that injury: stigma is always contingent. Chris Mounsey has coined the term "variability" to express discontent with the binary opposite of able-bodied/disabled, and this is a useful concept to keep in mind when exploring disfigurement: one person's disabling injuries, in medieval culture, might be another person's badge of honor, depending on what both did for a living or how both responded to their new faces.[47] In this book, the range of facial conditions considered as possible "disfigurements" ranges from common injuries such as scratches and broken noses to severe, potentially fatal head injuries with the capacity to leave permanent scarring and/or cognitive impairment. The facial "frame," that is, the hair and the ears, are also considered part of this visual compendium, and so "disfigurement" is used as shorthand for a broad and mutable range of conditions. Yet texts relating incidents of early medieval disfigurement present a much less fluid picture: whether inflicted legally or not, deliberately or not, disfigurement was intended to be visible, and/or perceived to be humiliating.[48] It also falls into a number of repeating categories: shaving and hair-cutting, surface burning and branding, the removal of all or part of a facial feature (nose, eyes, ears), injury by blade, and injury by projectile. The very few cases that fall outside these categories are, by definition, written up as exceptional. The authors of texts detailing the very few exceptions, discussed later in the book, took great pains to *justify* why a disfiguring injury should not be read negatively.[49]

The underlying message is the same: the disfigured potentially formed what anthropologists would term an "out-group"—and their stigma might be overlain with a heavy veneer of moral opprobrium—these people are disfigured, our authors argue, because of some fault of their own or others. This contention will be explored further in Chapter 4. Yet unlike other stigmatized medieval groups, *the* disfigured do not feature in early medieval texts *as a group or category*—in contrast to *the* blind, *the* lame, *the* poor or *the* leprous, for instance. This has contributed to their relative invisibility in scholarly studies to date, despite the sheer quantity of examples (set out chronologically in Appendices 1 and 2, below) in texts of the period.

## Sources and Resources

So where do we capture the "flicker of revulsion" in medieval texts? Does it even exist? The study examines a wide range of sources in order to trace moments of acquired disfigurement, the contexts within which they were reported, and the language used to report both perpetrators and victims. These include law codes, early and later; chronicles and annals; hagiographic texts; medical texts; archaeological remains; and iconography. Whilst the occasional example will be drawn from the works of the medieval literary imagination (one cannot explore facial disfigurement and ignore the riches of early Irish myths, or tales such as Marie de France's *Bisclavret*, for example), such texts are discussed at the point of citation, and so are not analyzed collectively here.

### Law Codes

Western Europe in the early Middle Ages was a patchwork of formative polities, whether the multiple small kingdoms of early Irish society, the very similar territories surrounding *trefi* in Wales, or the successor states (duchies, kingdoms and principalities) to Roman rule in England and the continent. Byzantium, by contrast, was a fully-formed empire, albeit one with wildly-fluctuating borders between 500 and 1200CE. A common thread running through all of their histories, however, was the urge to legislate, or to set down in writing the laws of their region, or to revise existing codes. This was not—or at least not entirely—a product of the conversion to Christianity, and some early laws have clear signs of incorporating older practices within the overarching rhetoric of peace brought about by compensation for injury.

The social realities of civil life in the early medieval West and Byzantium, and the often intricately detailed frameworks for that civil society set out by numerous laws rarely intersected, however. Laws were always a work in progress, designed more to reflect the aspirations of the ruler to authority vested in his/her own body and/or conferred by God than to actively regulate every aspect of her/his subjects' lives. It would be all too easy to dismiss the law as essentially the intellectual, text-based activity of court cultures, concerned to project a certain image of rulership whose pedigree stretched back to the Roman Empire, but unenforceable and largely unenforced. The continuous process of excerpting, reordering and adding to the legal corpus made visible by generations of legal historians certainly does not convey much sense of justice in action.

Indeed, law codes may not even represent contemporary attitudes toward violence or aspire to its control. In a series of articles and his last book, Patrick Wormald raised the important question of the purpose of medieval legislative texts, particularly their copying and preservation. For the Frankish kings, he suggested, recopying and preserving the ancient Salic laws was about reinforcing Frankish identity, and co-existed with supplemental law-giving in the form of capitularies which often seemed to respond to specific cases.[50] Such practices were not confined to the Frankish world, of course; Wormald argued that the "ideological climate of King Alfred's Wessex belonged to the Carolingian zone," and that England was by no means isolated from the intellectual currents of the continent in the tenth and eleventh centuries. Successive kings of England (or, rather, their clergy, such as Wulfstan of York) revised and renewed the laws of their predecessors.[51] This urge to revise and add to the law, ultimately deriving from Roman models and continued as well in the kingdoms within Wormald's "olive belt," that is, southern Europe, was particularly (and unsurprisingly) demonstrated by Byzantine emperors as well, who issued Novels or new laws to add to the old, rather than attempting new codifications.[52] Each new ruler seems to have been unable to resist the temptation to tinker, amend and add laws that "seemed good," as numerous preambles to extant law codes make clear.

Yet these introductions, setting out the why and wherefore of the new code, were of course as much a rhetorical performance of kingliness or imperial dignity as they were representative of an actual ruler's aspirations. The ideological value of setting up the ruler as legislator exceeded the practical impact of the laws themselves. In an important recent article, Geoffrey Koziol has used capitulary evidence from the end of

Charlemagne's reign in the early 800s to demonstrate that not only could early medieval central government, such as it was, not regulate its citizens' lives, it did not seek to do so, but set up models of right behavior, effectively asking the people to discipline themselves, rather than expect state intervention.[53] Charlemagne and his successors, however, still engaged in the work of codifying and re-issuing Frankish laws and, as the Carolingian empire expanded, newly-subject peoples were also "given" written codes of law by their Frankish rulers.

Turning to the content of laws, therefore, we need to keep in mind this ideological frame, even if subsequent writers have argued for a more nuanced approach than Wormald's.[54] In the laws of early medieval Western European kingdoms, it is most obvious in extended, and almost ubiquitous, sections on the body: corporeal injuries down to specific teeth in the mouth were tariffed with specific fines, conveying the sense of a pervasive justice system which literally could reach into every orifice.[55] Lengthy tariff lists set out what payment in money or value of chattels (or female slaves) was due to the victim of an assault, and this was dependent not only on which part of the body had been injured, but also how seriously (did the wound heal?) and often taking into account the social status of the victim as well (male or female, slave or free).

The close attention to the body paid in the early medieval law codes has already attracted the attention of medieval historians.[56] Textual similarities between different codes, however, such as a memorable cluster judging the size of bones retrieved from a skull injury by the sound they made in various receptacles, caution against their literal reading.[57] These parallels, occurring in laws from Francia, Italy, Frisia and Wales, suggest that borrowings took place over space and time. Either way, they provide a substantial body of evidence for concern with the head and face in early medieval culture. For our purposes, the value of using these legal sources lies not so much the question of whether such laws were ever put into practice, as in the ideological framing of the face and body that they reveal.

## Chronicles and Annals

Not surprisingly, many of the contemporary and later reports of deliberate disfigurement in chronicles and annals (accidents being something of a rarity in the texts) appear to share the ideals and moral frameworks laid out in the laws. Blows to the face, whether or not disfiguring, seem to have been serious enough to merit recording, especially if the victim was of high status.[58] Some of their evidence has been cited in previous works dealing with cruelty and atrocity in medieval society, or in studies of extreme emotions such as anger. Some, such as the tit-for-tat disfiguring atrocities committed during the later Albigensian crusade, have become emblematic of that entire enterprise, obscuring the less sensational stories of the spread of the friars and the imposition of French royal power in the region.[59] Often, such episodes have been read literally to reinforce stereotypes of medieval society as extremely and unrelentingly violent, rather than being read with a critical eye as to what the author's purpose was in constructing his (or occasionally, her) report. Keeping in mind that most reporters were working within a clerical or even monastic environment, extreme violence is used, more often than not, to point up the lack of judgment, or downright cruelty, of the perpetrator, and is written up by authors to evoke pity for the victim.

At the most extreme end of this spectrum of violence is a late, but emotive example reported by Rolandinus of Padua for the year 1259. Having captured the city of Friuli, Ezzelino da Romano:

> ... ordered, that the unfortunate people of Friuli, male and female, great and small, clerics and laypeople, and all of those cut down and injured, should bear the rage of Ezzelino throughout Lombardy and the March. It did not profit the innocent children that they had not sinned, rather, whilst the old and the young were exposed to a triple penalty, mutilated in their eyes, noses and feet, the infants and innocents suffered a quadruple penalty, for having lost their noses and feet at Ezzelino's order, they were blinded in their eyes and their genitals were cut off. This extreme cruelty was perpetrated by Ezzelino at the end of June in the aforementioned year of our Lord.[60]

Rolandinus makes it clear how his readers should react to his report—whatever the exact circumstances of Ezzelino's treatment of the Friulians, his cruelty is written in language evoking Herod's massacre of the innocents, and designed to provoke shock and revulsion. Already condemned as a heretic in a letter of Pope Alexander IV a year earlier,[61] Ezzelino could be used by Rolandinus as an archetype of evil. Indeed, it might be argued that mass mutilation had become something of a generic plot device by the thirteenth century[62]—the man capable of this, it is implied, is beyond redemption.

Whilst falling outside the period under review in this study, Rolandinus's passage is useful for pointing up the framework within which medieval chroniclers largely operated. His subtle evocation of a parallel between Ezzelino and Herod was a common trope, and often made explicitly by clerical writers to decry rulers as tyrants.[63] Gregory of Tours, for instance, calls King Chilperic (d. 584) "the Nero and Herod of our time" for his cruelty in punishing crimes.[64] Clerical authors, though, could and did draw upon a whole range of Old Testament *exempla* to frame their chronicles. Whilst some may protest their veracity or are sprinkled throughout with conscious references to their reliability, including references to authors consulted, records used and the oral reports of reliable witnesses, their writing was shaped by the generic, biblical frameworks visible in those same earlier works. As Guy Halsall comments, referring to reports of violence, "Neither writer nor reader expected the *minutiae* of what actually happened to bog down a written account, or to take precedence over the display of knowledge of classics, scripture or the writings of the Church Fathers (patristics). The 'True Law of History [*lex vera historiae*]' was moral, not empirical."[65] Antonella Liuzzo Scorpo and Jamie Wood concur that many narratives of violence were written in a "scriptural mode," offering ready-made rhetorical devices for description, but also a set of tropes around forgiveness and redemption.[66]

With regard to disfigurement, the Levitical ban on mutilated priestly bodies was never far from the mind, especially in reports of injured rulers or clergy. We shall meet numerous cases of rulers "removed" from power through facial mutilation and/or blinding, and a range of responses to such acts by our authors, running from the just punishment of a usurper or tyrant to a quasi-hagiographical martyrdom. Thietmar of Merseberg's early eleventh-century account of the blinding of Boleslav III of Bohemia (d. 1037), for example, lies on the former end of this spectrum.[67] Moreover, whilst the "mark of Cain" does not appear to have been a reference point in accounts of disfigurement (the Bible is, after all, somewhat ambiguous about what the mark or sign was), its interpretation as sparing his life but thereafter identifying him as a murderer was an influential rationale in medieval justice schemata—a mark of infamy, rather than swift execution, conveyed the message of royal authority, and extended beyond murder to such offences as treason and theft.[68]

This common framework for the Christian texts under review is most apparent if we compare across centuries: Rolandinus's horror at Ezzelino the tyrant in the thirteenth century echoes almost perfectly Anna Komnena's twelfth-century depiction of the Norman Robert Guiscard (d.1086), or Amatus of Montecassino's account of the cruelty of Prince

Gisulf II of Salerno (d.1077), and Gregory of Tours' condemnation of Merovingian kings who imposed mutilations unjustly in the sixth century.[69] Facial disfigurement, as we shall see, was more often than not presented by chroniclers as a measure of the evil or lack of control of medieval rulers or their servants.[70] Every episode, therefore, was highly ideological: it was used to think with, rather than being widely prevalent as a practice in medieval Europe and Byzantium. Those reports of actual harm, I suggest, need to be examined with an eye to the writer's purpose in reporting them, as none are without political or moralizing message, and some, like Rolandinus's account of Ezzelino, test the boundaries of credibility. It is not enough to take the descriptions of such violence as evidence that medieval society was driven by violent acts, and the terror evoked by multiple or group disfigurements should not lead us to the conclusion that all disfigurement was understood in this way. These are specific instances set out within pre-determined frameworks of good and evil, and deployed for specific purposes in the texts. If our writers had been interested in the phenomenon of disfigurement in and of itself, we should surely have more reports of accidents, or injuries caused by fire, one of the great hazards of medieval life, but until the advent of coroners' reports in later medieval Europe, we do not. Individuals with acquired disfigurements had to have a special story in order to be recorded at all; many cases to be considered were drawn from the social elite, for whom status trumped their newly-damaged features. The rest, if they existed in any substantial numbers, remain outsiders in that their lives and experiences—and the responses of others to their disfigurement—were not thought worth setting down in writing.

### Hagiographic Texts

The exception to this statement regarding the visibility of disfigured people is the hagiographic genre, where some *do* appear in more than brief detail. Historians of medicine have long mined such texts as indicators (and, in earlier works, evidence) of medieval attitudes toward sickness and cure,[71] and early work on medieval disability, too, plundered the rich sets of examples of impairment in medieval saints' lives to explore this theme.[72] But what credence should we give to the punishments inflicted by saints that were targeted at the face? What are we to make of eyeballs popping out in the *Book of Sainte Foy*, for example?[73] This seems a dangerous field to enter into if we are in search of the lived experience of victims of disfigurement—the supernatural nature of the punishments largely excludes them from consideration (just as I have excluded other conditions deriving, in medieval eyes, from the will of God). Hagiography does, however, shine a more direct light on the ideological frames that inform our supposedly reliable chroniclers; we might say that there is little to choose between them in terms of mindset. In building the case for this or that saint's holiness, hagiographic texts often tangentially incorporate important types of disfigurement that other sources omit. In the present study, hagiographic texts are used to inform our analysis of the ideology and rhetoric of disfigurement in three specific contexts.

The first is the Byzantine Empire during the two periods of iconoclasm, when a purge was decreed of all figurative icons as idolatrous. Hagiography of this period presents the stories of monks resisting the decree, and being punished with various atrocities targeted at their faces and bodies. The tortures seem chiefly to precede execution, but not always, suggesting that the punishments are exemplary and designed to be read and understood by those encountering the victims. As far as I am aware, however, there has not been any consideration of the apparent link between erasure of icons and erasure of facial features in the punishments of the iconodules (icon-supporters). This despite the fact that icons, like living faces, were understood as far more than an aesthetic image.[74]

The second context is the Anglo-Norman world of the eleventh and twelfth centuries, where saints are reported as repairing the damage of unjustly-inflicted mutilations. Strikingly, texts from this period echo the Byzantine examples in their motifs: tyrannical or misguided rule inflicting a terrible punishment, and the hagiographer explicitly criticizing that decision. Here, though, the saints put things right. Thus Thomas Becket from beyond the grave assisted Ailward of Westoning, restoring the man's eyesight and testicles after their mutilation, and the miracles of St Wulfstan of Worcester give a lengthy account of the mutilation, and subsequent cure by Wulfstan (d.1095), of Thomas of Elderfield, wrongly blinded and castrated in 1217.[75] Both of these episodes are well-known and have been discussed in numerous contexts, particularly the sensationalism with which the mutilations themselves are presented: heightened language, the horror of Thomas of Elderfield's eyeballs and testicles being used as footballs.[76] Rather neglected, by contrast, is the careful and possibly equally-suspect account of the moment when Ailward realized that he could see, for embedded in the text here is an account of the care that had been applied to his now-empty eye-sockets. This, to my knowledge, has not been considered in studies of early medieval medicine and surgery, and deserves further attention.[77]

The third area in which hagiography is helpful is in providing material on the mutilation of female faces, saintly or otherwise. Disfigurement, it will be argued, is a highly-gendered concept, but where it has been discussed in previous studies, it has been seen as part and parcel of a series of mutilations inflicted chiefly on the male body, resulting in damage to the masculine identity. This is not surprising: the vast majority of cases documented in all types of source are of disfigured men. Chapter 5, however, will turn its attention to the minority of incidents concerning women. Hagiographic texts are valuable here because of their discourse on the dangers of female beauty. In Ruth Mazo Karras's words, "there was a strong strand in medieval thought that wanted women to internalize the blame for men's desires."[78] Whilst this is a familiar trope to historians of medieval Europe, insufficient attention has been paid to the ways in which hagiography and legal sources locate the danger chiefly in the female *face* (as opposed to bodily form), and come to startlingly similar (and radical) conclusions as to solving this problem. Whilst laws threatened facial mutilation to destroy any further chance of adulterous women being considered attractive, female saints' lives embraced the practice enthusiastically as a model of the ultimate sacrifice in order to defend chastity and virginity. Beginning with early medieval examples of extreme mortification and mutilation in the face of barbarian threat,[79] the theme was taken up again in hagiography of the twelfth and thirteenth centuries, precisely the period when judicial mutilation, too, was at its height and did not baulk at the idea of defacing a female felon.

### Medical Texts

The early Middle Ages are commonly dismissed as the period where the medical knowledge of antiquity—in particular its theoretical groundings—was almost completely lost in Western Europe, and its surviving texts are often highlighted as at best empirical and at worst the product of ignorance and superstition. Even studies purporting to explore medieval medical practice focus their attention on a period when text-based knowledge was again circulating and being translated.[80] In challenging this outlook, Peregrine Horden has demonstrated that the problem lies not only in a relative dearth of texts in comparison with the riches of the later Middle Ages, but also in an uneven field of study of those texts.

Anglo-Saxon medicine, for example, is very well-explored in comparison with the outputs of continental scriptoria.[81] Early Byzantine medicine, similarly, is well-documented and has been the subject of several studies.[82] Yet there is another problem underlying the dismissal of the early Middle Ages, and that is the privileging of intellectual medicine over its practice. Medical *knowledge* was sometimes conceptualized as separate from medical *practice*, as the letters of the tenth-century polymath and teacher Gerbert of Aurillac (d. 1003) make clear. In one missive, to an unknown recipient looking for advice on a kidney stone, Gerbert responds: "Do not ask me to discuss what is the province of physicians, especially because I have always avoided the practice of medicine even though I have striven for a knowledge of it."[83] In fact Gerbert's letters are suffused with medical analogies, as we shall see, and he did sometimes deign to offer advice, for all his protestation to the contrary. Yet he was an exceptional case: his book-collecting activities in fact give us a picture of the early medieval monastic world and its circulation and copying of texts. We can sometimes track the dissemination of knowledge, but medical texts will not show us the doctor at work.

How, then, can surviving medical texts assist in exploring responses to acquired disfigurement? We have already noted Bald's *Leechbook* as a valuable text for studying surgical procedures for congenital disfigurement such as hare lip. In terms of treating head injury, however, it is rather less detailed than some of the legal sources introduced above. And because surgery, as we shall see, was considered a subordinate, even separate, skill to medicine, dealing with surface injury rather than underlying symptoms and etiology, it may not show up even in specifically medical texts. As the study progresses, it will become apparent that early medieval medical interventions are noted not so much in medical texts, as in non-medical material where the practice of the doctor is often surprisingly well-documented.

### Archaeological Evidence

This practice is also particularly visible in human cemetery remains. The science of osteoarchaeology is well-established, and has provided historians of medicine with rich details of the ravages of malnutrition, some diseases, gradual mechanical wear and tear, and acquired physical injury as these manifest themselves on the human skeleton.[84] The head has attracted some attention in these studies, not least because there is a growing sample of early medieval cranial injuries that show clear signs of surgical intervention, including various forms of trepanation. This accords well with the evidence of legal sources describing procedures to reduce the pressure on the brain, carried out by the doctor (*medicus*) in the case of trauma to the skull. The implication of the archaeology is that early medieval surgery was considerably more sophisticated than has been thought hitherto: unlike the limbs, that arguably could be treated by anyone with a modicum of experience in the care of injured animals, the need for specialist care to the head may expose the early medieval surgeon at work. Archaeology can also, as we have already seen, reveal differentiation (or not) in the treatment of the impaired dead; more importantly for our purposes, archaeologists are increasingly able to determine whether an injury to the head or face was pre-, peri- or post-mortem. The first category is key here—some people might live for lengthy spells after sustaining a major wound that leaves evidence in the bones, and this prompts speculation as to what kinds of lives they might have led.[85]

### Iconography

The evidence of iconography has already been alluded to in the depictions of rulers' facial hair and in consideration of Byzantine iconoclasm. But neither of these engages directly with the problem of disfigurement in medieval Europe. In fact, early medieval images (on parchment, panels or in stone sculptures) were largely unconcerned with the depiction of lived experience, still less with the depiction of those whose distorted or damaged features might have left them in a liminal position within their communities. (This is, of course, the central assumption to be tested within the present study.) In fact, we are dealing with a dearth not only of disfigured faces, but an almost complete absence of individual facial likenesses at all.[86] Stephen Parkinson explains:

> Medieval artists and patrons were... aware of the possibility of producing images whose appearance resembled that of their human models, but they chose not to do so. This was partly as a result of the belief that appearances were incapable of conveying a thing's essential nature, a widespread opinion in the early middle ages.[87]

This link between the visual image and the nature of the subject, he goes on, began to emerge only in the later Middle Ages, when much more naturalistic portraits begin to be made in paint and stone. Unsurprisingly, this coincided with Western Europe's rediscovery of physiognomy, offering ways to make a direct link between appearance and character traits.

In fact, whilst the physically impaired or the poverty-stricken might be portrayed in standardized representations of saints (physical impairment usually indicated by the presence of a wooden crutch or crawling-box),[88] facial distortion or disfigurement is reserved, when it appears at all, for allegorical portrayals of sin or vice.[89] (The female face appears, for example, in characterizations of vices such as *luxuria*.) That is, their value as evidence for *actual* disfigurement is negligible. Yet, just as the chroniclers and hagiographers drew upon biblical motifs to frame their narrative, so arguably the medieval judicial (and extrajudicial) practice of slicing off ears had its inspiration in accounts of the arrest of Christ, when the servant of the High Priest, Malchus, is physically attacked by Simon Peter, and this particular scene appears both in manuscripts such as the Winchester Psalter (c.1150) and in later medieval paintings such Duccio Boninsegna's *Christ Taken Prisoner* (1309–10), now in the Museo dell'Opera del Duomo in Siena. Malchus's face is already distorted and ugly in many depictions: his lost ear (which Christ, even then, restores to its place) cannot disfigure him any further.

Iconography has, however, been explored by Umberto Eco in his twin publications on beauty and ugliness. Utilizing works of art from antiquity to the modern day, he seems to have been able to complete his project on beauty far more satisfactorily than its counterpart on ugliness. Whilst "ugly" and "disfigured" are not precisely the same, the medieval texts that Eco consulted were not concerned to analyze ugliness itself, since for them it simply represented the inverse of beauty. As early as the seventh century, however, there is an important distinction made in Isidore of Seville's *Etymologies* between beauty as ornamentation and beauty as utility—a damaged body or face, therefore, might be interpreted in highly multi-valent ways. Thomas Aquinas would take up this problem in his *Summa Theologiae* in the thirteenth century, equating mutilation with ugliness and lack of use.[90]

Another reason to persist with visual images, even if they do not give us literal renditions of disfigured faces, is that sometimes they seem to serve as stand-ins for the power of the person they portray. A statue of the Frankish King Lothair (r. 954–86) was decapitated on the same day as Louis XVI lost his head in 1793.[91] Icons of Byzantine emperors occupied a liminal space between straightforward portrait and saintly image; they were both, and neither. But their power was sufficient that faces might be removed and repainted during regime changes; the icon was a framework of power, only the occupant needed replacing.[92] Imperial politics also lay at the heart of another iconographic source, coinage. Here, though, the idealization of the ruler seems to have trumped his or her actual physical appearance, and so the noseless Emperor Justinian II of Byzantium, for example, is shown without blemish. We shall return to his case as an example of how his disfigurement was treated in written sources.

## APPROACHES TO DISFIGUREMENT

Our sources, then, are numerous but recalcitrant. They are not directly concerned with the question of acquired disfigurement and its effects. Many of the examples discussed in the book will in fact center on the *moment* of disfigurement, the action of a just or unjust assailant, rather than its aftermath, and the present study cannot be considered a comprehensive survey of all cases of disfigurement in the early Middle Ages. Only a tiny minority of these reports can be read literally as a record of the incidence of facial disfigurement, but they can more profitably be mined for their assumptions about facial damage. For our purposes, one way of unlocking this evidence is to apply questions generated by modern studies of interpersonal and societal relations, testing the modern assumption that facial damage changed a person's life for the worse. Each of the following chapters, therefore, takes a concept generated by modern sociological, anthropological and gender-inflected research as a starting point in its exploration of medieval texts about the damaged face.

Chapter 2, The Face, Honor and "Face," asks the question "What is a face, and how does it function in social relations?" This may be a somewhat disingenuous entry point, yet it is an important one to pose since several recent medieval studies play on the multiple meanings of the word "face" to imply not only the physical features of a person, but that deeper sense of personhood we met in Groebner's discussion above. Giorgio Agamben and François Delaporte have both interrogated the face as a surface, connected (or not) to the person behind or beneath.[93] Stephen Pattison, too, has reflected upon the relationship between the physical and metaphorical face.[94] To "lose face" is a well-used phrase, but whilst it may function in the modern western world as shorthand for a humiliation of sorts, or loss of dignity, in many cultures it has a far greater specificity of meaning, and conceptually is the very glue binding together and regulating social relations.[95] This demands a certain care in the use of the term—which has not been apparent within historical studies—when utilizing it to convey loss of status in medieval culture. Even then, the metaphorical loss of face might or might not involve loss of or damage to *physical* facial features (hence Groebner's play on the term in *Defaced* and in his associated article): the potential for confusion is therefore apparent.[96] Associated with the idea of face, but not exactly coterminous with it, is that of honor. Whilst we shall discuss the meanings of honor in detail below, it is important to flag up here the strong association visible in the early medieval sources between the physical face and personal honor, although couched in different terms for men and women. Whilst it might be assumed that damage to women's faces would have been more devastating to their chances of social acceptance, in fact most of the source material indicates that it was *men* who had more to lose from disfigurement. The reasons for this will be explored later.

Chapter 3 further investigates the troubled connection between many cases of disfigurement and claims to authority expressed in medieval legal sources. Framing this discussion will be a consideration of Giorgio Agamben's work on sovereign power[97]: whilst early medieval law codes universally condemned interpersonal violence and poured particular opprobrium on damage inflicted to the head and face, medieval rulers reserved the right to inflict exactly the same kinds of damage as punishment for transgressions against the law, particularly in cases of repeated theft, adultery or treason. When such punishments became frequent or unjustified, however—when, in Agamben's formulation, the exceptional became the norm—medieval writers report them as atrocities, making clear to readers that such behaviors were unacceptable, despite the ruler's special status as constituting, rather than being bound by, the law.

The flipside to honor, in most medieval discussions, was shame. This introduces the theoretical framework explored in Chapter 4, the idea of disfigurement as stigma. Elaborated in detail by Erving Goffman in the 1960s, and influential on generations of sociologists and historians since, stigma is a powerful analytical concept with which to explore medieval disfigurement. As Goffman points out, a stigmatizing condition could be visible or invisible, the product of a person's own actions or inflicted upon her or him by the wider social group. Different categories of stigma have been elaborated by subsequent studies, and their negative inflections explored in detail. But what is particularly interesting about stigma for a medievalist is the fact that the marks of shame, *stigmata*, had an entirely different valence in later medieval Christian society, as the privileged marks of God's favor toward an earthly recipient. The chapter will therefore investigate the biblical ambivalence toward marking of any kind.

The fifth chapter will take a gendered approach to disfigurement in terms of its disempowering function, but will then examine in detail the minority of documented cases of disfigured women. How do these reports differ from those dealing with men? Was a woman's face only equated with beauty and marriageability, and/or an asset put at risk by transgressive behavior? Given the strong tradition within hagiography of the earlier and later Middle Ages of women disfiguring themselves when under threat of sexual assault or unwanted marriage, to what extent were these ideas typical of the contexts within which such texts were produced? In what circumstances were men's and women's faces treated similarly, and what were the major differences? This chapter will explore issues such as visibility and modesty among women: even with a disfigured face, was it possible for a woman to "pass" more easily because she would in any case be required to partly conceal her head with wraps or a hood? Throughout the chapter, "gender" will be understood as a web of power relations between not only men and women, but within each group. I have suggested elsewhere that the power to disfigure a woman signaled not so much a man's authority over her, but his position vis-à-vis other men, for whom control over their households and family was central to their own masculinity.[98] This will be developed further as the chapter progresses.

The question of how visible a disfigurement might be brings us to the vexed question of the medieval and modern gaze, examined in Chapter 6. "Ways of seeing" as an approach, pioneered by John Berger in the 1970s, has been largely confined to the field of art history since then, though here it offers an entry point into visual representation and consumption. More germane to the present study is Rosemarie Garland-Thomson's groundbreaking work on staring.[99] We have already touched upon the fact that medieval artwork of this early period did not seek to depict the fleshly figure realistically, but how do the sources portray the act of looking at other people? This chapter seeks to find out whether the "flicker of revulsion" can be detected in descriptions of the disfigured. Modern neuropsychological studies about face perception assist here in setting out the evolutionary parameters of the human gaze. Face perception is—and according to the studies always has been—a key element in social interaction, the first point of contact between humans. Medieval texts abound with descriptions of faces, and the later rediscovery of the pseudo-science of physiognomy concentrated attention on the facial features like never before. A key question in this chapter will be how a disfigured face might fit into or disrupt existing schemata for facial description: did political considerations, for example, trump historical accuracy when it came to depictions or descriptions of the disfigured elite?

The theoretical chapters will enable the study to examine the ways in which disfigurement was presented by the medieval sources, and suggest some reasons why the representation took certain forms. Chapter 7 distills remaining examples of actual disfigurement or disfiguring head injury, and examines the evidence from texts and archaeology that suggest ways in which disfigured individuals and/or their carers might seek solutions to their damaged appearance, whether through concealment or actual treatment. Included here will be the rare cases documenting a "rehabilitation" of sorts, whether medical or moral. Just as there was a spectrum of disfigurement in our sources, so the level of perceived need for help might vary considerably. We have already briefly considered clothing around the head and face; to this might be added cosmetics, self-isolation (the likely route of the stigmatized individual, according to Goffman) and medical or surgical treatments to repair wounds and/or restore the skin blemished by injury or burns. The evidence for all of these is scant, and likely only to be encountered in tangential references, but striking medical metaphors on wound care in the pastoral letters of clergy suggest that knowledge was not actually lost, simply transferred into a different conceptual arena. We return full circle to the problem we set out with, the ideological framework within which early medieval writing was produced and consumed: exploring the face as a focus may shed significant new light on the processes of its production.

## Notes

1. Muscular dystrophy sufferer Denis Creegan, "Adapt or succumb," in *Stigma: the Experience of Disability*, ed. Paul Hunt (London: Geoffrey Chapman, 1966), 114. [The nature of each author's disability preceded his or her essays.]
2. Consider the case of Bibi Aisha, discussed in Patricia Skinner, "The gendered nose and its lack: 'medieval' nose-cutting and its modern manifestations," *Journal of Women's History*, 26.1 (2014): 45–67, whose nose was cut off by her husband's relatives and whose reconstructive surgery, courtesy of an American philanthropic foundation, was delayed by the need to give her counseling. See also the

cases featured in Channel 5 TV series *Making Faces,* aired in October 2012, following the maxillofacial unit at Birmingham's Queen Elizabeth Hospital in the UK: http://www.channel5. com/shows/making-faces [accessed 29 July 2015].

3. Kumaran Shanmugarajah, Safina Gaind, Alex Clarke and Peter E. M. Butler, "The role of disgust emotions in the observer response to facial disfigurement," *Body Image,* 9 (2012): 455–461.

4. William Ian Miller, *The Anatomy of Disgust* (Cambridge, MA: Harvard University Press, 1997), 27.

5. For example Katie Piper (attacked with acid), *Beautiful* (London: Ebury Press, 2011); Tina Nash (whose partner gouged out her eyes), *Out of the Darkness* (London: Simon and Schuster, 2012); James Partridge (burns), *Changing Faces: the Challenge of Facial Disfigurement* (London: Penguin, 1990). This is just a sample from the UK alone. Veterans: Suzannah Biernoff, "The rhetoric of disfigurement in First World War Britain," *Social History of Medicine,* 24.3 (2011): 666–685; Edward Bishop, *McIndoe's Army: the Story of the Guinea Pig Club and its Indomitable Members* (London: Grub Street, 2004); Falklands War veteran Simon Weston, *Going Back: Return to the Falklands* (London: Penguin, 1992).

6. E.g. the *1914FACES2014 Exeter* Project: http://blogs.exeter. ac.uk/1914faces2014/ [accessed 13 February 2014]. Biernoff, "The rhetoric of disfigurement," 668.

7. Sander Gilman, *Making the Body Beautiful: a Cultural History of Aesthetic Surgery* (Princeton/Oxford: Princeton University Press, 1999); D. Reisberg and S. Habakuk, "A history of facial and ocular prosthetics," *Advances in Ophthalmic Plastic Reconstructive Surgery,* 8 (1990): 11–24.

8. Quoted at length in Biernoff, "Rhetoric," 671. Biernoff comments that the directness of Muir's prose would probably be replaced nowadays with a "more sensitive (and more euphemistic) treatment of disfigurement."

9. Erving Goffman, *Stigma: Notes on the Management of Spoiled Identity* (Englewood Cliffs, NJ: Prentice-Hall/London: Penguin, 1963); Henri Tajfel, "Intergroup relations, social myths and social justice in social psychology," in *The Social Dimension,* ed. H. Tajfel, II (Cambridge: Cambridge University Press, 1984), 695–716. Durkheim's theory of *anomie,* a breakdown of social norms

resulting in deviant behavior, was expounded in his *De la division du travail social [The Division of Labour in Society]* (Paris: Presses universitaires de France, 1893).

10. Even recently, archaeologists E. and G. Craig have commented that "facial disfigurement had the strong potential to result in disability in the early medieval period": "The diagnosis and context of a facial deformity from an Anglo-Saxon cemetery at Spofforth, North Yorkshire," *International Journal of Osteoarchaeology*, 23 (2013): 631–9, at 636.

11. The trauma is vividly captured in a series of portrait paintings by Mark Gilbert, of patients before, during and after surgeries, commissioned by surgeon Iain Hutchinson for the *Saving Faces* charity, most recently exhibited in *Saving Faces* at the University of Exeter, 25 February to 25 March 2015. See also Rosemarie Garland-Thomson, *Staring: How We Look* (Oxford: Oxford University Press, 2009), 6–7, featuring Gilbert's portrait of the late Henry de Lotbiniere.

12. Michael McVaugh, *The Rational Surgery of the Middle Ages* (Firenze: SISMEL-Edizioni del Galluzzo, 2006).

13. See Emily Cock, "'Lead[ing] 'em by the nose into public shame and derision': Gaspare Tagliacozzi, Alexander Read and the lost history of plastic surgery, 1600–1800," *Social History of Medicine*, 28.1 (2015): 1–21, with references to earlier literature; the conference *Modified Bodies and Prosthesis in Medieval and Early Modern England*, held at the University of Sussex in May 2014 (publication in preparation). See also Naomi Baker, *Plain Ugly: the Unattractive Body in Early Modern Culture* (Manchester: Manchester University Press, 2010).

14. Peregrine Horden, "What's wrong with early medieval medicine?" *Social History of Medicine*, 24.1 (2011): 5–25, succinctly dissects the reasons for the neglect of the earlier period. See also the special issue of *Social History of Medicine*, 13.2, co-edited by Horden and Emilie Savage-Smith, dealing with *The Year 1000: Medical Practice at the End of the First Millennium*. A welcome exception to the rule is the work of Clare Pilsworth, *Healthcare in Early Medieval Northern Italy: More to Life than Leeches* (Turnhout: Brepols, 2014), which takes a holistic view and rejects the distinction between "learned" and "practical" medicine.

15. E.g. *The Final Argument: the Imprint of Violence on Society in Medieval and Early Modern Europe*, ed. Donald J. Kagay and L. J. Andrew Villalon (Woodbridge: Boydell, 1998); John Gillingham, "Killing and mutilating political enemies in the British Isles from the late twelfth to the early fourteenth century: a comparative study," in *Britain and Ireland 900–1300: Insular Responses to Medieval European Change*, ed. B. Smith (Cambridge: Cambridge University Press, 1999), 114–134; D. Baraz, *Medieval Cruelty: Changing Perceptions from Late Antiquity to the Early Modern Period* (Ithaca, NY: Cornell University Press, 2003); P. Freedman, "Atrocities and the execution of peasant rebel leaders in later medieval and early modern Europe," *Medievalia et Humanistica*, n.s. 31 (2005): 101–113; *Violences souveraines au Moyen Âge*, ed. F. Feronda *et al.* (Paris: PUF, 2010); Daniel Lord Smail, "Violence and predation in later medieval Mediterranean Europe," *Comparative Studies in Society and History*, 54.1 (2012): 7–34. Rather more sophisticated readings of violence in texts are offered by Albrecht Classen, *Violence in Medieval Courtly Literature: a casebook* (New York: Garland, 2004), and the contributors to *Violence and the Writing of History in the Medieval Francophone World*, ed. Noah D. Guynn and Zrinka Stahuljak (Cambridge: D. S. Brewer, 2013) and *History-Writing and Violence in the Medieval Mediterranean*, ed. Antonella Liuzzo Scorpo and Jamie Wood, special issue of *Al-Masāq: Journal of the Medieval Mediterranean*, 27 (2015).

16. On judicial procedures see Mitchell Merback, *The Thief, the Cross and the Wheel: pain and the spectacle of punishment in medieval and renaissance Europe* (London: Reaktion Books, 1999); Klaus van Eickels, "Gendered violence: castration and blinding as punishment for treason in Normandy and Anglo-Norman England," *Gender and History*, 16.3 (2004): 588–602.

17. Piers Mitchell, *Medicine in the Crusades: Warfare, Wounds and the Medieval Surgeon* (Cambridge: Cambridge University Press, 2004). And see below, Chap. 7.

18. *Framing Medieval Bodies*, ed. Sarah Kay and Miri Rubin (Manchester: Manchester University Press, 1994). The diversity of the field even a decade or so in was examined critically by Caroline Bynum, "Why all the fuss about the body? A medievalist's

perspective," *Critical Inquiry*, 22 (1995): 1–33, at 5: "despite the enthusiasm for the topic, discussions of the body are almost completely incommensurate – and often mutually incomprehensible – across the disciplines." Recent studies include *Fleshly Things and Spiritual Matters: Studies on the Medieval Body in Honor of Margaret Bridges*, ed. Nicole Nyffenegger and Katrin Rupp (Newcastle: Cambridge Scholars Press, 2011) and *Disembodied Heads in Medieval and Early Modern Culture*, ed. C. G. Santing, B. Baert and A. Traninger (Leiden: Brill, 2013).

19. Miri Rubin, "The person in the form: medieval challenges to bodily 'order'," in *Framing Medieval Bodies*, 100–122, at 101.

20. Martin Porter, "A persistent fisnomical consciousness, c.400BC–c.1470CE," in *id.*, *Windows of the Soul: The Art of Physiognomy in European Culture, 1470–1780* (Oxford: Oxford University Press, 2005); *Seeing the Face, Seeing the Soul: Polemon's Physiognomy from Classical Antiquity to Medieval Islam*, ed. Simon Swain (Oxford: Oxford University Press, 2007).

21. Irina Metzler's two wide-ranging surveys, *Disability in Medieval Europe: Thinking about Physical Impairment during the High Middle Ages, 1100–1400* (London and New York: Routledge, 2006) and *A Social History of Disability in the Middle Ages: Cultural Considerations of Physical Impairment* (London and New York: Routledge, 2013) laid out the groundwork with an impressive array of examples; Edward Wheatley, *Stumbling Blocks before the Blind: Medieval Constructions of a Disability* (Ann Arbor: University of Michigan Press, 2010), challenges the monolithic approach to specific impairment by illustrating how fluid the category of "blindness" could be. The deaf are rather less represented, only featuring in S. de Vriendt, "Doven in de middeleeuwen: drie vragen aan mediëvisten," in *Een School spierinkjes: Kleine opstellen over Middelnederlandse artes-literatuur*, ed. W. P. Gerritsen, Annelies van Gijsen and Orlanda S. H. Lee (Middeleeuwse studies en bronnen, 26, Hilversum: Verloren, 1991), 168–171, and several studies on the deaf Theresa de Cartagena. See also Kristina L. Richardson, *Difference and Disability in the Medieval Islamic World: Blighted Bodies* (Edinburgh: Edinburgh University Press, 2012); *Disability in the Middle Ages: Reconsiderations and Reverberations*, ed. Joshua Eyler (Aldershot: Ashgate, 2010); and *The Treatment of Disabled Persons in Medieval Europe*, ed. Wendy Turner and Tory Vandeventer Pearman (Lampeter: Edwin Mellen, 2010).

22. Norbert Elias, *The Civilizing Process, vol 1: The History of Manners,* trans E. Jephson (Oxford: Blackwell, 1969, original German edition 1939). Although thought of as a recent phenomenon, perhaps influenced by the translation of Elias' work into English, the current wave of studies was preceded over a century ago by Henry Osborn Taylor, *The Medieval Mind: A History of the Development of Thought and Emotion in the Middle Ages,* 2 vols (London: Macmillan, 1911; repr. Cambridge, MA: Harvard University Press, 1959 and 1962). The topic has been promoted strongly by Barbara H. Rosenwein: see *Anger's Past: The Social Uses of an Emotion in the Middle Ages,* ed. Barbara H. Rosenwein (Ithaca, NY: Cornell University Press, 1998); Barbara H. Rosenwein, "Writing without fear about early medieval emotions," and Carolyne Larrington, "The psychology of emotion and the study of the medieval period," *Early Medieval Europe,* 10 (2001): 229–234 and 251–6 respectively; Barbara H. Rosenwein, "Worrying about emotions in history," *American Historical Review,* 107 (2002): 821–845; *ead.,* "Identity and emotions in the early middle ages," in *Die Suche nach den Ursprüngen: Von der Bedeutung des frühen Mittelalters,* ed. Walter Pohl (Vienna: VÖAW, 2004), 129–137; *ead.,* "Histoire de l'émotion: méthodes et approches," *Cahiers de civilisation médiévale,* 49.193 (2006): 33–48, and *ead., Emotional Communities in the Early Middle Ages* (Ithaca, NY: Cornell University Press, 2006). The last decade has seen a flurry of research across Europe: *Codierungen von Emotionen im Mittelalter/Emotions and Sensibilities in the Middle Ages,* ed. Stephen C. Jaeger and Ingrid Kasten (Berlin: De Gruyter, 2003); *Histoire de la Vergogne [History of Shame],* a special issue of *Rives Méditerranéennes,* 31 (2008); *Le sujet des émotions au Moyen Âge,* ed. Damian Boquet and Piroska Nagy (Paris: Editions Beauchesne, 2009); *Politiques des émotions au Moyen Âge,* ed. Damian Boquet and Piroska Nagy (Florence: SISMEL-Edizioni del Galluzzo, 2010). The establishment of the Australian Research Council Centre of Excellence for the History of the Emotions (Europe 1100–1800) at the University of Western Australia in 2011 has provided an institutional base for much research since then.

23. Horden, "What's wrong," who highlights the contrast between the well-developed study of Anglo-Saxon texts in comparison with

continental Latin manuscripts; Clare Pilsworth, "'Can you just sign this for me John?': Doctors, charters and occupational identity in early medieval northern and central Italy," *Early Medieval Europe*, 17 (2009): 363–388; Patricia Skinner, *Health and Medicine in Early Medieval Southern Italy* (Leiden: Brill, 1997). And see above, note 14. The potential of legal texts for the history of medicine is illustrated by the essays in *Medicine and the Law in the Middle Ages*, ed. Wendy Turner and Sara Butler (Leiden: Brill, 2014), although the bulk of the material discussed here is later medieval.

24. See below, note 85.
25. Paul Edward Dutton, *Charlemagne's Mustache and other Cultural Clusters of a Dark Age* (New York: Palgrave Macmillan, 2004), especially the eponymous first essay, 3–42 and notes, 201–9; Robert Bartlett, "Symbolic meanings of hair in the middle ages," *Transactions of the Royal Historical Society*, 6th series, 4 (1994): 43–60; Miller, *Anatomy of Disgust*, 54–58, discusses the horror of excessive hair or hair out of place. As we shall see in Chap. 2, facial hair matters.
26. The term of course comes from R. I. Moore, *The Formation of a Persecuting Society* (Oxford: Blackwell, 1987, 2nd ed., 2007). As manifestations of these harsher attitudes we might cite studies that examine how civic authorities dealt with the disabled and begging poor, demanding evidence of their disability: Sharon Farmer, *Surviving Poverty in Medieval Paris* (Ithaca, NY: Cornell University Press, 2002); Metzler, *Social History*, Chap. 4. On the intersection of poverty and disability, see also Ephraim Shoham-Steiner, "Poverty and disability: a medieval Jewish perspective," in *The Sign Languages of Poverty*, ed. Gerhard Jaritz (Vienna: VÖAW, 2007), 75–94, developed in *id.*, *On the Margins of a Minority: Leprosy, Madness and Disability among the Jews of Medieval Europe* (Detroit: Wayne State University Press, 2014).
27. *The Dark Side of Childhood in Late Antiquity and the Middle Ages*, ed. Katariina Mustakallio and Christian Laes (Oxford: Oxbow, 2011); Mayke de Jong, *In Samuel's Image: Childhood Oblation in the Early Medieval West* (Leiden: Brill, 1996); Dudley Wilson, *Signs and Portents: Monstrous Birth from the Middle Ages to the Enlightenment* (London and New York: Routledge, 1993); John Boswell, *The Kindness of Strangers: the Abandonment of Children*

*in Western Europe from Late Antiquity to the Renaissance* (Chicago: Chicago University Press, 1988).

28. *L'Enfant et la vie familiale sous l'Ancien Régime* (Paris: Plon, 1960). Translated into English by Robert Baldick as *Centuries of Childhood: A Social History of Family Life* (New York: Vintage, 1962); the *Annales de Démographie historique* for 1973 was a special issue on *Enfance et sociétés*, responding to Ariès. More recent challenges are Barbara Hanawalt, *Growing up in Medieval London: The Experience of Childhood in History* (New York and Oxford: Oxford University Press, 1995) and Nicholas Orme, *Medieval Children* (New Haven, CT: Yale University Press, 2003).

29. Sally Crawford, *Childhood in Anglo-Saxon England* (Stroud: Sutton, 1999), 95.

30. Craig and Craig, "Diagnosis and context of a facial deformity."

31. Edward Wheatley, *pers. comm.*, is currently preparing a study on this subject.

32. Most notably castration, with which disfigurement has an entangled history: see *Castration and Culture in the Middle Ages*, ed. Larissa Tracy (Cambridge: D. S. Brewer, 2013).

33. Targeting children and infants, as we shall see later in this chapter, was used as a way to mark the perpetrator as evil beyond redemption.

34. Cf. the comments in Biernoff, "Rhetoric of disfigurement."

35. Valentin Groebner, *Defaced: the Visual Culture of Violence in the Later Middle Ages* (New York: Zone, 2004), 76.

36. A useful survey of the disease's effects in the past, identified by archaeological evidence, is Keith Manchester, "Medieval leprosy: the disease and its management," in *Medicine in Early Medieval England: Four Papers*, ed. Marilyn Deegan and D. G. Scragg (Manchester: Centre for Anglo-Saxon Studies, 1987), 27–32.

37. *Acta Sanctorum*, vol. XI, 20 April, Vita Ven. Oda Praemonstratensis c.V.20, p. 776. See Patricia Skinner, "Marking the face, curing the soul? Reading the disfigurement of women in the later middle ages," in *Medicine, Religion and Gender in Medieval Culture*, ed. Naoë Kukita Yoshikawa (Woodbridge: Boydell, 2015), 287–318, for a fuller discussion of Oda. Timothy S. Miller and John W. Nesbitt, *Walking Corpses: Leprosy in Byzantium and the Medieval West* (Ithaca, NY: Cornell University Press, 2014), 6–9, discuss definitions of the disease.

38. Elma Brenner, "Recent perspectives on leprosy in medieval western Europe," *History Compass*, 8.5 (2010): 388–406; *ead., Leprosy and Charity in Medieval Rouen* (Woodbridge: Boydell, 2015); Luke Demaitre, *Leprosy in Premodern Medicine* (Baltimore: Johns Hopkins University Press, 2007); Carole Rawcliffe, *Leprosy in Medieval England* (Woodbridge: Boydell, 2006); Guenter P. Risse, *Mending Bodies, Saving Souls: a History of Hospitals* (Oxford: Oxford University Press, 1999), Chap. 4 on leper hospitals and seclusion; Peter Richards, *The Medieval Leper and his Northern Heirs* (Cambridge: Brewer, 1977). A recent, major archaeological find relating to the disease is reported by Simon Roffey and Katie Tucker, "A contextual study of the medieval hospital and cemetery of St Mary Magdalen, Winchester, England," *International Journal of Paleopathology*, 2.4 (2012): 170–180.

39. Skinner, "Marking the face," highlights the case of Margaret of Cortona.

40. This incomplete statistical exercise is intended simply to illustrate the fluidity of terminology when searching for disfigured people, and does not reflect the range of examples ultimately found (for which see below, Appendix I).

41. *Leges Langobardorum*, ed. F. Bluhme, Rothari c. 341, in *MGH LL*, IV, ed. G. H. Pertz (Hannover: Hahn, 1868); Matthew: *MGH SS*, XXVIII, *Ex Rerum Anglicarum Scriptoribus saec. XIII*, ed. F. Liebermann and R. Pauli (Hannover: Hahn, 1888), 119.

42. E. H. Freshfield, *A Manual of Later Roman Law: the Ecloga ad Procheiron Mutata* (Cambridge: Cambridge University Press, 1927), 138; *Ο ΠΡΟΧΕΙΡΟΣ ΝΟΜΟC: Imperatorum Basilii, Constantini et Leonis Prochiron*, ed. C. E. Zachariae v. Lingenthal (Heidelberg: Mohr, 1837), 153. I have been unable to identify the root verb for ἀποσφαλτιώσας – is it related to ἀποψῖλόω, meaning to strip of hair or make bald (and implying therefore that it is the *beard*, not the person, who is "destroyed")?

43. *Leechdoms, Wortcunning and Starcraft of Early England*, ed. O. Cockayne, 3 vols (London: Longmans and Green, 1864–6), II, 53, 77–81 (blotches), 59 (hare lip). And see below, Chap. 7.

44. See the essays in *Why the Middle Ages Matter*, ed. Celia Chazelle *et al.* (New York: Routledge, 2012); and from a feminist and economic perpective Judith Bennett, "Less money than a man would take," in her *History Matters: Patriarchy and the Challenge of*

*Feminism* (Philadelphia: University of Pennsylvania Press, 2006), 82–107; and Skinner, "Gendered nose."

45. Miller, *Anatomy of Disgust*, 11; *id.*, *Humiliation and Other Essays on Honor, Social Discomfort and Violence* (Ithaca/London: Cornell University Press, 1998), 197.

46. Richard Horton, "Offline: the moribund body of medical history," *The Lancet*, vol 384, issue 9940 (2014), 292. Carsten Timmermann, "Not moribund at all! An historian of medicine's response to Richard Horton," *The Guardian*, 4 August, 2014, online at http://www.theguardian.com/science/the-h-word/2014/aug/04/not-moribund-historian-medicine-response-richard-horton [accessed 14 August 2014], unfortunately missed the opportunity to include the premodern in his rebuttal of Horton's case. For this see Pratik Chakrabarti, Graham Mooney and Patricia Skinner, "Editorial," *Social History of Medicine*, 27 (2014): 629–631.

47. Chris Mounsey, "Variability: beyond sameness and difference," in *The Idea of Disability in the 18th Century*, ed. Chris Mounsey (Plymouth: Bucknell University Press, 2014), 1–30.

48. I have explored this issue from the point of view of the early medieval warrior in Patricia Skinner, "Visible prowess? Reading men's head and face wounds in early medieval European sources to 1000CE," in *Wounds and Wound Repair in Medieval Culture*, ed. Kelly de Vries and Larissa Tracy (Leiden: Brill, 2015) 81–101.

49. See below, Chap. 4, for examples.

50. Patrick Wormald, *The Making of English Law: from Alfred to the Twelfth Century*, vol 1 (Oxford: Blackwell, 1999), 44: "it was by memorizing them that crystallising *gentes* fixed the identity of their particular law."

51. *Ibid.*, 46 and 124 (quote). Wormald explicitly updated his earlier essays on the subject in this book and in his collection of essays, *Legal Culture in the Early Medieval West: Law as Text, Image and Experience* (London: Hambledon, 1999).

52. Although the intensity of legislation varied widely between individual emperors, as is made clear by the contributions to *Law and Society in Byzantium: Ninth-Twelfth Centuries*, ed. A. Laiou and D. Simon (Washington: Dumbarton Oaks, 1994).

53. G. Koziol, "Leadership: why we have mirrors for princes but none for presidents," in *Why the Middle Ages Matter*, 183–198.

54. E.g. Charles Insley, "Rhetoric and ritual in late Anglo-Saxon charters," in *Medieval Legal Process: Physical, Spoken and Written Performance in the Middle Ages*, ed. Marco Mostert and Paul Barnwell (Turnhout: Brepols, 2011), 109–121. Wormald's work is reviewed and built upon in *Early Medieval Studies in Memory of Patrick Wormald*, ed. Stephen Baxter, Catherine Karkov, Janet Nelson and David Pelteret (Aldershot: Ashgate, 2009).

55. See below, Appendix 2, for a list.

56. Most notably the work of the late Lisi Oliver: "Sick maintenance in Anglo-Saxon law," *Journal of English and German Philology*, 107.3 (2008): 303–326; *ead.*, "Protecting the body in early medieval law," in *Peace and Protection in the Middle Ages*, ed. T. B. Lambert and D. Rollason (Durham: Centre for Medieval and Renaissance Studies, 2009), 60–77; and *ead.*, *The Body Legal in Barbarian Law* (Toronto: Toronto University Press, 2011).

57. Specifically, Alemannic laws from the seventh and eighth centuries in *Leges Alamannorum*, Pactus I.4 and Leges A, LVII.4 and B, LIX.4, ed. K. A. Eckhardt, *MGH LL nat. Germ.*, V.1 (Hannover: Hahn, 1966); Rothari's edict for the Lombards, dated 643, c. 47, in *Leges Langobardorum*, ed. F. Bluhme, *MGH LL*, IV, ed. G. H. Pertz (Hannover: Hahn, 1868); *Lex Frisionum*, XXII.71, ed. K. de Richthofen, in *MGH LL*, III, ed. G. Pertz (Hannover: Hahn, 1863). Compare the compilation of Welsh laws attributed to the tenth-century King Hywel Dda, where the bone makes a sound when falling into a copper basin: *The Laws of Hywel Dda The Book of Blegywryd*, tr. M. Richards (Liverpool: Liverpool University Press, 1964), 64. Clearly size mattered in all these cases. According to Rolf H. Bremmer, Jr, "'The children he never had, the husband she never served': castration and genital mutilation in medieval Frisian law," in *Castration and Culture*, 108–130, the extraordinarily detailed provisions of Frisian law are unlikely ever to have been put into effect.

58. E.g. when the citizens of Rome ejected their newly-elected pope John XIII in 965, according to Benedict of Soracte, "some hit his head and others gave him slaps in the face [*alii percutiebant caput eius, alii alapas in facies eius percutiebat [sic]*": *Benedicti S. Andreae Monachi Chronicon*, in *MGH SS*, III, ed. G. H. Pertz (Hannover: Hahn, 1839), 719.

59. Below, Chap. 4, note 8.

60.  ...fecit, quod infelix illa gens Friolana, mares et femine, magni et parvi, clerici et laici, generaliter omnes cesi et deformati, per Lonbardiam et marchiam signum deferunt Ecelinice rabiei. Nichil quoque profuit parvulis innocentibus non peccasse, immo, cum triplicem penam senes et iuvenes paterentur, oculis naribus et pedibus mutilati, infantes et innocentes penam quadruplicem habuerunt, nam Ececlini iussu naribus et pedibus deformati, cecati sunt oculis et parvis genitalibus sunt exsecti. Fuit autem hec Ecelini ultima perpetrata crudelitas in predicto anno Domini [1259], mense Iunii circa finem: *Rolandini Patavini Chronica* XI.17, ed. P. Jaffé, in *MGH SS* XIX: *Annales Aevi Suevici*, ed. G. H. Pertz (Hannover: Hahn, 1866), 136.

61.  *MGH Epp Saeculi XIII e Regestis Pontificum Romanorum Selectae*, ed. C. Rodenberg, III, letter 481 (Berlin: Weidmann, 1894), 445–6.

62.  Similarly, Frederick II's treatment of (presumably mercenary) Genoese archers, "manu et oculo mutilati" after his capture of Milan in 1245 is written up as an act of cruelty: *Bartholomaei Scribae Annales*, s.a. 1245, in *MGH SS*, XVIII, ed. G. H. Pertz (Hannover: Hahn, 1863), 219.

63.  It appears to have gained particular popularity as a motif in texts and iconography of the twelfth century: Einat Segal, "Sculpted images from the eastern gallery of the St-Trophime cloister in Arles and the Cathar heresy," in *Difference and Identity in Francia and Medieval France*, ed. Meredith Cohen and Justine Firnhaber-Baker (Farnham and Burlington: Ashgate, 2010), 67–69, highlights the motif in chronicle evidence from the century; other creative uses are discussed by John Marlin, "The Investiture Contest and the rise of Herod plays in the twelfth century," *Early Drama, Art and Music Review*, 23 (2000): 1–18, and Miriam Anne Skey, "The iconography of Herod in the Fleury Playbook and in the visual arts," in *The Fleury Playbook: Essays and Studies*, ed. C. Clifford Flanigan, Thomas P. Campbell and Clifford Davidson (Kalamazoo: Medieval Institute, 1985), 120–143.

64.  *Gregorii Episcopi Turoniensis Libri Historiarum X*, ed. B. Krusch and W. Levison, *MGH SS Rer Merov.*, I (Hannover: Hahn, 1951) [hereafter *GT*], Bk VI, 46.

65.  Guy Halsall, *Warfare and Society in the Barbarian West, 450–900* (London: Routledge, 2003), 1–2.

66. Antonella Liuzzo Scorpo and Jamie Wood, "Introduction: history-writing and violence in the medieval Mediterranean," *Al-Masāq*, 27 (2015): 1–6, at 5.

67. *Thietmar Mersebergensis Episcopi Chronica*, ed. Robert Holtzmann, *MGH SSRG* n.s. IX (Berlin: Weidmann, 1935) [hereafter *Thietmar*], V.30.

68. On the ambiguity of the passage in question, and its subsequent history, see Ruth Mellinkoff, *The Mark of Cain: An Art Quantum* (Berkeley: University of California Press, 1981).

69. Anna: see below, Chap. 6; Amatus: see below, Chap. 4, note 84; Gregory: above, note 64.

70. I explore Norman historiography on this theme in Patricia Skinner, "The Political uses of the body in Norman texts," paper read at *People, Texts and Artefacts: Cultural Transmission in the Norman Worlds of the Eleventh and Twelfth Centuries*, Ariano Irpino, Italy, 20–22 September 2013. A publication of this conference, and its follow-up at Cambridge in 2014, is planned.

71. E.g. Valerie J. Flint, "The early medieval *medicus*, the saint – and the enchanter," *Social History of Medicine* 2.2 (1989): 127–145; Darryl Amundsen, *Medicine, Society and Faith in the Ancient and Medieval Worlds* (Baltimore: Johns Hopkins University Press, 1996); Patricia Skinner, "A cure for a sinner: sickness and healthcare in medieval southern Italy," in *The Community, the Family and the Saint: Patterns of Power in Early Medieval Europe*, ed. J. Hill and M. Swann (Leeds/Turnhout, Brepols, 1998), 297–309; Clare Pilsworth, "Medicine and hagiography in Italy, 800–1000," *Social History of Medicine*, 13.2 (2000): 253–264.

72. Metzler, *Disability in Medieval Europe*, has an appendix of cases from three sample hagiographic texts.

73. *The Book of St Foy*, tr. Pamela Sheingorn (Philadelphia: University of Pennsylvania Press, 1995), 50.

74. See the essays collected in *Icon and Word: the Power of Images in Byzantium*, ed. Anthony Eastmond and Liz James (Aldershot: Ashgate, 2003). On iconoclasm, Leslie Brubaker and John Haldon, *Byzantium in the Iconoclast Era c.680–850: a History* (Cambridge: Cambridge University Press, 2011), noting at 199 their warning that much of the hagiography of persecution ("the *myth* or *legend* of opposition [to iconoclasm]") was constructed after the final

restoration of icons in the ninth century. For examples of punishments, see below, Chap. 3.

75. The Wulfstan episode is quoted at length and extensively discussed by Wheatley, *Stumbling Blocks*, 175–179 and considered by van Eickels, "Gendered violence," 595. Becket: The *Miracula* of Benedict of Peterborough, reproduced in *English Lawsuits from William I to Richard I, volume II: Henry II and Richard I*, ed. R. C. Van Caenegem (London: Selden Society vol 107, 1991), case 471B, 509–514. And see below, Chap. 7.

76. See, e.g. Larissa Tracy, "'Al defouleden is holie bodi': castration, the sexualization of torture and anxieties of identity in the *South English Legendary*," in *Castration and Culture*, 94–6.

77. The passage will be discussed below in Chap. 7.

78. Ruth Mazo Karras, *Sexuality in Medieval Europe: Doing unto Others* (New York: Routledge, 2005), 39.

79. On the earlier cases, Jane Tibbetts Schulenberg, *Forgetful of their Sex: Female Sanctity and Society c.500–1100* (Chicago: Chicago University Press, 1998), 145–8 (Eusebia of Marseilles, Ebba of Coldingham and Oda of Brabant). On later cases Claire Marshall, "The politics of self-mutilation: forms of female devotion in the late middle ages," in *The Body in Late Medieval and Early Modern Culture*, ed. Darryl Grantley and Nina Taunton (Aldershot: Ashgate, 2000), 11–22, and Skinner, "Marking the face." Armando R. Favazza, *Bodies under Siege: Self-mutilation and Body Modification in Culture and Psychiatry* (2nd ed., Baltimore: Johns Hopkins University Press, 1996), explores self-mutilation both as religious practice and as mental illness from antiquity to the modern day.

80. E.g. *Practical Medicine from Salerno to the Black Death*, ed. Luis Garcia-Ballester, Roger French, Jon Arrizabalaga and Andrew Cunningham (Cambridge: Cambridge University Press, 1994).

81. Horden, "What's wrong?" For Italy, Pilsworth, *Healthcare*, 74–104, illustrates the value of examining individual, early manuscripts on their own terms.

82. Notably the work of Timothy Miller, *The Birth of the Hospital in the Byzantine Empire* (Baltimore: Johns Hopkins University Press, 1985); Miller and Nesbitt, *Walking Corpses*; see also *Symposium on Byzantine Medicine: Dumbarton Oaks Papers*, 38, ed. John Scarborough (Washington: Dumbarton Oaks Research Library, 1985); Peregrine Horden, "The earliest hospitals in Byzantium,

western Europe and Islam," *Journal of Interdisciplinary History*, 35 (2005): 361–389.

83. *The Letters of Gerbert with his Papal Privileges as Sylvester II*, trans. Harriett Pratt Lattin (New York: Columbia University Press, 1961), 187, Letter 159 (Rheims, 1 March 989).

84. The classic studies are Charlotte Roberts and Keith Manchester, *The Archaeology of Disease*, 3rd ed. (Stroud: Sutton, 2005), and Tony Waldron, *Palaeopathology* (Cambridge: Cambridge University Press, 2008); see also D. J. Ortner, "Human skeletal paleopathology," which inaugurated the *International Journal of Paleopathology*, 1 (2011): 4–11.

85. Archaeological examples, several of which either show signs of healing or surgical intervention: E. T. Brødholt and P. Holck, "Skeletal trauma in the burials from the royal church of St Mary in medieval Oslo," *International Journal of Osteoarchaeology*, 22.2 (2012): 201–18 (undated material); Piers Mitchell *et al.*, "Weapon injuries in the twelfth century crusader garrison of Vadum Iacob castle, Galilee," *International Journal of Osteoarchaeology*, 16.2 (2006): 145–155; P. Patrick, "Approaches to violent death: a case study from early medieval Cambridge," *International Journal of Osteoarchaeology*, 16.4 (2006): 347–354; Raphael Panhuysen, "Het scherp van de snede: sporen van geweld in vroegsmiddeleuwse Maastricht," *Archeologie in Limburg*, 92 (2002): 2–7, where two cases of blade injuries to the skull showed signs of healing. (I thank Professor Panhuysen for assisting me in gaining access to this valuable article.)

86. Willibald Sauerländer, "The fate of the face in medieval art," in *Set in Stone: the Face in Medieval Sculpture*, ed. Charles T. Little (New York: Metropolitan Museum, 2006), 3.

87. Stephen Parkinson, "Sculpting identity," in *Set in Stone*, 120–1.

88. As an illustrative example, British Library MS Royal 13 B VIII, f. 30v (late Twelfth -early thirteenth century English compilation) features a crippled man using hand stools.

89. Lepers, whose moral status was ambivalent, are portrayed, however: Christine M. Boeckl, *Images of Leprosy: Disease, Religion and Politics in European Art* (Kirksville, Missouri: Truman State University Press, 2011). Her examples include the depiction, 32, of Christ healing a leper on the *Codex Aureus of St Emmeram*, dating to c.870. It is notable that the leper's arms and legs are covered in raised dints to represent the disease, but his face, whilst fashioned with holes and lumps, remains entirely recognizable (*ibid.*, 33).

90. Umberto Eco, *On Beauty*, tr. A. McEwan (London: Secker and Warburg, 2004), 111 (Isidore and Thomas); Umberto Eco, *On Ugliness* (London: Harvill Secker, 2007).
91. Stephen K. Scher, "Iconoclasm: a legacy of violence," in *Set in Stone*, 20.
92. Antony Eastmond, "Between icon and idol: the uncertainty of imperial images," in *Icon and Word*, 73–85.
93. Giorgio Agamben, "The face," in *id.*, *Means without End: Notes on Politics*, tr. V. Binetti and C. Casarino (Minneapolis: Minnesota University Press, 2000) [originally published as *Mezzi senza fine* (NP: Bollati Boringhieri, 1996)], 91–100; François Delaporte, *Anatomy of the Passions*, tr. S. Emanuel (Stanford: Stanford University Press, 2008) [originally published as *Anatomie des passions* (Paris: PUF, 2003)].
94. Stephen Pattison, *Saving Face: Enfacement, Shame, Theology* (Aldershot: Ashgate, 2013).
95. P. Christopher Earley, *Face, Harmony and Social Structure: An Analysis of Organizational Behavior across Cultures* (Oxford: Oxford University Press, 1997), offers a useful overview.
96. Groebner, "Losing face, saving face?"
97. Giorgio Agamben, *Homo Sacer: Sovereign Power and Bare Life*, tr. Daniel Heller-Roazen (Stanford: Stanford University Press, 1998) [Italian publication Torino: Einaudi, 1995].
98. Skinner, "Gendered nose."
99. John Berger, *Ways of Seeing* (London: Penguin, 1972, repr. 2008); Garland-Thompson, *Staring*.

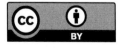

# CHAPTER 2

# The Face, Honor and "Face"

## What Is a Face?

What is a face and what is it for? Is it the assembly, in regular order and conforming to an ideal type, of features making up a whole? Does it encompass the whole head or simply the eyes, nose and mouth? And does the face function as more than a facade, instead expressing a deeper sense of personhood and identity epitomized by its mobility, the ability to express emotion and connection through the movement of its subcutaneous muscles and nerves? Humans are programmed to look at faces almost from birth. The face conveys the ability not only to recognize a person, but also to make judgments on whether s/he belongs to a particular community and what clues s/he is giving off through her/his expression as to her/his willingness to be included in social interactions. All this information is encoded within scrutiny of less than a second, looking first at the eyes and then working downwards.[1] Experiments in cognitive development have concluded that, despite the need for faces to be differentiated in order to recognize individuals, the face that is *too* different causes confusion:

This chapter is partly based on papers given at the conference *European Perspectives on Cultures of Violence*, held at Leicester University in June 2013, and at the North American Association for Welsh Culture and History meeting at the Royal Military Academy, Kingston, Ontario, in July 2014. My thanks are due to Simon Sandall and Huw Osborne, who organized these meetings, and the delegates who offered pertinent avenues to follow up.

© The Author(s) 2017
P. Skinner, *Living with Disfigurement in Early Medieval Europe*,
DOI 10.1057/978-1-137-54439-1_2

normal interaction demands that all the frontal features (i.e. eyes, nose and mouth) be present in order that the scrutiny is not interrupted by a hole where there should not be one, or asymmetrical halves of the face.

The elements of the face (including the ears and hair) are worth examining in detail, since the value accorded to each, both monetarily in legal compensation, and metaphysically in terms of their function and potential, reveals both a hierarchy of facial features and of their associated senses. Of these sight was by far the most precious. The eye, after all, was a window or portal to the soul—nothing would be more horrifying, according to Miller, than "to think of poking it out."[2] But the eyes are also expressive— they count as an active element in facial expression, whether through dilation of pupils, opening or closing of eyelids, shedding tears or frowning. Miller again: "Eyes represent us at our most vulnerable and most beautiful..."[3] Sight was commonly used as a metaphorical device by medieval clerical writers—the eleventh-century chronicler, Bishop Thietmar of Merseberg (d. 1018), for example, refers twice to physical blindness in association with "inner vision," and Gerald of Wales (d. 1223) comments that a man who had been blinded by the saint for spending a night in the church with his dogs decided to go on a pilgrimage to Jerusalem, "for he did not wish to allow his spiritual light to be extinguished as his eyes had been."[4] We could multiply examples of this clerical *topos*, and will return to sight as a sense in Chapter 6.

The nose arguably played more of a role in medieval discourse than has been recognized. At the center of the face, the nose provides a relatively immobile structure, a centering tool for assessments of symmetry, a still part of the face to contrast with the mobility and expressiveness of eyes and mouth. Although the Freudian correlation of the nose with the penis does not contribute much to our understanding of its importance in the Middle Ages, a damaged or cut-off nose clearly had profound effects on the person so injured, as legal sources make clear.[5] They are, however, all aesthetic: the potential loss of ability to smell or taste, associated with major damage to the nostrils that funnel aromas up to the olfactory receptors, is never referred to.

The mouth, lips and tongue were all susceptible to disfiguring injuries, and mutilating any or all of its parts could inflict speech impediments or even muteness. The aesthetic qualities surrounding teeth, particularly in legal texts, seem to relate to their presence or absence. Occasionally, authors refer to the drawbacks of having bad teeth; Thietmar, for instance, reports that his deceased colleague had not been able to chew food due to an "infirmity" of his teeth, and had been restricted to drinking for nour-ishment.[6] None, however, seem to comment on the spectacle of rotten teeth. As the authors of a recent study on medievalism in modern film-making comment wryly, "when the actors smile, aesthetic anachronisms shine across the screen in their perfectly straight teeth gleaming with the striking whiteness typical of Hollywood stars but mostly alien to the pre-orthodontic milieus of earlier centuries."[7] Silencing of speech through the mutilation of the tongue, while outwardly invisible, may represent one of the worst disfigurements of all in this orally driven society.[8]

Extending outwards from the circle formed by the face were the ears. Although less horror seems to have accompanied deafness than blind-ness, the absence of ears and the consequent potential to impair hearing was noted, as we shall see in Chapters 4 and 5. However, the ear was also connected, in early medieval medical thought, with the testes: a cut-off ear, the repository of sperm, could represent an ersatz—and much more visible—castration.[9] Given the small number of mutilations relating to women overall in the sample collected here, it is hard to determine whether ear-cutting was gender-specific. It is, however, suggestive that the majority of cases I have found have been of men, and that in one instance featuring a man and a woman punished together, only the man was muti-lated in this way.[10]

A missing ear, of course, might be disguised by growing out the hair. This too was freighted with symbolism, and some authors use hair practices to interpret the customs of other peoples. Thietmar reports, for example, that among the "faithless" Liutici, hair cut from the top of the head was the sign of peace-making and atonement for disagreeing with others in assembly.[11] As Robert Bartlett demonstrated in a classic article, and Paul Dutton has commented more recently, hair (head or facial) was a signifi-cant element in elite social identity: its owner's status was often indicated by its presence, abundance, color, or lack.[12] Notker the Stammerer, writ-ing in the latter half of the ninth century, tells a convoluted story about the embarrassment caused by red hair.[13] In his *Ten Books of History*, written in stages during the latter half of the sixth century, Gregory of Tours pro-vides evidence for the importance of long hair to the Merovingian kings of Francia. His account of the first Frankish king Clovis (r. 481–511) sees the new king having his opponent Chararic and Chararic's son tonsured and made clerics, but "As they were threatening to grow their hair again... he had their heads cut off." Later on King Theodovald (r. 548–555), is described as withdrawing from the political contest; having "no wish for earthly dominion... with his own hands he cut his hair short."[14] The end of Merovingian rule is famously reported in Einhard's oft-cited ninth-century report: when King Childeric III was deposed in c.751, "his hair was cut and he was shut up in a monastery." Dutton argues that the Carolingians *deliberately* cultivated a short-haired, mustached appearance partly to distinguish themselves from the long hair encoded within the honor of their Merovingian predecessors.[15] A later example of hair removal in a Byzantine context is reported by the eleventh-century author Amatus of Montecassino; Theodwin, disgraced oppressor of the abbey and exiled when he and his master fled to Constantinople, was shaved of his beard and hair, "a great disgrace amongst the Greeks," and kept his head covered with an otter's skin.[16]

## SURFACE AND DEPTH

The relationship between the surface features of the face and the underlying personality has formed the subject of philosophical enquiries, notably by Giorgio Agamben and François Delaporte, and discussion from a theological standpoint by Stephen Pattison.[17] Made up of "active" and "passive" elements, respectively the eyes and mouth and the ears, nose and cheeks, the face "is always suspended on the edge of an abyss," threatening to open up and reveal "the amorphous background," according to Agamben.

Agamben's characterization of what lay beneath the skin reflects an ancient tradition: medieval authors, too, drawing upon the works of earlier Church Fathers, contrasted the possibly deceptive outward beauty of the skin with the inside "understood as a vile jelly, viscous ooze or a storage area for excrement."[18] Luke Demaitre comments that medical practitioners viewed the skin as "at best, a screen onto which internal reality was projected and, at worst, an obstacle veiling the secrets of the body."[19] Thus, puncturing or breaking down the skin risked revealing the true nature of what lay beneath: if "pus, running sores [and] skin lesions... were a regular feature of medieval life," nevertheless *deliberately* damaging and breaking open the face could still be seen as an act of cruelty and rashness, evoking both pity and disgust.[20] What came out of a face naturally, however—blood from a nosebleed, vomit, spit—did not hold such horror provided it was not used to insult another (for example, by vomiting over them or spitting at them).[21] A nosebleed is carefully set apart in legal sources as a normal event, somewhat unusually given other blood taboos visible in the same texts. (The postmortem nosebleed of Bishop Syrus of Genoa features as a key event in establishing his cult, according to his later *vita*.)[22] Even before it took on major Eucharistic significance, blood was a substance evoking strong responses. Bettina Bildhauer explains, "The idea that spilt blood cries to heaven comes from Genesis 4:10, which states that Abel's blood, shed by Cain, cries to God for vengeance."[23] The work of Mary Douglas has been influential on medieval historians interested in exploring the leakiness of the female body (and, in the form of involuntary ejaculation, that of men as well), but the face, with its multiple orifices and delicate surface, perhaps presented the most fragile container of all.[24]

For Agamben, "the face is at once the irreparable being-exposed of humans and the very opening in which they hide and stay hidden." It is also "the only location of community," a communicating entity that is more than simply the sum of its outward expressions (what Agamben terms "visages") or physical resemblance. In his short, dense essay on the subject, he rejects the commodification of the physical face and its co-option into state systems of control, and instead proposes a metaphysical notion of face based upon language and behavior, the essence of person-hood expressed within—but more tangibly beyond—the facial features. Rosi Braidotti comes to similar conclusions about the body as a whole, stating that it forms "an interface, a threshold, a field of intersection of material and symbolic forces...a surface where multiple codes of power and knowledge are inscribed."[25] The views of both commentators have profound implications for how we might understand disfigurement: physical injury here, by definition, is an injury to the visage or surface, potentially limiting the ability to be expressive or be recognized, rather than to the social being to whom it belongs. But the *meanings* of such visible injuries, constituted by language, penetrate and are inscribed upon the person, and might also affect the ability and/or choice of that person to remain "being-exposed" or "to hide and stay hidden." The dividing line—if such exists—between the physical surface and "face" as an expression of social status, might be very fragile. With this thought in mind, let us turn to definitions of "face" as a social phenomenon.

## HONOR AND "FACE"

The concept of "face" has, in many studies, been used as a synonym for honor, and applied rather uncritically. Richard Watts defines "face" as a "metaphor for individual qualities and/or abstract entities such as honor,

respect, esteem and the self, etc."[26] "Losing face" is often used as a popular shorthand for "honor impugned," whether or not the physical face
is implicated in the process of injury.[27] Yet modern anthropological and
psychosocial studies have pointed out that there is a clear distinction
between honor cultures and face cultures, and this distinction is used to
form the basis for analysis of medieval texts in this chapter. It is fair to
say that after its heyday in the 1960s and 1970s, the value of sociological
and anthropological research has rather receded from the study of early
medieval societies, and some historians write with explicit hostility toward
such methodology.[28] Certainly there has been something of a backlash
against the easy assumptions of some anthropologically informed work
published in the 1980s and 1990s, by scholars within and outside the
Anglo- and Francophone worlds.[29] Yet Max Gluckmann's seminal work
on feud, published in 1955, clearly laid a trail for understanding the reciprocal nature of violence in early medieval society,[30] and the essays collected
by Peristiany in 1966 have an enduring value for understanding the ritual
character of honor in close-knit communities, even for studies contrasting other societies with the Mediterranean region that was its focus.[31]
As Geoffrey Koziol points out, however, social anthropology has moved
on somewhat since these studies and "the subject [of ritual] has become
more than a little passé."[32] Here, though, I am less interested in ritual
*per se* and more concerned with how the disfigured face was constituted
and understood within the culture of early medieval society, and how it
functioned as a marker of status. Using disfigurement as an entry point,
I suggest that honor remains a useful category to work with, but that it
was not the only way in which social interactions were regulated in early
medieval society. Lurking alongside "honor," it is possible to discern a
largely unspoken and unwritten culture of "face." Some definitions are
therefore required.

Honor culture, according to social anthropologist Julian Pitt-Rivers, is
"the value of a person in his own eyes, but also in the eyes of his society"—
and it has to be actively claimed through words and actions.[33] Cultures of
honor, according to psychologists Angela Leung and Dov Cohen, "tend
to originate in 'lawless' environments" and consist of "a competitive environment of rough equals."[34] It is interesting to note that they cite the
work of William Ian Miller on feuding in saga Iceland to illustrate their
point, and indeed they imply that medieval culture was an honor culture
*par excellence*. In short, participants in an honor culture care about their

own reputation and repeatedly test it—horizontally—against that of their peers.[35] Moreover, according to Pitt-Rivers again, "The victor in any competition for honor finds his reputation enhanced by the humiliation of the vanquished."[36] Miller highlights the role of mutilation in this humiliating process—victims were meant to live mutilated and shamed, and therefore were uncompromisingly hostile to their mutilators, just waiting for an opportunity to return the insult.[37]

Face culture, on the other hand, still links the individual's status to the opinion of others but, unlike honor culture, face relies upon knowing one's place within a relatively rigid hierarchy, and paying due and correct deference to one's superiors—preserving their face as well as one's own—while ensuring the same from one's inferiors.[38] The contrast here is obvious: a participant in a face culture has as much (if not more) social capital tied up in ensuring harmonious *vertical* relationships, prioritizing the face of others in order to maintain one's own, and sensitive to perceived slights from social inferiors.[39] What I find tremendously useful about these distinctions is their clarity—while individuals within each of these cultures might not adhere tightly to the rules, the cultural categories outlined offer historians a way into exploring why violence does, or does not, occur, and what its likely outcomes might be.

Studies of early medieval Western Europe have tended to focus on honor as the means by which social capital was gained and lost.[40] Studies of the feud, or early medieval laws, or medieval literary tales, have emphasized reciprocity amongst equals, whether violent or within a gift-giving framework, as the glue underpinning early medieval social relations. A fantastically bloody example of how this pervades literature is the feud-fest that is *Raoul of Cambrai*, an epic poem of the late-twelfth/early-thirteenth century that sets its story in an earlier period. *Raoul* is essentially a tale of reciprocity without satisfactory resolution. Indeed, a recent study of the poem has commented that it "fails to ever truly end."[41] During the course of the poem, however, the physical face recurs again and again as a site for attacking honor and punishing betrayal, whether it is Raoul threatening to blind and mutilate the barons who fail to heed his summons (line 850), or hitting Bernier's head and drawing blood (lines 1535–1540), or threats to "pull out the whiskers" of Guerri the Red (lines 1864, 3991). When Gautier cuts off Bernier's ear, however, the latter cries "If I don't avenge myself I'll never be happy again!" (lines 4832–4).[42] In this literary text the message is explicit: you get hurt, you respond in kind.

## CASE STUDY: THE CELTIC WORLD

Yet there were territories—particularly in Celtic Europe—where it seems as if social relations were organized, or at least legislated for, in a more fluid, nuanced way. Focusing on face-related injuries and terminology in the sources from these regions, however, it becomes apparent that the restoration of honor between equals does not adequately explain some of the transactions we can see.

The key material to consider here is medieval Welsh law, in which the payment given in compensation for insult and injury, normally termed *sarhaed*, was occasionally termed *wynebwerth*, or "the worth of the face."[43] A variant of this, *wynebwarth* or "shame of the face," also occurs in some of the surviving manuscripts. Dafydd Jenkins notes a particular association in the Welsh Law of Women between the use of *wynebwerth* and offenses relating to sexual misbehavior in marriage, but comments that elsewhere it seems as a term to be earlier than, and interchangeable with *sarhaed*.[44] The complex history of the Welsh laws has of course attracted the attention of generations of scholars, and debate still centers on the vexed question of whether, or how, the surviving, mainly thirteenth-century manuscripts or Books, that claim their origins in the laws of King Hywel in the tenth century, truly reflect the earlier medieval legal situation.[45]

Here, however, the intention is to explore the idea of "face price" (a concept shared, as we shall see, with the legal cultures of other Celtic peoples) and to broaden out into a wider consideration of the physical face as a site of honor and shame in medieval Welsh society.[46] By exploring visible facial and head wounds in early Welsh laws and literature, we can see a distinction played out within a medieval society along gendered lines ("gender" here expressing unequal power relations, rather than specifically male-female interactions), and suggest that *wynebwerth* and *sarhaed* may not be as interchangeable as has sometimes been thought. The semantic entanglement between the two terms becomes even less helpful when we consider the relationship between the appearance of the physical face, and how facial injury or difference could impact a person's social standing or honor. Consider this triad from one of the earliest versions of the law in South Wales, which also appears in similar form from the northern text the *Book of Iorwerth*:

> There are three conspicuous scars on a man: a scar on his face is worth 120d; a scar on the back of his right hand 60d; a scar on the back of his right foot 30d.[47]

Facial scarring, it is implied, damaged honor more than less visible scars, and attracted a higher compensatory payment. Parallel examples of the damage a scar could do can be found in other legal collections, for example, a payment of twelve shillings for leaving a sunken scar called a *sipido* in early ninth-century Frisian law,[48] or the 16 *solidi* payable for nose and ear wounds "healing to a scar" in the even earlier, seventh-century edict of the Lombard King Rothari in Italy.[49]

Now while facial scarring *might* be read as a badge of bravery in warfare, the assumption in lawcodes was that the victim of interpersonal violence was shamed by his scar. There are many indications in early lawcodes, however, of medical attention being available and paid for by the perpetrator (and one of the three "legal needles" in Welsh law was of course that of the medic to stitch wounds).[50] Yet the shame remains: in the early Irish medico-legal code *Bretha Déin Chécht*, the shame of the public scar is made explicit, as a blemish on the face exposed its victim to public ridicule—hence, the law states, a fine has to be paid for every public assembly the victim has to endure with facial disfigurement.[51]

Literary tales from Wales and Ireland reinforce this sense of public shame. Although their use as historical sources is debatable,[52] they provide some illustrations of how disfigurement and shame intersected in early Irish society. In the Irish mythic tale *The Wooing of Étaín*, for example, Mider tries to break up a pack of squabbling boys:

> a sprig of holly was hurled at him, and it put out one of his eyes. Mider returned to the Macc Óc, his eye in his hand, and said, "...I have been shamed; with this blemish I can neither see the land I have come to nor return to the land I have left."[53]

This being a mythical tale, the Macc Óc in fact sees to it that Mider's eye is healed "without shame or blemish." The Welsh tales making up the Mabinogion and associated later materials (which reached their written form in the eleventh and twelfth centuries) are full of indicators of face and shame, some, it has been noted by other scholars, very close in language to the legal material.[54] In particular, "shame on my/thy/his beard" recurs in both earlier and later tales.[55] If a woman wished shame or a blemish on her husband's beard, she was essentially questioning his masculinity and had to pay a small fine (*camlwrw*) or suffer a beating on her body.[56] Presumably, injury to her head or face would be considered excessive, not to mention make visible what was essentially a domestic matter between spouses. (The beard, it might be noted, features prominently in the nick-names attributed to Arthur's men in *Culhwch and Olwen*, and in storylines about its removal/plucking or shaving.)[57]

Returning to the law, other aspects of facial dignity are visible. In the laws of Hywel as transmitted by the *Book of Iorwerth*, the king's door-keeper is charged with ensuring that the chief officers of the court are admitted without stopping them. If he does stop them (and the impli-cation here could be that he does so deliberately or that he does not recognize these prominent individuals), he is charged to pay them *wynebwerth*.[58] A judge's accuser is liable to pay *wynebwerth* if he falsely accuses the judge and loses.[59] As has already been noted, *wynebwerth* is also strongly associated with male-female relations. A woman could take her *wynebwerth* if she left her adulterous husband, or if she was raped.[60] A man's *wynebwerth* from his wife was among his "unclaimable things," and vice versa.[61]

In his legal survey, Thomas Glyn Watkin has noted the payment to the judge for his "loss of face," but did not elaborate on the meaning of this phrase.[62] What strikes me about *wynebwerth* payments, at least those discussed so far, is that they are indeed about loss of "face," but not loss of "honor." That is, far from being similar to *sarhaed*, *wynebwerth* seems to have been paid when the social status or position of the two parties was *already unequal* and then infringed—woman to man, doorkeeper to superior members of the court, petitioner to judge. The people paying were in effect recognizing that they had challenged someone higher up in the social hierarchy, which sounds very close to the idea of damag-ing their superiors' "face." *Sarhaed* might still be paid between people of unequal status, but it is striking that this is often by the senior party to the junior—hence a husband beating his wife for no reason was liable to pay her *sarhaed*, according to Iorwerth. But in acting so violently, I wonder whether the loss of honor implied is his, rather than hers?[63] I think it is no accident that a woman insulting her husband (as above) pays only a small fine or is beaten—her insult did not constitute *sarhaed*, as she was not her husband's social equal. A late version of a legal triad even makes this dis-tinction explicit: "the disgrace of *wynebwerth* is not as great as *sarhaed*."[64] Rees Davies has noted that the term *wynebwerth* does not appear in the court rolls, and suggests that by the fourteenth century it was an archa-ism.[65] My sense of this is that by the fourteenth century, the very specific and hierarchical meanings expressed by *wynebwerth* payments had been overtaken by (or subsumed within) the hierarchical values of chivalric culture. (The infiltration of romance elements into the later Welsh stories appended to the Mabinogion is another manifestation of this trend.)

To summarize then, *sarhaed* seems to have been a payment by social equals or superiors, and might buy back honor after a dishonorable act by the giver, as well as compensate the recipient. It was also a very public payment, and thought to concern more serious injuries (physical or social). *Wynebwerth*, by contrast, seems to have been a payment by social inferiors to their superiors to restore the latter's "face," did not reflect any honor onto the person paying, and was considered less serious, perhaps because of the lower status of that person. Essentially, the actions of a social inferior were being marked as less damaging to the recipient of *wynebwerth*; the challenge had to be compensated for, but it was not the same as a loss of honor between equals. The co-existence of these two, imperfectly defined payment systems, exposed by looking at real, physical faces and their conspicuous scars, suggests that medieval Welsh society had two strands of personal status running parallel to each other, "face" and "honor," and they were not the same.

If I am correct about the distinction between *sarhaed* and *wynebwerth*, then it would follow that we need to look carefully at evidence from other regions for similar labeling practices. In Ireland, the compensation for injury was termed *log n'enech* (literally: "the price of the nose").[66] Wendy Davies's study of Breton society reflects this when she reports on the settlement of a case in which "face was saved" between the abbot of Redon and his defaulting tenants.[67] Sarah Sheehan points up the "facedness" of terminology in old Irish for the gaining and loss of honor: *enech* for face/honor, but also words for physical blemishes and blots conveying a metaphorical injury as well: *ainim* and *on*. She emphasizes the role of mutilation and insult, totally humiliating the opponent in order to win honor among equals, in her analysis of the early Irish tale of the carving of Mac Dathò's pig.[68] Thomas Charles-Edwards states that, in Welsh and Irish society at least, we are dealing with honor "which must be publicly declared." He goes on, however, to distinguish "honor" from "status," the "hierarchy of social ranks," and discusses the very fine gradations of language and behavior required to preserve status—for which read "face"—in these communities. In essence, therefore, he is acknowledging the difference that can be picked up between horizontal and vertical relationships within these communities.[69]

Was Celtic society exceptional in this respect? Chapter 5 will take a gendered approach to responding, but here the focus is on broadening geographically. It is worth noting, of course, that the Celtic regions were by no means isolated from the rest of Europe, and ideas, as well as goods, percolated along trade routes extending as far as Francia, northern Spain and Italy.[70] Physical attacks leaving visible scars were dishonoring and required recompense. As will become apparent in this chapter, however, legal materials from England and continental Europe do not appear to have differently named categories of compensation, nor do they utilize face-related terminology to name compensation payments. The difference between "honor" and "face" in these medieval societies may still be visible, however, if we focus again on unequal relationships, but this time explore the indirect effect of mutilation as a shaming practice. In Ireland, an insult to a wife was also an insult to her husband, as "the value of her face was dependent upon the value of his."[71] What happens if we extend the idea of dependence further, and explore other parts of Europe?

## MODELING "FACE" AS AN ELEMENT OF ELITE MALE AUTHORITY

Christian authors in Medieval Europe had a clear idea of the social gradations of early medieval society, and one commonplace in texts describing the qualities of good lords and kings is that they offered protection to their dependents, especially the weak and vulnerable. How, though, did a good lord avenge injuries done to his subjects? Leaving aside the issuing of laws, which is the subject of the next chapter, we can see some hints in narrative sources. Notker suggests, in his portrait of the Carolingian King Louis the Pious (d. 840), that Louis appointed a man to stand in for him when justice had to be meted out on those injuring the poor. This justice, Notker says, consisted of "retaliation in kind for injuries and wounds received (*iniuriarium vel lesionum taliones*), and in more serious cases the cutting-off of limbs, decapitation and the public display of those executed."[72] The problems with this account are legion—by suggesting active and violent retribution for "injuries and wounds received," Notker elides completely the existing framework of laws in Francia that prescribed compensatory payments precisely to *avoid* retaliation (and, by inference, escalation of the violence). The image of Louis (or at least his representative) as an avenging warrior for his people is an interesting counterpoint to his reputation for piety, but in writing him this way Notker allows the image to trump the realities of Louis' relative *impotence* when faced with violent acts (not least from his own family).

To develop the theme of the ruler's "face" further, we can turn to a passage from Adam of Bremen's *History of the Church of Hamburg/Bremen*, completed in the 1070s but relating to an earlier episode. Referring to pirate attacks on the Saxon coast in 994, Adam says that the pirates severed the hands and feet and cut off the noses of their captives and cast them on the land "maimed and half-dead... Among them were some noble men who lived a long time after, *a reproach to the Empire* and a *pitiful spectacle for all the people* [my emphasis]."[73] There is an explicit criticism here—notably at a safe chronological remove from the actual events—of an emperor who did not defend his subjects, in particular (but not exclusively) the men who would be expected to make up his court. Adam's account is late, but we can compare his report with that of Thietmar, who was not only a contemporary witness to the troubles but almost ended up being traded for one of the noble hostages himself. Thietmar's three uncles, Henry, Udo and Siegfried were directly involved in fighting off the pirates. Udo was killed, but Henry and Siegfried were captured along with Count Adelgar. Thietmar reports that "the news of this quickly spread," underlining the severity of the situation.[74] Negotiations were opened by Duke Bernhard "who was nearby," to ransom the hostages, and resources began to be gathered for a payment, but Thietmar is curiously reticent about the emperor's own contribution to the collection. Eventually, part of the ransom was paid, and several of the hostages were released in exchange for stand-ins (Henry's son, Adelgar's uncle and cousin). Since Siegfried did not have any children, Thietmar's mother nominated first his brother, a monk, and then Thietmar himself to be substituted. In the event, Siegfried managed to escape before Thietmar was handed over. This action led to the pirates coming ashore, stealing all the women's earrings, and the mutilation and dumping of the remaining hostages, who included Thietmar's cousin Siegfried, Henry's son.[75]

Although the accounts of Thietmar and Adam differ slightly in their presentation of this episode, they share unease about the power of the ruler to prevent such atrocities. The emperor himself was not maimed, but his face was irreparably damaged—one might say mutilated by proxy—by the dishonoring of his men. Context is crucial here, however: the emperor in question was the child Otto III, whose rule from 983 onwards had been contested by Duke Henry of Bavaria, and for whom his mother, Theophanu, and grandmother, Adelaide, ruled successively as regents. (The insecurity of this decade is apparent in the letter-collection of Gerbert of Aurillac, one of Otto III's supporters and his tutor.) In 994, Otto was approaching his majority, but the weakness of his position is perhaps epitomized by the humiliation of his nobles. Adam's passage, of course, does not comment directly on this background, but he was surely inspired to reflect on the shortcomings of lords in his writings by the contemporary politics of his own day. Writing in the late eleventh century, he had witnessed the accession of King Henry IV of Germany, also as a minor, and Henry's subsequent hostile treatment of Adalbert, archbishop of Bremen and Adam's own patron. The text of Adam's third book, arguably, tries to save the "face" of his over-reaching ecclesiastical lord.

Can we see this motif of lordly failure elsewhere in the literature? In fact, it is a fairly common occurrence, used to highlight starkly the failure of protectors across time and place. So, for example, the future king of England, Cnut (r. 1016–1035), is famously reported as having mutilated the ears, noses and hands of his English hostages (to be more precise, the hostages sent to his father Sweyn in 1013 "from every shire" in the Danelaw, and from Oxford, Winchester, London and the west country, and placed in Cnut's charge), before putting them ashore at Sandwich in 1014. While the Anglo-Saxon Chronicle makes no explicit comment, the juxtaposition of this act with King Aethelred's return to England may not be accidental, symbolizing the latter's inability to resist the Danish invasions or protect his people.[76] Failure to protect also infuses the sixth-century author Jordanes' report, in his *Getica*, that the first wife of Huneric the Vandal was sent home to her father, Theodoric the Goth, with her nose and ears cut off, "because of the mere suspicion" that she was plotting to poison her father-in-law, Huneric's father, King Gaiseric.[77]

In all of these cases, the shame of the mutilations rebounds upon a third party, but does so, I suggest, in multivalent ways. Two of the attacks, reported in Jordanes and the Anglo-Saxon Chronicle, involve a present or future king dishonoring a social equal (another king) by harming those whom they are expected to protect (as father and ruler). But all three attacks also have the potential to challenge and harm the "face" of the ruler, in terms of undermining his superior status by calling into question his *ability* to perform his expected functions as ruler. This is most explicit in the attack by social inferiors (the pirates) upon their betters (the nobles) interpreted by Adam as a disgrace to the emperor, but arguably damaging the "face" of both the emperor and the nobles themselves. In all three cases, however, the vulnerability of the ruler is made explicit without his being touched at all, and in sociological terms this could be described as a "face-threatening act."[78] How can the ruler recover? One way was to manage the report of the incident. For all that she is the victim, Theodoric's daughter (whose mutilation is explicitly written up by Jordanes as sign of the Vandals' barbarity) was nevertheless associated in his account with the suspicion of treason. The blame for the incident is thus shifted partly onto her, for having provoked such suspicion. This does not exactly mitigate the insult to Theodoric, but it is arguably less damaging to him than the multiple mutilations of socially important men in the other two accounts. Jordanes, it must be admitted, had no reason to minimize the damage to Theodoric, but if his work does indeed draw from an earlier history by Cassiodorus, then the latter's position serving the king may be reflected here. The other two examples of weak kingship share a common context of external attack and the inability of the ruler to defend even his own territory (again, there is a contrast with the episode in Jordanes—Theodoric's daughter was in a foreign land when she was attacked).

A key question at this point is whether and how these three examples are represented—are they barbaric atrocities, something "others" do, or are they all calculated actions within a shared discourse of how to damage the prestige of lords? Guy Halsall addressed this question indirectly in his discussion of the debate about Viking attacks on Europe, arguing that the Viking "atrocities," written up largely by those on the receiving end of the attacks, were the result of a clash of cultures, and mutual incomprehension, rather than a calculated move by the raiders to destroy Christians or undermine long-accepted models of warfare in England and Francia.[79] As a culturally different group, Halsall argues, the Vikings of the ninth century could not be expected to understand or share the expectations of those whom they attacked. Notably, Halsall draws a distinction between these early waves of raids and the later Danish invasions, when physical proximity and conversion changed the game considerably. It is within this later context that Cnut's action can, indeed, be understood as a deliberate and knowing act.

Intriguingly, the potential for indirect harm also extended to the mutilation of animals, as Andrew Miller has recently pointed out.[80] Miller highlights the fact that numerous writers reported on the deliberate disfiguring of Thomas Becket's animals, and suggests that these highly visible actions were calculated to bring shame upon the archbishop. In Wales the laws attributed to Hywel penalized anyone putting out the eye or cutting the tail of the king's stag-hound, another highly visible challenge to royal authority.[81] Publicly damaging something owned, however, is a slightly different category—into which we should also place the injuries to slaves and the semi-free visible in the early medieval lawcodes discussed in the next chapter. Unlike the examples just discussed, the mutilation did not directly undermine the relationship between the mutilated and their lords. It did have the potential to sway the opinion of third parties, perhaps, and this may explain why financial compensation was still paid for injury. In an interesting variation on this, a later version of the story of Congal Cáech, the king of Ulster and Tara (r. c. 626–637), incapacitated and disqualified from his position by a bee-sting in the eye, has him demanding (in vain) that the eye of the beekeeper's son be put out as recompense for the bee's action.[82]

It might be objected that we do not need sociological theories of face to explain a common assumption in medieval literature that the ruler was expected to offer protection to his people (female rulers faced a problem here that none quite resolved). Yet the ideal ruler was often extolled as the protector only of those who could not fight and defend themselves—the clergy, women, children, the poor and sick. The dynamic visible in two of the three cases discussed here is somewhat different: the mutilated are men who would be expected to be able to fight, but are placed in an impossible position of vulnerability because their leaders are ineffectual and unable to assist them. Thietmar offers another example: his own nephew, Henry, seized and blinded a "distinguished but over proud soldier (*militem egregium set nimis superbum*)" of the bishop of Wurzburg "on account of the injuries he had suffered (*ob inlatas sibi iniurias*)." The bishop's men reported the incident to the king, who exiled Henry. Again we see an attack on an able-bodied man, damaging to the bishop, but reciprocated this time by the *bishop's* lord and thus perhaps revealing the relative weakness of the episcopal position when it came to responding to violent acts.[83]

If injury to followers can be described as a loss of face for the ruler, do the followers themselves have any role in preserving face, given that this is a hierarchical scheme whereby they would be expected not only to acknowledge and defer to superior status, but to work proactively in its defense? A quasi-hagiographic tale from the chronicle of St Peter's monastery near Halle in Germany reveals that insult to honor by a social equal could be the pretext to an act of disfigurement enacted by followers to save the face of their lord. The story, dating to the early twelfth century, centers on Conrad, count of Wettin, claiming that Henry, marquis of Meissen, was in fact a changeling of low birth ("the son of a cook"), whose father had arranged his exchange with the cook's wife. But what started as a verbal injury between "rough equals" also compromised their retinues: Henry "stirred up his supporters to avenge his injury (*ut suam iniuriam vindi-carent, omnibus suis fidelibus supplicavit*)." Meanwhile one of Conrad's followers, Heldolf, vowed, in front of the altar of St Peter's, to prove the truth of this insult or lose the health (*sanitas*) of his body. Almost immediately he was waylaid by two of Henry's servants and, unable to get his horse to move and escape them (the supernatural element), suffered mutilation of his eyes, nose, lips, cheeks and ears at their hands, and thus ended up as a permanent reminder that the story was false, his damaged face a testimony to the unwise vow he had made and proof that Henry was not a changeling.[84] Picking apart this story—we must remember above all that it appears in a chronicle designed to promote the power of the cult site at St Peter's—we might suggest that in making the accusation, Conrad put himself and his followers in a difficult position, at risk of retaliation for the insult. Indeed, Henry demanded that *his* followers take action. Heldolf, looking to save his master's face by invoking the saint's help to prove the story, misuses the altar and receives a terrible physical punishment from Henry's men, who in turn save the face of their lord and restore his reputation.

Heldolf's comprehensive mutilation is presented in the source as a just punishment, as well as an indictment of his lord's unwise challenge to Henry's reputation. In failing to sustain his claim against one who is proven *not* to be socially inferior, and in his additional failure to protect his follower, Conrad himself loses honor *and* face. Arguably, Heldolf's own face does not need to be the site of mutilation to get this message home—he could equally well have been struck directly by the saint with a punishment such as muteness or paralysis for his brash boast—but the physical face here is the most visible target for Henry's followers. And they not only mutilate, but also totally destroy Heldolf's features (this is an extreme example by the standards of the texts I have explored). At the beginning of this chapter we considered the physical face as a composite, expressive and capable of communicating with others actively and passively. Heldolf's fate is to lose his ability to "be" Heldolf: now his face communicates a story. The veracity of the tale is less important than the moral lessons to be learnt about respect, for one's equals, one's betters and, crucially, for the saint, always at the top of the medieval hierarchy.

It has become apparent in this chapter that the physical face and the metaphorical one are intimately interconnected in the accounts of damage and its recompense. Although the concept of injury is semantically linked to facial features only in the Celtic languages, the potential for social disgrace or humiliation through facial injury reverberates through-out Latin texts as well. The facial features were easy targets, and highly vis-ible once damaged. A damaged face arguably did not bring the same levels of impairment as a serious injury to body or limb (unless the victim's eyes were attacked, on which see below, Chapter 6) but the social disability associated with the disruption of the facial features was potentially much greater. Materially speaking, facial damage had to be pretty severe before it prevented someone from continuing to work.

Here, though, the class of the victim matters as well. Almost all of the examples we have discussed were of high status: the hostages mutilated by Cnut were clearly chosen and "sent from every shire," and in order to function effectively as hostages they had to have some recognizable value to those who sent them. Yet, a careful reading of the meanings of honor and face has also revealed that the careful preservation of vertical social ties entailed reciprocal responsibilities: a lord gained face by protecting his subjects, and honor by interacting appropriately with his equals; his subjects shared responsibility in defending and preserving his face through their actions.[85] Yet when Henry stirred up his followers to avenge the insult done to him by Conrad, it is notable that they are not simply pre-sented galloping off and attacking Conrad himself. Such violence from social inferiors would not have been appropriate and would have been punished severely, and might in fact have further *dis*honored Henry, fan-ning the rumor that he was little better than his servants. Returning to Agamben, the exposed abyss of Heldolf's face stood as a symbol for what happened when evil words and deeds were let out in public, and when supernatural aid was sought for an unjust assertion.

## NOTES

1. Vicky Bruce and Andy Young, *Face Perception* (London and New York: Psychology Press, 2012) and see below, Chap. 6.
2. William Ian Miller, *The Anatomy of Disgust* (Cambridge, MA: Harvard University Press, 1997), 90.
3. William Ian Miller, *Eye for an Eye* (Cambridge: Cambridge University Press, 2006), 29.
4. *Thietmar Mersebergensis Episcopi Chronica*, ed. Robert Holtzmann, *MGH SSRG* n.s. IX (Berlin: Weidmann, 1935), Book VII, chapters 55 and 67 [hereafter *Thietmar*]; Gerald of Wales, *Journey through Wales*, I.1, tr. L. Thorpe (London: Penguin, 1978), 77–8.

5. On Freud and noses, see the discussion in Jay Geller, *On Freud's Jewish Body: Mitigating Circumcisions* (New York: Fordham University Press, 2007), esp. 96.

6. *Thietmar*, VI.64.

7. Tison Pugh and Angela Jane Weisl, *Medievalisms: Making the Past in the Present* (Abingdon: Routledge, 2013), 83. And see below, note 16 of this chapter.

8. Loss of speech through a stroke merited comment, even if it was to draw a moralizing lesson: Orderic Vitalis, *Ecclesiastical History*, ed. Marjorie Chibnall, 6 vols, III (Oxford: Oxford University Press, 1972) [hereafter *Orderic*], Book IV.ii.310, reports Archbishop John of Rouen, made mute by a stroke, sent by God to curb his pride, which he survived for a further 2 years.

9. Danielle Jacquart and Claude Thomasset, *Sexualité et savoir médical au moyen âge* (Paris: PUF, 1985), 46 n. 2. This association does not appear to have been picked up in the recent volume *Castration and Culture in the Middle Ages*, ed. Larissa Tracy (Cambridge: D. S. Brewer, 2013).

10. But see below, 00, the case of Theodoric's daughter, and cf. the mutilations of women in Chap. 5.

11. *Thietmar*, VI.25.

12. Robert Bartlett, "Symbolic meanings of hair in the Middle Ages," *TRHS*, ser.6, 4 (1994): 43–60. See also Conrad Leyser, "Long-haired kings and short-haired nuns: writing on the body in Caesarius of Arles," *Studia Patristica*, 24 (1993): 143–150; Paul Dutton, *Charlemagne's Mustache and other Cultural Clusters of the Dark Ages* (New York, Palgrave Macmillan, 2004).

13. Notker, *Gesta Karoli, MGH SS rer. Ger. n.s. 12*, ed. H. Haefele (Berlin: Weidmann, 1959) [hereafter *Notker*], I.18. And see below, Chap. 6, for discussion.

14. *GT*, II.41 and III.18. English translation: Gregory of Tours, *History of the Franks*, tr. Lewis Thorpe (London: Penguin, 1974), 156 and 182.

15. *Einhardi Vita Karoli Magni*, ed. O. Holder-Egger, *MGH SS rerum. Germ.*, XXV (Hannover: Hahn, 1911) [hereafter *Einhard*], I.1. English translation: Einhard and Notker the Stammerer, *Two Lives of Charlemagne*, tr. L. Thorpe (London, Penguin, 1969), 55. Dutton, *Charlemagne's Mustache*, 22–3.

16. *History of the Normans*, II.13, tr. Prescott N. Dunbar with introduction by G. A. Loud (Woodbridge: Boydell, 2004), 68.

17. Giorgio Agamben, "The face," in *id.*, *Means without End: Notes on Politics*, tr. V. Binetti and C. Casarino (Minneapolis: Minnesota University Press, 2000), 91–100 [originally published as *Mezzi senza fine* (NP: Bollati Boringhieri, 1996)]; François Delaporte, *Anatomy of the Passions*, tr. S. Emanuel (Stanford: Stanford University Press, 2008) [originally published as *Anatomie des passions* (Paris: PUF, 2003)]; Stephen Pattison, *Saving Face: Enfacement, Shame, Theology* (Farnham/Burlington, VT: Ashgate, 2013), 77–84.

18. Miller, *Anatomy of Disgust*, 52 and 89 (quote).

19. Luke Demaitre, "Skin and the city: cosmetic medicine as an urban concern," in *Between Text and Patient: The Medical Enterprise in Medieval and Early Modern Europe*, ed. Florence Eliza Glaze and Brian K. Nance (Florence: SISMEL-Edizioni del Galluzzo, 2011), 97–120, at 104; M. McVaugh, "Surface meanings: the identification of apostemes in medieval surgery," in *Medical Latin from the Late Middle Ages to the 18th Century: Proceedings of the ESF Exploratory Workshop in the Humanities organized under the supervision of Albert Derolez, Brussels, 3–4 September 1999*, ed. W. Bracke and H. Deumans (Brussels: ESF, 2000), 13–29.

20. Miller, *Anatomy of Disgust*, 53.

21. Nosebleed: e.g. *The Laws of Hywel Dda (The Book of Blegyrwyd)*, tr. M. Richards (Liverpool: Liverpool University Press, 1954), 106; spitting: Johan Goudsblom, "Public health and the civilizing process," *Milbank Quarterly*, 64.2 (1986): 161–188, at 164; Miller, *Anatomy of Disgust*, 145, relates a particularly lengthy episode on vomiting in the sagas.

22. Cited in Clare Pilsworth, *Healthcare in Early Medieval Northern Italy: More to Life than Leeches* (Turnhout: Brepols, 2014), 120.

23. Bettina Bildhauer, *Medieval Blood* (Cardiff: University of Wales Press, 2006), 46.

24. Mary Douglas, *Purity and Danger: an Analysis of Concepts of Pollution and Taboo* (2nd edition, London: Routledge, 2002); on leaky women see the late medieval examples explored by Sarah A. Miller, *Medieval Monstrosity and the Female Body* (New York: Routledge, 2010); on involuntary ejaculation Conrad Leyser, "Masculinity in flux: nocturnal emission and the limits of celibacy

in the early middle ages," in *Masculinity in Medieval Europe*, ed. D. M. Hadley (London: Longman, 1998), 103–119.

25. Rosi Braidotti, *Patterns of Dissonance: A Study of Women in Contemporary Philosophy* (Cambridge: Polity Press, 1991), 219.

26. Richard J. Watts, *Politeness* (Cambridge: Cambridge University Press, 2003), 119–122, citing the influential work of sociologist Erving Goffman.

27. Valentin Groebner, "Losing face, saving face: noses and honour in the late medieval town," *History Workshop Journal*, 40 (1995): 1–15; Sarah Sheehan, "Losing face: Heroic discourse and inscription in flesh in *Scéla Mucce Meic Dathó*," in *The Ends of the Body: Identity and Community in Medieval Culture*, ed. Suzanne Conklin Akbari and Jill Ross (Toronto: Toronto University Press, 2013), 132–152.

28. See Bernard S. Bachrach's comments in *Early Carolingian Warfare: Prelude to Empire* (Philadelphia: University of Pennsylvania Press, 2001), 86: his main objection, it seems, was the categorizing of early medieval society as in some way "primitive."

29. *Negotiating the Gift: Premodern Figurations of Exchange*, ed. A. Giladi, V. Groebner and B. Jussen (Göttingen: Vandenhoeck and Ruprecht, 2003); Philippe Buc, *The Dangers of Ritual: Between Early Medieval Texts and Social Scientific Theory* (Princeton: Princeton University Press, 2002). And see the response to Buc, in particular, by Geoffrey Koziol, "Review article – The dangers of polemic: is ritual still an interesting topic of historical study?", *Early Medieval Europe*, 11 (2002): 367–388.

30. Max Gluckmann, "The peace in the feud," *Past and Present*, 8 (1955): 1–14. Its influence is visible, for example, in the essays collected in *The Settlement of Disputes in Early Medieval Europe*, ed. Wendy Davies and Paul Fouracre (Cambridge: Cambridge University Press, 1986), and in William Ian Miller, *Bloodtaking and Peacemaking: Feud, Law and Society in Saga Iceland* (Chicago: Chicago University Press, 1990).

31. *Honour and Shame: the Values of Mediterranean Society*, ed. J. Peristiany (Chicago: Chicago University Press, 1966). See the contrast drawn by William Ian Miller between Mediterranean and northern societies' use of shame, particularly in relation to women, in *Humiliation and other Essays on Honor, Social Discomfort and*

*Violence* (Ithaca and London: Cornell University Press, 1998), 118. Unfortunately, Miller also collapses the useful distinction between honor culture and face culture when, in talking about shame as the opposite of honor, he states "All of us care about maintaining face," 9.

32. "Review article – The dangers of polemic," 367.

33. Julian Pitt-Rivers, "Honour and social status," in *Honour and Shame*, ed. Peristiany, 21–77, quote at 21.

34. A. K.-Y. Leung and D. Cohen, "Within- and between-culture variation: individual differences and the cultural logics of honor, face and dignity cultures," *Journal of Personality and Social Psychology*, 100.3 (2011): 507–26, at 509–510.

35. Miller, *Anatomy*, 144 makes the same point.

36. Pitt-Rivers, "Honour," 24. He goes on to note the prime importance of rituals surrounding the head and face (whether crowning, slapping or decapitating) within the honor system.

37. *Bloodtaking and Peacemaking*, 197.

38. Leung and Cohen, "Within- and between-culture variation," 510.

39. The notion of "social capital," of course, is another idea drawn upon heavily by medieval historians from the social sciences, in particular the work of Pierre Bourdieu, *Outline of a Theory of Practice* (Cambridge: Cambridge University Press, 1977).

40. Most recently, Peter Baker, *Honour, Exchange and Violence in Beowulf* (Woodbridge: Boydell, 2013); Dana Polanichka and Alex Cilley, "The very personal history of Nithard: family and honour in the Carolingian world'" *Early Medieval Europe*, 22 (2014): 171–200. The flipside to honor, shame, has also received recent, welcome attention: *Shame between Punishment and Penance: the Social Uses of Shame in the Middle Ages and Early Modern Times*, ed. Bénédicte Sère and Jörg Wettlaufer (Florence: SISMEL-Edizioni del Galluzzo, 2013).

41. Andrew Cowell, "Violence, history and the Old French epic of revolt," in *Violence and the Writing of History in the Medieval Francophone World*, ed. Noah D. Guynn and Zrinka Stahuljak (Cambridge: D. S. Brewer, 2013), 19–34, at 33.

42. All line references are to *Raoul de Cambrai*, ed. and tr. Sarah Kay (Oxford: Clarendon Press, 1992).

43. T. M. Charles-Edwards, *The Welsh Laws* (Cardiff: University of Wales Press, 1989), 41.

44. *The Laws of Hywel Dda: Law Texts from Medieval Wales*, tr. Dafydd Jenkins (Llandysul: Gomer Press, 1986), 392.

45. Charles-Edwards, *Welsh Laws*, provides a useful summary of the scholarship and main problems of the manuscripts.

46. Thomas Glyn Watkin's recent survey of Welsh legal history, from an avowedly legalistic rather than social perspective, reminds us that Wales was by no means isolated from the rest of Europe in the early middle ages: T. G. Watkin, *The Legal History of Wales* (Cardiff: University of Wales Press, 2007), 28–29, 40.

47. *The Legal Triads of Medieval Wales*, Cyfn mss U3, V3, W3 and Z4, 83, ed. Sara Elin Roberts (Cardiff: University of Wales Press, 2007). Iorwerth parallel: *Laws of Hywel Dda*, II.8, tr. Jenkins, 97.

48. *Lex Frisionum, Additiones Sapientium* III.34, ed. K. de Richthofen, in *MGH LL III*, ed. G. Pertz (Hannover: Hahn, 1863).

49. *Leges Langobardorum*, Rothari 55 and 56, ed. F. Bluhme in *MGH LL*, IV, ed. G. H. Pertz (Hannover: Hahn, 1868). Full details of laws in Appendix 2, below.

50. X63 from the earlier Cyfn tradition, elaborated on in Q94 in the extended triad collection of a fifteenth-century Blegwryd manuscript: Roberts, *Legal Triads*, 75 and 139.

51. *Bretha Déin Chécht*, clause 31, cited in Fergus Kelly, *A Guide to Early Irish Law* (Dublin: Dublin Institute of Advanced Studies, 1988), 132

52. A typically robust defense of utilizing literary sources is Miller, *Bloodtaking*, 45.

53. *Early Irish Myths and Sagas*, tr. with an introduction and notes by Jeffrey Gantz (London: Penguin, 1981), 42.

54. *The Mabinogion*, tr. Gwyn Jones and Thomas Jones (London: Everyman, 1949).

55. *Branwen daughter of Llŷr*: Heilyn son of Gwyn "shame on my beard if I do not open the door [to Cornwall and Aber Henfelen]" (*ibid.*, 33); *The Lady of the Fountain* (one of 3 later, Romance tales): the maiden to Owein, taking ring she has given him: "Thus does one do with a false treacherous deceiver, to bring shame on thy beard" (*ibid.*, 144); *Peredur son of Efrawg*: Peredur allegedly says "may I lose all face if I go back to Arthur" (*ibid.*, 156), though this does not correspond with the Welsh in at least one manuscript; in the same text Peredur insists on sharing food, "if not, shame on

my beard" (*ibid.*, 162); an old man says "shame on my porter's beard" when Peredur traps his tame lion (*ibid.*, 169).

56. Case law or *Damweiniau*, in *Laws of Hywel Dda*, tr. Jenkins, 52. Not on her head: *Laws of Hywel Dda*, tr. Richards, 67.

57. *Mabinogion*, tr. Jones and Jones, *Culhwch and Olwen*. Nicknames of Arthur's men: Llawfrodedd "the bearded," Nodawl "cut-beard," *ibid.*, 86; Uchdryd "cross-beard" and Rhynnon "stiff-beard," *ibid.*, 98. Plucking a beard from Dillius the Bearded – has to be done whilst he is alive with wooden tweezers, *ibid.*, 99, and the act itself on the stunned man in a pit, *ibid.*, 106; Ysbadadden's death preceded by Cadw son of Prydein, who "came to shave his beard, flesh and skin to the bone, and his two ears outright," *ibid.*,113.

58. *Laws of Hywel Dda*, tr. Jenkins, 26.

59. *ibid.*, 141.

60. *ibid.*, 46, 51. A revision to Iorwerth stated that if she claimed *wynebwerth* three times without leaving her adulterous husband, or put up with his behavior without claiming *wynebwerth*, she lost the right to the payment and was considered a shameful woman: *ibid.*, 53.

61. *ibid.*, 61; *Legal Triads*, ed. Roberts, X10, 45.

62. *The Legal History of Wales*, 71.

63. Similarly, triad Q24 in *Legal Triads*, ed. Roberts, 105, illustrates sexual offences against a woman attracting *sarhaed* – but whose honor was offended, hers or her family's? Beating in Iorwerth: *Laws of Hywel Dda*, tr. Jenkins, 53.

64. *Legal Triads*, ed. Roberts, Q166, 175.

65. R. R. Davies, "The status of women and the practice of marriage in late-medieval Wales," in *The Welsh Law of Women: Studies presented to Professor Daniel A. Binchy on his 80th Birthday*, ed. Dafydd Jenkins and Morfydd Owen (Cardiff: University of Wales Press, 1980), 93–114, at 99. Sarah Elin Roberts follows this chronological scheme when she states, *Legal Triads*, 309, that *wynebwerth* was "the earliest word for honour price."

66. Wendy Davies, "Anger and the Celtic saint," in *Anger's Past: the Social Uses of an Emotion in the Middle Ages*, ed. B. H. Rosenwein (Ithaca and London: Cornell University Press, 1998), 191–202, at 199: Irish *lóg n'enech*, Welsh *wynebwerth*. See also Kelly, *Guide*, 8.

67. Wendy Davies, *Small Worlds: The Village Community in Early Medieval Brittany* (Berkeley: University of California Press, 1988), 149.

68. Sheehan, "Losing face," 134.
69. Thomas Charles-Edwards, "Honour and status in some Irish and Welsh prose tales," *Eriu*, 29 (1978): 123–141.
70. Watkin, *Legal History*, 28–9, surveys some of the Welsh evidence.
71. Charles-Edwards, "Honour and status," 138.
72. *Notker*, II.21, ed. Haefele, 91, tr. Thorpe, 170.
73. *Magistri Adam Bremensis Gesta Hammaburgensis Ecclesiae Pontificum*, II.xxxi, ed. Bernhard Schmeidler, *MGH SS rer. Germ.*, II (Hannover and Leipzig: Hahn, 1917), 29:...*pyratae mox in furorem versi, omnes, quos in vinculis tenuerunt, meliores ad ludibrium habentes, manus eis pedesque truncarunt ac nare precisa deformantes ad terram semianimes proiciebant. Ex quibus erant aliqui nobiles viri, qui postea supervixerunt longo tempore, obprobrium imperio et miserabile spectaculum omni populo.* English translation: *Adam of Bremen, History of the Archbishops of Hamburg-Bremen*, tr. Francis J. Tschan with introduction and notes by Timothy Reuter (New York: Columbia University Press, 2002), 75–6.
74. *Thietmar*, IV.23: *fama volante mox dilatatur*.
75. *Thietmar*, IV.24–25.
76. *The Anglo-Saxon Chronicle: a revised translation*, C (D, E) for 1013 and 1014, ed. Dorothy Whitelock (London: Eyre and Spottiswoode, 1961), 92–93.
77. Jordanes, *Getica*, Bk XXXVI, tr. C. C. Mierow (Princeton: Princeton University Press, 1915), 184: Accessed at: http://people.ucalgary.ca/~vandersp/Courses/texts/jordgeti.html [17 September 2012]. On Jordanes as an author, see W. Goffart, *The Narrators of Barbarian History* (Princeton: Princeton University Press, 1988), 20–111, and A. H. Merrills, *History and Geography in Late Antiquity* (Cambridge: Cambridge University Press, 2005), 100–169.
78. A term made popular by Erving Goffman: see below, Chap. 4.
79. Guy Halsall, "Playing by whose rules? A further look at Viking atrocity in the ninth century," *Medieval History*, 2.2 (1992): 3–12. See, however, the disclaimer by the author at http://600transformer.blogspot.co.uk/2013/07/playing-by-whose-rules-further-look-at.html [Accessed 2 October 2014].
80. Andrew G. Miller, "'Tails' of masculinity: knights, clerics and the mutilation of horses in medieval England," *Speculum* 88 (2013): 958–995. He erroneously follows Klaus van Eickels, "Gendered

violence: castration and blinding as punishment for treason in Normandy and Anglo-Norman England," *Gender and History*, 16.3 (2004), 588–602, however, in attributing this practice to a Norman import.

81. *Laws of Hywel Dda*, ed. Richards, 61.
82. Kelly, *Guide*, 239.
83. *Thietmar*, IV.21.
84. *...sicque illis irruentibus captus, et oculis, naso, labiis, lingua, auribus mutilatus, proprie ma勒diccionis effectu visus est. probasse, quod Henricus marchio non fuerit pro femina commutatus*: *Chronicon Montis Sereni*, ed. E. Ehrenfeuchter, *s.a.* 1126, in *MGH SS*, XXIII, ed. G. Waitz (Hannover: Hahn, 1874), 140.
85. I am using "his" here advisedly: as I will suggest in Chap. 5, women's 'face' may have been differently understood.

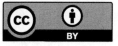

# CHAPTER 3

# Disfigurement, Authority and the Law

The previous chapter touched upon some of the legal evidence for damage to the face and head, and began to tease out the possible social categories that such evidence revealed. In particular, the indirect association of violence inflicted on subjects, and the potential damage this caused to the ruler, was the basis of my argument that medieval society was not simply an honor culture, but had more subtle vertical gradations of personal status that equate closely with the modern definition of face culture. In this chapter, the legal material will be mined more deeply to define how injury was conceptualized, and how the ruler, whose laws ostensibly existed to prevent violence escalating, was also able to claim a sovereign right to inflict violence in specific circumstances. Toward the end of the chapter, a later sample of material from court cases will offer some idea of how injuries were presented by their victims.

The sheer preponderance of violent injuries and punishments in the medieval laws and accounts of judicial proceedings might be responsible for some of the shriller assessments of the medieval period as one of unmitigated violence and brutality.[1] The core thesis of Michel Foucault's influential *Discipline and Punish* (which in turn built on earlier work by Johan Huizinga, Norbert Elias and, more pertinently for medieval history,

---

This chapter is based on a paper titled "Envisaging violence: the rhetoric and reality of medieval disfigurement in Europe and Byzantium, c.800–1200," given at the Medieval Academy of America meeting in Knoxville, Tennessee, in March 2013. I am grateful for the comments received at that meeting.

P. Skinner, *Living with Disfigurement in Early Medieval Europe*,
DOI 10.1057/978-1-137-54439-1_3

Marc Bloch)—that the corporal display and uncontrolled, emotion-driven savagery of the medieval period was replaced by more "rational" forms of punishment such as imprisonment in the modern era[2]—whilst disputed and discredited by subsequent research,[3] is still highly influential in shaping perceptions. Studies of medieval violence per se, whilst not always accepting such a viewpoint, do little to radically shift the paradigm. Miller comments of Elias that he "paints a caricatured view of the Middle Ages in which civility was at a minimum and shame and disgust over bodily functions pretty much non-existent," but goes on to suggest that "It is a trait of great works to be able to be proven wrong in particulars and still manage to offer a truth about the larger picture."[4] Sean McGlynn terms Foucault "misleading" but prefaces his work with the statement "we should not let the stories of brutality in this study be blunted by the wearing-down of the centuries."[5] Medievalists do not, it seems, have to go far to find juicy examples of violence and coercion, perpetuating the image of a time when brutality served as a deterrent to transgression. Yet what is striking about much of this work is that, first, it tends to read the sources too literally, taking accounts of violence and extreme cruelty as emblematic of medieval society as a whole (Guy Halsall's introduction to *Violence and Society in the Early Medieval West*, one of the few volumes to focus on our period, suggests that "Violent relationships can often be seen as a discourse structured around shared norms"); and, secondly, it largely relates to the later medieval period.[6] As Lucy Grig points out, accounts of violence and torture elicit strong, often negative, responses from those studying them, obscuring the fact that such accounts are not neutral and have a specific purpose that closer reading can reveal. She comments, "The Catholic church asserted its authority through narrative, through the power of the story, as much as by any other means."[7] Her acute observation has a broader application, well beyond the late antique martyrologies that she was using as examples. Randall Collins has commented, in an influential and much-cited essay on cruelty, that our job as researchers is not so much to judge and justify the violence of an age, but to try to gain access to the discernible patterns and meaning of that violence.[8] Work on the early Middle Ages, such as the majority of essays in the 1998 volume *Anger's Past*, in fact found that the violent expression of that emotion was not as spontaneous or uncontrolled as Elias, in particular, had argued.[9] Early medievalists, again utilizing insights gained from the social sciences, identified clear parameters and rituals determining and circumscribing violent acts and *how they were reported by writers*. Expressions of horror and disgust, therefore, might be targeted at the actions of a perpetrator, rather than the eventual appearance of the victim. It is also easy to assume that what was going on in the later Middle Ages must have had its roots in earlier practices, but a careful reading of just some of the abundant legal material, taking as its entry point material relating to injuries and mutilations of the head and face, suggests that whilst the values enshrined in the early medieval laws did have wider purchase (at least, according to the reports of other members of the same, literate class), they are not at all reliable as evidence for levels of violence in early medieval society.

## LAWS AND INJURIES

The early medieval lawcodes issued in Europe from c.650 to c.1050 contain multiple clauses dealing with injuries to the face and head, as well as to other parts of the body, listed in often minute detail, as is well known. Appendix 2 gives something of a sense of their content and extent, as well as their remarkably similar nature. Specific elements of the laws' concern with the treatment of wounds will be discussed later in Chapter 7.

What the raw statistics reveal, however, is the fact that in almost all cases, the perpetrator of the injury was fined rather than physically punished. This is not a straightforward, talionic legal system of reciprocal injury—an eye was not given for an eye, a tooth did not replace a tooth.[10] There also seems to be an increasing elaboration of clauses, with ever-finer detail, in later codes. The *Lex Frisionum*, "given" by the Carolingians to the Frisians soon after Charlemagne's imperial coronation in 800CE, is a positive panoply of personal injury, with the head and face covered by nearly thirty individual—but possibly not original—chapters.[11] It is useful to examine the categories of injury alongside each other, however, because some are clearly not related to bodily harm so much as bodily appearance or personal interactions.[12] There are, for instance, numerous clauses about hair, whether cutting, pulling or shaving it.[13] Not just hair, but beards, mustaches and even eyebrows were featured, damage to which incurred a penalty.[14] Teeth, too, feature in many of the codes, with damage or removal of the front teeth, those most visible, incurring higher fines than damage to the back teeth.[15]

These injuries might literally be termed superficial, but honor in these codes—understood here as the horizontal status of an individual face-to-face with his or her social peers—was explicitly linked to unblemished personal appearance, and damage to this carried with it a penalty to be paid to avoid reprisal. Shame (*turpis*) accompanied injury, as several clauses point out.[16] Furthermore, in some codes the tariff for injury was broken down into still more detail by assessing the social rank of the victim in order to determine the appropriate compensation.[17] Where slaves and the semi-free were injured, for example, the injury was really to their master, and the latter certainly received the compensation payment for his/her slave being out of action. Whilst some of the Germanic codes owed much to their late Roman predecessors in ideas and ideals of personal honor—compare Emperor Justinian's sixth-century *Digest* chapters on "Contumelies and Defamatory Writings"[18]—the emphasis on physical appearance as a marker of honor seems a feature of post-Roman legal culture.[19] The *Lex Frisionum*, by far the most explicit on this matter, included a clause punishing any mutilation of the face that was visible at twelve feet away. As we have seen, the tenth-century compilation of Welsh laws attributed to Hywel Dda, similarly, was concerned with compensation for the "conspicuous scar" to the face, that is, one which would elicit inquiry as to what had happened.[20]

That personal appearance as the heart of the legal framework is emphasized when we turn to what might, medically, seem more serious head injuries—cutting off noses and ears, gouging eyes, or hitting the head so hard that skull and brain were exposed and/or broken. Despite the obviously disabling, and potentially life-threatening, nature of these injuries, the monetary penalties were not substantially higher than for the "superficial" group: the earliest Frankish law fines exposing the brain, cutting off an ear or knocking out a tooth are all at 600d or 15 *solidi*. The *Lex Frisionum* fined the same amount for exposing the skull or knocking out a front tooth.[21] The examples of mismatched injuries carrying the same penalty could multiply, but what this seems to suggest is that the actual affront—and potential for revenge—contained in an action was at the core of legislators' priorities, rather than the after-effects of specific injuries on the victim. (Only if a wound ran continuously is there any reference to the perpetrator paying for ongoing medical assistance.)[22] The apparent illogicality (to modern eyes) of the fines is a warning not to "substitute for what the evidence actually said and did more modern notions of what it should have been saying or doing."[23]

Before leaving this subject, it is worth highlighting that in some law-codes, at least, injuries that left a permanent impairment were recognized and fined more heavily. Edward Wheatley's categories of "blindness" come to mind as we find a reference in the Alemannic laws to seeing "as if through glass"—partial sight epitomized.[24] Deafness resulting from a blow to the head or injury to the ear, muteness and speech impediment were also noted.[25] To reiterate, however, such clauses are numerically far outweighed by those concerned with appearance. Shame, however, is not the same as disgust: the legislators do not dwell on disfigurement, nor do they make any judgment apart from assessing the status of the victim and the potential for disordering revenge.

Just as the earlier law codes seem to have borrowed from each other, so later prescriptions might echo the earlier ones. The *Ecloga ad Procheiron Mutata*, a compilation made for the Greek-speaking subjects of the Norman kings of Sicily and southern Italy in the twelfth century, combines clearly Byzantine elements with a section (Chap. XXXI (XVIII)) on interpersonal violence, which orders compensation for the victim for hitting on the head, blinding, splitting the nose, knocking out teeth, breaking the arm (for which a doctor is to be called), and "injuring a neighbor's beard so as to disfigure him."[26] The concern for appearance here, and the injuries listed, suggests that the compiler was familiar not only with Byzantine law, but possibly also with the earlier Lombard laws that still had great purchase in parts of the South.

## Mutilation as Punishment – and Redemption?

Whilst the laws ostensibly punish violent behavior through fines on the one hand, some also assert the ruler's right to inflict facial mutilation as punishment, most frequently in criminal cases such as theft or treason, also extending to other acts of betrayal such as adultery. There is a flipside, therefore, to the injury tariffs: serious corporal punishment—such as branding, slitting of the nose and loss of ears—was threatened for certain offences, raising the possibility of permanent physical impairment and/or social disablement if actually carried out. The sixth-century Bishop Gregory of Tours, whose History of the Franks is regularly mined for examples of early medieval violence, reports mutilations as punishment for treason: the would-be assassins of King Childebert II (d. 595), he says, were deprived of their ears and noses and let out to become "an object of ridicule."[27] Notker's account of Louis the Pious's enforcer, discussed earlier, envisaged corporal injuries being meted out.[28] The Lombard king Liutprand's laws of 726 included shaving and branding on the forehead and face as the penalty for repeated theft, although such corporal punishment was in fact unusual within the Lombard codes.[29] The eighth-century *Ecloga* of

Byzantine Emperors Leo III and Constantine V prescribed blinding for a thief stealing from a church, the removal of perjurers' tongues, and the cutting off or slitting of the nose for sexual offences, including adultery and incest.[30] Despite these laws being superseded in Byzantium by the legislative activity of Emperor Basil I (r. 867–886), their influence was felt later in the West through the partial transmission of the *Ecloga ad Procheiron Mutata*.[31] This possibly explains why nose-slitting and removal recur in the Sicilian laws of Frederick II, inspired by and building on the earlier Norman kings' rulings.

In the period between these early and later manifestations of Byzantine law in southern Europe, however, we find similar prescriptions of mutilation in the laws of King Cnut (r. 1016–1035) for England:

> A woman who commits adultery with another man whilst her husband is still alive, and is found out, shall suffer public disgrace, and her husband will have all her property, and she will lose her nose and ears. If she denies it and fails to purge herself, let a bishop take control and punish her severely.[32]

Nose-cutting of women is in fact visible as a penalty well beyond the end of the period under review here. And whilst we have no early medieval court cases showing the injury tariffs discussed earlier being brought to bear on offenders, it is not difficult to find examples in the chronicles and capitularies of rulers mutilating their subjects, whether justly (following plots) or not.[33] Charlemagne's second capitulary of Thionville (805), for example, ordered that those assisting in sworn conspiracies be condemned to cut each other's noses off, a fate Jinty Nelson described as "savage" and "ghastly," and which Paul Edward Dutton interprets as demonstrating the Carolingians "at their most secretive and anxious."[34]

Here, an extreme act (and to cutting off the nose and ears could be added other judicial sentences such as blinding, branding or tattooing the face) was appropriated by the ruler and permitted because he (and in some cases she) *was* the ruler, demonstrating Giorgio Agamben's distinction between the sovereign as constituting power (and thus outside the law) and the constitution and laws of the state over which s/he ruled.[35] Agamben highlights, usefully for our purposes, the *potential* use of force by the sovereign—it is available but only used and visible when forced upon the ruler by the transgressor—it is therefore entirely exceptional and to be used circumspectly.[36] Medieval authors recognized the difference: Gregory of Tours presents himself explaining to the Frankish

King Chilperic I that "if any one of our number has attempted to overstep the path of justice, it is for you to correct him. If on the other hand, it is you who acts unjustly, who can correct you?"[37] Excessive force by rulers, therefore, often finds its way into our sources in the context of condemnation of exceptional or extreme (to the observer) practices and/or accounts of unjust (again, in the eyes of the observer) persecutions. In the same passage condemning Chilperic's injustice, Gregory cites the case of Gailen, servant to Chilperic's opponent Merovech, who is mutilated gratuitously as punishment for having deprived Chilperic of the opportunity to kill Merovech himself: they cut off his hands, feet, ears and nose, and tortured him cruelly before killing him "in the most revolting fashion [*infiliciter negaverunt*—here the translator's own distaste shows through]."[38] Gregory's huge history, with its numerous instances of violent acts by Frankish kings and their subjects, makes it hard to judge whether the successors to the Merovingian kings were less prone to such acts, or whether the apparent drop in cases is simply due to differences in source material. Nevertheless, the threat of violence was a crucial tool for keeping the peace, a role that the Carolingians emphasized in their projection of royal authority, and the ambivalence surrounding violence as reported by clerical chroniclers is visible.[39]

King Cnut in England, too, exemplifies "good" and "bad" mutilation: as king his threat to mutilate adulteresses was legitimate, but several years earlier his actions in mutilating a group of Anglo-Saxon hostages was remembered in the Anglo-Saxon Chronicle as a highly illegitimate act.[40] The treatment of the face and head, the most visible parts of the body, seems to have acted as an index for reporting such excess. For example, Pope Nicholas I, addressing a letter of 106 chapters to the Bulgarians in 866, specifically condemned the practice whereby Bulgarian judges beat confessions out of suspected thieves by blows to the head and pricking with iron implements. A confession, he pointed out, was not valid in human or divine law unless it was voluntary.[41] Similarly condemned as excessive behavior (at least in hagiographical texts) is the iconoclast Byzantine Emperor Leo V's order that saints Theodore and Theophanes be tattooed with a twelve-line indictment of their errors on their faces, the last three lines of which read:

> They did not abandon their lawless stupidity.
> Therefore with their faces inscribed as evil-doers,
> They are condemned and driven forth again.[42]

Arguably these men, known to posterity as the *"graptoi* [inscribed]," got off lightly, compared with the 342 holy men imprisoned with St Stephen the Younger (d. 764/5) and described thus:

> some with cut off noses, others with their eyes gouged out, some with their hands cut off for writing in favor of icons, others with no ears, whipped, others with their hair shaved, most having their honorable beards soaked in pitch and burnt.[43]

The latter two cases, however, fit into Lucy Grig's formula relating to accounts of torture: the sufferings undergone by these supporters of icons simply reinforced their moral superiority and the righteousness of their case.[44]

Why would rulers act in this way? Collins defines mutilation as "punishment not by death, but by life at its lowest level." It is interesting that he characterizes it as a behavior typical of "iron age (agrarian) societies which are highly-stratified around a patrimonial form of government."[45] If mutilation does indeed reinforce hierarchy, we are again seeing hints of the "face" culture posited in Chapter 2. Again, however, we are mainly dealing with threat rather than action: even the idea of being mutilated surely had the power to terrify subjects into submission. Miller suggests that threatening punishments, as most lawcodes did, would have little effect if not carried out occasionally to make the threat believable.[46] Agamben's formulation of the *potential* power of the ruler is clear to see in the threatened punishments in law. If the idea of mutilation was to shame the victim, however, the treatment of Gailen reported by Gregory of Tours seems almost gratuitously cruel. Gregory reserves his disgust, however, for the perpetrators, not the spectacle of the victim.

Yet the fact that we are, for the most part, only dealing with rhetorical threats raises another problem. In Cnut's laws for England, at least, Wormald has demonstrated that the penalty quoted above for adultery (although not the principle of mutilating itself) was an addition by Archbishop Wulfstan of York (d. 1023). Wulfstan was active in drafting laws for both Cnut and his predecessor Aethelred, driven by a strong sense of moral reform, and he would have been well aware of the biblical precedent of nose-cutting as a punishment for adultery.[47] Several commentators have highlighted the persistence of Old Testament models for medieval behavior: G. R. Evans has commented that the separation between law and theology visible in the modern university curriculum would have been unintelligible to the medieval student. For Evans, "The primary authority for medieval scholars is the Bible, and it was not necessary to stretch interpretation to take that to be a text with something to say to lawyers." Patrick Wormald adds, "...it is hard to exaggerate (though easy for a modern mind to overlook) the impact of the Old Testament as a prescriptive mirror for early medieval societies."[48] The underlying justification for commuting death sentences to mutilation, after all, was Ezekiel 33.11: "I have no desire for the death of the wicked. I would rather that a wicked man should mend his ways and live." The nasal mutilation of the Egyptian prostitute Oholibah, threatened in Ezekiel Chapter 23, surely inspired not one, but three separate codes of law from different parts of Europe: eighth-century Byzantium, eleventh-century England, and twelfth/thirteenth-century Norman and Hohenstaufen law in the Kingdom of Sicily, all of which prescribed facial mutilation for sexual transgressions.[49] As Collins points out, far from being a suppressant for such cruelty, "Medieval Christianity... is not an aberration from the main pattern, but the pattern itself."[50]

## CASE STUDY: BYZANTINE DISFIGUREMENTS

This link between law and biblical precedents was particularly apparent in Byzantium. The lawmaking activities of the Byzantine emperors were increasingly driven by religious zeal as the secularized concerns of Justinianic legislation made way for an image of the emperor as an "instrument of God."[51] Old Testament precedent also underpinned a facet of Byzantine political behavior that appears to have spread westward, namely the blinding or disfiguring of political opponents, an echo of the Levitical ban on disfigured men acting as priests and, by extension, holding a position of authority.[52] Blinding and nose-cutting were favored means of disposing of political opponents, and the latter as a political act reached a peak in seventh- and eighth-century Byzantium. The cutting off of the nose of an incumbent emperor, Justinian II (r. 685–95, 705–11), may however have been a cut too far, if his restoration after a ten-year hiatus is any indicator.[53] The fascination with and repetition of Justinian's story apparent in western authors such as Paul the Deacon (writing in the late eighth century) and Agnellus of Ravenna (early ninth century) suggests that even if they were used to the idea of mutilation as a loss of honor, the reality was a rather rarer occurrence. Paul's colorful account paints a picture of the restored emperor seeking vengeance for his injury every time his nasal orifice dripped:

when he was restored to power, every time he wiped away a droplet of snot with his hand, he ordered that one of those who had opposed him should be slaughtered.[54]

whilst Agnellus highlights that Justinian lost his nose and ears, and replaced both with gold prosthetics.[55]

It is striking, however, that after the bloodiness of the eighth and ninth centuries, blinding and tonsuring seem to have replaced nose-cutting as a political tool.[56]    Blinding, of course, could be accomplished without the shedding of blood, and this may explain the apparent change (conversely, it could still be a bloody business).[57] The evidence of the chronicler Michael Psellos (1018–96) seems to underscore the transition and a distaste for bloodiness—he reports the Bulgar usurper "Dolianus" being captured by prince Alousianus: "He arrested Dolianus, cut off his nose and blinded his eyes, using a cook's knife for both operations."[58] The detail of the cook's knife is, I think, revealing, the unplanned and "barbaric" removal of Dolianus's features a fitting way for these "Scythians" to be united under one ruler. For Psellos, such mutilations are what Others do. But they were also things that characterized a ruler out of control: his report of Constantine VIII's brief reign (c.1025–8) is peppered with references to "cruel punishments," "uncontrolled anger," "awful tortures" and arbitrary and indiscriminate punishments:

> it was not a question of temporary restrictions, or of banishment, or of prison; his method was to punish malefactors on the spot, with blinding of the eyes by a red-hot iron... quite apart from the fact that, in one case, he was dealing with apparently flagrant crime, in another with minor delinquency.[59]

Psellos goes on to report other, later blindings, such as that of the exile John Orphanotrophos, in whose downfall "evil followed evil"—blinded in prison, he was then banished and executed. Basil Skleros, he says, "had the misfortune to be deprived of his sight." It is clear that Psellos is troubled by blindings: when Constantine IX went against his oath to show clemency when faced with rebellion, and ordered the blinding of Tornikios and Vatatzes "on the spot" (an echo of the earlier Constantine's tyranny?), one of the rebels "emitted a cry of anguish," whilst the other "merely remarked that the Roman empire was losing a valorous soldier, straightway lay down on the ground, face upwards, and *nobly* submitted to his fate [my emphasis]."[60] As we shall see in Chapter 6, Psellos uses this structuring tool of contrasting behaviors in the face of adversity again, when he reports at length on an episode to which he was an eyewitness.[61]

Reports of blinding in certain Byzantine texts, for example that of Anna Komnena (writing in the first half of the twelfth century), are so matter-of-fact as to suggest that this became something of a norm. Komnena dwells at length on some examples and reports a variety of methods in her numerous cases.[62] In fact, such episodes occur frequently in Byzantine texts of this period. Alexander Kazhdan notes how the judicial mutilations and unjust punishments contained in the later account of Nicetas Choniates (d. 1215/16) have been read as evidence of "Byzantine depravity." Instead, he argues, we should note that the chronicler is actually concerned with the preservation of human life, and that mutilations were in fact a merciful alternative to execution.[63] Geneviève Bührer-Thierry has made much the same point for earlier medieval examples in the West,[64] but it is also clear that earlier western authors shared assumptions about this being a "Byzantine" practice, if a strange story in Notker is indicative. Recounting an embassy from Charlemagne to the Byzantine emperor, Notker relates that the envoy breached strict Byzantine protocol at a dinner, opening himself up to punishment by death. Given a last request by the emperor, the envoy asked that anyone who had *seen* him being disrespectful should lose their *own* eyes. Not surprisingly, his challenge silenced his accusers, and thus were the "empty-headed sons of Hellas beaten in their own land."[65] Such punishments had to be justifiable: some cases attracted particular opprobrium in contemporary and subsequent histories because they could not be presented as legitimate punishment. The Byzantine empress Irene's blinding of her son Constantine is a case in point. It stood out because she was both woman and mother perpetrating this act, for all that she had her apologists. As we shall see in Chapter 5, gender sometimes intersected with discussions of "right" and "wrong" instances of disfigurement.

## POPES, SAINTS AND MUTILATION

Visible mutilation was associated with breaches of trust, and thus intimately connected with the codes of honor expressed in the injury tariff lists. To mutilate someone judicially (or politically) had the same meaning: it was a shaming act, regardless of how severe the actual bodily injury was. Thietmar reports that in retaliation for the killing and humiliation of envoys sent to negotiate Otto III's marriage to Theophanu, Otto II's men Gunther and

Siegfried captured and blinded some Greeks in Calabria, and seized the tribute being collected for the Byzantine emperor.[66] In essence the attacks on servants (envoys, subjects) fit our pattern of inflicting face-damaging injury to the rulers concerned. Rather less easy to justify, however, were attacks on churchmen. Twenty years later, Emperor Otto III's troops cut off the hands and ears and blinded the eyes of Pope John XVI when they deposed him in 998. For at least three more years (the date of his death is uncertain), he lived as a prisoner in the abbey of Fulda. John's case is illuminating on a number of levels: surviving his awful injuries, he could easily have become a focus for sympathy, particularly given his elevated status as pope. Killing him was not an option, but permanent removal to a closed community ensured that his potential as a living martyr was contained. Radulf Glaber's report of the mutilation (written within living memory of the event) makes it clear that he thought the punishment justified: he calls John, who had been installed by the Crescenzi family of Rome after the deposition of Otto's candidate, a pope of "little authority [*male securum*]" whose amputated hands were "almost sacrilegious [*manus quasi sacrilegas*]."[67] Not surprisingly, the episode is reported in several texts: John the Deacon's Venetian history, for example, elaborates that John was deprived of his eyes, nose, ears and tongue, and thus "shamed [*deturpatus*]" he was shut away, but only after being deprived of clerical office and publicly displayed in Rome riding facing backwards on a mule.[68]

Here a false pope—and opponent of the Emperor—was written up as getting his come-uppance, yet as Gerd Althoff points out, Otto's actions have been interpreted as unusually brutal, and opportunities had presented themselves for a peaceful settlement between the emperor and his Roman subjects.[69] An earlier pope, Leo III (r. 795–816), was also the victim of an assault to his face, but here it was his *legitimate* authority as pope that was being questioned, and reports of the incident all play up his suffering in order to introduce Charlemagne as his protector. Whilst Einhard simply reports that Leo suffered attempted blinding and cutting out of his tongue, forcing him to flee to Charles for help, Notker gives a more extended version that, according to his modern translator, shows him to have been "better-informed" about the incident. In Notker's account, Leo's assailants tried to put his eyes out but lost heart. Unsuccessful in their attempt to gouge his eyes, they then slashed him across the face with a knife. God restored Leo's damaged eyesight and, "As a sign of his innocence, a shiny scar, as white as driven snow, ran across his dovelike eyes, in the shape of a very thin line."[70] Far from being "better-informed," Notker's account appears to be developing the story of Leo into a quasi-hagiographical account, and it is I think no accident that a substantial proportion of the evidence for judicially-mutilated faces occurs in narrative, particularly hagiographic, texts. We have already met Paul the Deacon and Agnellus of Ravenna fantasizing about the noseless Byzantine emperor, Justinian II. The *topos* of the unjustly mutilated saint, or the saint rescuing/restoring an unjustly mutilated victim, recurs across both eastern and western texts. But there is an important difference to note here. The original mutilation in each case was intended to dishonor, or punish, the victim for challenging the authority of the ruler. How it was subsequently *read* and reported, however, lies at the heart of any methodological issue of tracking medieval disfigurement. For Notker, the recorders of icon-worshipping monk-saints under both periods of iconoclasm in Byzantium (and, for that matter, the author of an account of the leader of the anti-episcopal movement in Milan in the eleventh century), mutilation not infrequently preceded or was equated with martyrdom, guaranteeing some form of veneration.[71] But the point to note is that the texts celebrating their actions included the mutilation *at all*: it clearly functioned as a way to heighten the reader's devotion to the emergent cult. Physical dishonor meant nothing next to spiritual cleanliness. Turning to instances of saints restoring mutilated victims (familiar, no doubt, to students of Thomas Becket's miracle repertoire),[72] hagiography provides the earliest evidence of the use of facial mutilation to punish in England, as a law of Edgar, prescribing blinding, removal of ears, slitting of the nose, scalping and amputation of hands and feet for a convicted thief, is cited to preface a story of St Swithun's restoring of a near-dead, innocent victim of such multiple injuries.[73] Again, the practice itself mattered little to the hagiographer, only the unjust circumstances of the specific case.

## RHETORIC TO REALITY—AND BACK

The link between facial appearance and honor in the early Middle Ages can, I think, be securely argued. But what of the practical effects of disfigurement or perceived impairment? The stigma attached to visible difference, if not outright disgust, has already been hinted. Blindness is an interesting case in point. We read that the onset of blindness in an intended bride, for instance, could be cited as the reason to break off an engagement in Lombard law "on account of her weighty sins"; it is also identified as a blemish sufficient to disinherit a person in early Welsh laws, with the justification that "no one who is blemished can fully accomplish the service of the land due to the king in courts and hostings."[74] Here the physical impairment leads to loss of social position and potentially, loss of honor. Thus, striking out the eye of a one-eyed person, rendering him or her completely sightless, is also equated in Lombard law with social, if not actual, death.[75]

Thus far it has been evident that the Byzantine Empire provides many of our early examples of mutilation, and Janet Nelson, citing Mark McCormick, suggests that it was a Byzantine practice imported into the West in the sixth and seventh centuries.[76] Others, however, contend that the use of mutilation in western polities spread with the expansion of Norman power in the West and had its origins not in the East, but Scandinavia. Klaus van Eickels suggests that the danger of killing one's distant kinsman in Scandinavian society precluded the use of the death penalty and favored mutilation as a substitute.[77] In fact, blinding of traitors appears also to have had Biblical sanction: Gregory of Tours quotes Proverbs 30:17, "The eye that mocketh at his father, the ravens of the valley shall pick it out."[78]

It has in fact become something of a commonplace to blame the expansion of Norman power in the eleventh and twelfth centuries for a concomitant rise in recorded examples of judicial mutilation and instances of cruelty and disfigurement. Van Eickels' consideration of castration and blinding in Normandy and Anglo-Norman England accepts unproblematically the report of William the Conqueror replacing execution in some cases with mutilations such as these.[79] Edward Wheatley has drawn a contrast between blinding as a common punishment in France and Normandy, and its relative rarity in England.[80] He notes the increase of blinding as a punishment in England after 1066,[81] and attributes its introduction into southern Italy and Ireland to the Norman arrival.[82] A closer look, however, suggests that the connection between the arrival of the Normans and the introduction and/or increase in mutilation is wrong. Blinding as a political tool was already present in southern Italy by the ninth century, according to Erchempert.[83] In Ireland, for example, much has been made of the fact that old Irish laws do not mention it, whilst it is documented for the first time in 1224, but the absence of a judicial procedure does not mean the absence of mutilation as such.[84] As I have shown elsewhere in more detail, the weight of written sources relating the rise and establishment of Norman power may have exaggerated the sense of Norman "injustice" surrounding mutilations, and when such episodes occur, they are often presented as extremes of behavior going beyond the acceptable parameters.[85]

Unlike the king, men like William Talvas, guilty of blinding and castrating William of Giroie, were not permitted to step outside the law.[86] Norman authors such as William of Malmesbury in fact preserve accounts of such mutilations prior to the Conquest in both Normandy and England.[87]

These, like many Norman "mutilation" texts, offered the opportunity for writers of hagiography to develop the theme further. The Worcester monks, for example, made much of their saint, Wulfstan, curing the wrongly-blinded and castrated Thomas of Elderfield.[88] Key to the episode is injustice—Thomas loses a judicial duel engineered by one George, and is blinded and castrated by the victor and his associates. This may explain John Hudson's assertion that mutilations might be carried out not by a professional executioner, but by the person whom the convicted person had injured. However, this is an extract from a hagiographical text, which emphasizes the cruelty and injustice of the blinding and castration recounted. Could its perpetration by a layperson with no expertise simply be to heighten the horror?[89] Whilst judicial duels might well pit accuser and defendant against each other (as in the case of Geoffrey Baynard against Count William of Eu),[90] the extremity of outcome in Thomas's case may explain why it made a good subject for a miracle story. The problem with this type of evidence is obvious. I would argue that it was the infrequency of use of mutilation in Norman society that led Norman authors to report episodes in detail when they did occur. To return then to Agamben's formulation of political authority, many of the cases reported by Norman authors feature precisely as moments of exception, when either a legitimate ruler, or a challenger to that rule, stepped beyond the boundaries of the "normal" to inflict bodily injuries so terrible that they merited recording and condemnation. A later example of stepping outside the boundaries is the case of Berchtold, bishop of Passau, who was deposed c. 1251 on account of his "reprehensible" life, and his offence to his clergy, including having one of them blinded and mutilated in his nose and ears. Bernard, the Krems chronicler who records this, leaves us in no doubt as to his unsuitability as a pastor.[91]

## WHAT HAPPENED NEXT: DISFIGUREMENT IN THE COURTS

The rich evidence of the lawcodes, and rather more ambiguous accounts of narrative sources, show that the right to disfigure and mutilate was, in theory, tightly controlled and reserved to the ruler in medieval society. The missing piece of the puzzle, however, is to trace the impact of disfiguring head injuries on the lives of victims. Sensory impairment features as a potential outcome, but records of dispute settlements before 1200 relate almost exclusively not to personal injury cases but disputes over property.[92]

As a postscript to this discussion of disfigurement and the law, however, there exists rich evidence available from Angevin England which, although it strictly falls well outside our chronological parameters, nevertheless demonstrates some of the issues surrounding illegal injury. Early medieval court cases do not, as a rule, concern personal injury (although violence might accompany claims to land and be deployed deliberately and strategically in disputes), but some of the procedures visible in the thirteenth-century evidence from England suggest elements of continuity, as well as one significant change.[93]

Sitting in session in 1201, the English justices of the Cornish Eyre court heard a number of cases relating to interpersonal violence resulting in severe head injuries and/or facial disfigurement. At this court, the victim needed to plead "as a maimed man [*ut homo maaimatus*]" as well as describing the injury. Serlo of Ennis-Cavem did just this when he accused two men of beating him [*verberaverunt*] and seriously wounding him [*graviter vulneraverunt*] so that three bones were extracted from his head. Furthermore, the jurors who presented the case confirmed that Serlo had shown his fresh wounds at the county court, and that his injuries were as described. The first-named assailant was condemned to the ordeal of hot iron, with the second to be put to the same ordeal once the outcome of the first was known.[94] A similar judgment was passed on Robert of Penwithen, whom Eadmer of Penwithen, also pleading as a maimed man, accused of wounding him so that *twenty-eight* pieces of bone had been removed from his head. However, Eadmer subsequently withdrew his case.[95]

Although the Cornish roll also includes more mundane accounts of head wounds,[96] the striking detail of bone removal in these cases (there are four other, similar, accounts, including one of a female victim) points to something more than simple rhetoric.[97] It is noteworthy that none of the survivors of these serious head wounds was deemed able-bodied—the injury was simply too permanent (the bone in the skull was unlikely to regenerate to replace fully the hole that breakage and removal had left) to make a full recovery.[98] The dry court record gives little indication of how debilitated such victims were, but the prospect of living with head injury may have been worse than death itself. At best, an injury in which the integrity of the skull was compromised was disfiguring, painful and constantly at risk of infection, requiring constant care in terms of wound dressing. (The basic care of such a wound appears in the *Leechbook* of Bald: "if the brain is exposed take the yolk of an egg, mix a little with honey and fill the wound. Bind it up with tow and let it alone..."[99]) At worst, the victim might also have suffered brain injury with its associated problems of loss of motor or memory skills, behavioral changes or sensory deprivation.[100] Such symptoms were not, it seems, deemed necessary to record, even assuming they were verbally articulated, but rehearsal of the injuries at both county and royal court may have helped the victim to extract compensatory payments from her/his assailants, addressing their economic hardship if not their healthcare needs.

Court rolls were not, of course, written up to provide information for the social history of medicine in the Middle Ages. In most cases, the information provided about the head wound itself is sketchy, since it was the outcome of the wounding (death, maiming, permanent disability) that determined the actions of the court against the assailant. This apparently distances the court rolls from earlier codes of medieval law that, whilst they too sought to keep the king's peace, were also often concerned with financial compensation for lengthy incapacitation and medical care for the victim. In Angevin England, such a settlement would presumably have been out of court (and some of the examples to be discussed seem to hint at this), as the judicial process was only concerned with the compensation payable to the king for breach of his peace. Yet some of the ideas contained within both sets of records are strikingly similar. The early medieval lawcodes have largely been dismissed as documents of practice in several parts of Europe, and most comprehensively in England, but their extremely detailed categories of head injury, and the measures taken to judge the severity of the wound in fact offer assistance in interpreting the later, more laconic court roll entries.

Another problem with the court roll evidence is its selectivity. The itinerant royal justices were dependent for their information on the accounts of the local juries with whom they interacted; for a case to reach the Eyre court at all it had to be classed as a felony or breach of the king's peace. This serves as a filter for the injuries encountered in the records, for only the most serious accusations were likely to progress this far up the justice system. Contemporaries were well aware of this fact: although the process of bringing cases was through the local jury, it is clear that in some cases the description given by the plaintiff of his serious injuries (women's claims relating to non-sexual violence are very much rarer) was designed to draw attention to a grievance, rather than describe his actual physical state.[101] An example of the limits of the evidence is therefore appropriate before examining the information it provides.

At Coventry (Warwickshire) in 1221, the king's justices in Eyre heard an accusation against Robert, nephew of the chaplain at Ryton (Warwickshire), that he had wounded a certain Robert, son of Roger, and fled. The report continues:

> Robert still lies ill of these wounds and it is not known whether he can recover [*convalescere*] or not. This deed was done recently and therefore let it stand over until the coming of other Justices.[102]

It is not uncommon for reports of wounding in the Eyre rolls to be this unspecific, but here the justices were clearly not satisfied that the case warranted their attention as yet. The case was adjourned, therefore, to determine the outcome of the injuries: would Robert die or recover, and if he did, would he still be maimed? If he healed completely, the matter could be resolved without the formalities of a court hearing; wounding appeals were often withdrawn on payment of compensation, although the appellant might suffer a fine for wasting the court's time.

Many head and face wounds were written up equally briefly, particularly when they resulted in death. Thus, for example, three quarters of the cases dealing with head injury recorded in the crown pleas of the Shropshire Eyre of 1256 were concerned with fatalities.[103] The format of each entry is brief, but consistently includes the location of the injury, the weapon used to inflict it (ranging from sticks and staves to axes and a flail), and the length of time it took the victim to die, thus:

> 494. Philip son of Jordan of Rowton struck Nicholas Crawe of Acton on the head with a Danish axe [*hachia Danech*] so that he died the next day.
> 501. Edward of Brockton struck William son of Robert of Brockton on the head with a stake [*palo*] so that he died three weeks later.

In all of these cases the assailant fled, and the court was concerned with the amount of their chattels and the actions (or lack of action) taken by local communities to arrest him. Fines were exacted for this neglect, and for burial of the dead man without a coroner's view. Arguably, therefore, the record was less concerned with the actual fate of the victim: although the number of days survived (from none to 21, with most dying within five days) is recorded, its purpose was to ensure accuracy of the details linked to the legal process rather than any indication of care received before death. No reference is made to the latter at all.

Accidental deaths by head wounds were also noted, but still viewed as a breach of the king's peace if a perpetrator could be identified.[104] Thus when "William son of Robert Seys, a boy of 8 or 9 years, threw a javelin [*veru*] which by accident struck Thomas of Worthen below the eye, so that he died eight days later," the boy was still outlawed and his village fined for not apprehending him.[105] Whether the assailant was in fact of an *age* at which he could be held criminally responsible, however, is debatable: his action in throwing the javelin was apparently sufficient to condemn him. Another accident befell Thomas son of Richard the chaplain, whose brother William "struck [him] down to the brains [*usque ad cerebrum*]" trying to hit another William, son of Matilda. Thomas died immediately, and his brother promptly fled and was outlawed.[106]

The cases just discussed imply that a serious head wound in this period was viewed as unlikely to be survivable, and/or that death might be slow and lingering (as in the case of the two victims who took three weeks to die). This may have influenced the judges' attitudes when confronted with someone who did survive to tell his tale and bring a case. When this happened, however, the justices, like their colleagues in Coventry, were concerned to ensure that a genuine case could be established. A plea from Yorkshire, dating to 1218, was dismissed by the justices because the victim (whose case was brought by his son) had neither died nor lost his sight.[107] Another in Cornwall in 1201 was dismissed because the victim (whose brother brought the case) had recovered and not sued.[108] Back in Shropshire, William Tuppe's appeal, that John son of Reysent had robbed him and given him a wound "seven inches deep and three inches long" in his left shoulder with a Welsh knife and another "in the right shoulder three inches deep and one inch wide," was dismissed when another alleged assailant, Richard of Wottenhall (accused of a inflicting a sword wound in William's arm), pointed out that William had not mentioned the detail of his wounds or the robbery in the shire court. (Both John and Richard were, however, fined for using bladed weapons.) Similarly, Walter of Wottenhull's claim that Thomas of Willaston had hit him on the head with a stick was dismissed when the jurors stated that Thomas was only responding to an earlier assault by Walter. In both cases, fines were exacted.[109] A third plaintiff, Simon of Preen, who claimed he had been injured in the back and head with a sword and in the stomach with an arrow, had his appeal annulled when reference was made to the coroners' rolls.[110]

At the heart of these cases, there lurked the suspicion that the plaintiff was making a false or at the very least exaggerated appeal, hence the reference back to earlier written records; the specific details of William

Tuppe's claim were ultimately his undoing when earlier records showed he had not been so precise in his original claim. Why, then, had he cited the length and depth of his wounds in the Eyre court? One reason might well have been the fact that in order to secure a hearing at all, the non-fatal wounds he had suffered had to be (or sound) sufficiently serious to merit the attention of the royal justices. This suggestion is supported by a case heard in Berkshire in 1248, which is strikingly similar to William's in its language and outcome. Robert of Denmead claimed that Richard son of Gillian had given him a four-inch long wound in the head with a fork [*furca*], that Henry Redulf had given him a two-inch wound in the head with a hatchet, and that both had robbed him of a silver clasp and a dagger, whose exact value was stated. In their defense, the two accused pointed to the fact that Robert had not brought his case to the county court, and that previously he had accused Richard of using the hatchet, not Henry. The case was dismissed on these inconsistencies, but all three were again fined.[111]

The key to understanding the process of treating head wound cases seems to lie in the Yorkshire and Berkshire cases discussed above: if there was no permanent damage, then the plaintiff had little to complain about. It is noteworthy that Robert of Denmead offered to prove his claims "by his body as the court sees fit." This indicates that he was prepared to suffer the ordeal or a judicial duel with his opponents (as opposed to displaying his injuries) and thus was not permanently maimed by the alleged attack. Ironically, therefore, he undermined his claim by his physical fitness. In contrast, a certain Hereward's willingness to undertake a judicial duel with his assailant at the Lincolnshire Eyre of 1202, having previously shown his fresh wounds to the coroners and county court, does not appear to have damaged his credibility.[112] In these cases and others, the judicial ordeal or duel played an important part in providing proof of guilt, but it was not always the assailant who was put to the iron.

There are plenty of other cases from around England in the early thirteenth century that use similar language of "maiming" and/or record that the fresh injuries had been inspected by the local jury before the case came to before the justices of the Eyre. In Lincolnshire in 1202, for example, Astin of Wispington accused Simon of Edlington of putting out his eye (*et ei oculum eruit*) so that he was maimed of it (*ita quod maimatus est illo oculo*). (Simon was given the choice of who should undergo the ordeal, and not surprisingly elected that Astin should do so. The case was settled out of court and both parties fined).[113] The Cornish cases, however, seem to be unique in their detailed account of removal of pieces of skull, and thus raise the question of where this particular element had originated. Although the detail of specific injuries had a long documentary history in English lawcodes, it appears that concern with the severity and effects of head wounds was of continental origin. The Frankish *Lex Salica* specifically refers to head injuries exposing the brain, and those causing the three bones of the skull to protrude, provisions that found their way into later Carolingian legislation. The *Lex Frisionum*, another Carolingian compilation from the early ninth century, went into even greater detail, with no less than 23 provisions relating to head injuries, including exposure and fracture of the skull and exposure of and damage to the brain membrane (the *dura mater*).[114]

Its appearance in the Eyre roll suggests that either the justices, or more likely the clerk recording the case, had some familiarity either with such legal traditions, and/or with medical procedures. The "legal revolution" of the twelfth century might not have converted English courts to an entirely Roman model of justice—although corporal mutilations and branding to the face were clearly replacing older, compensatory modes of settlement—but it had encouraged study of the law, and there is no reason to exclude a continued interest in excerpting and compiling early medieval materials as part of this process. The compiler of the *Leges Henrici Primi* had certainly trawled through early Frankish law to supplement his pre-Norman content.[115] But the twelfth century had also seen an upsurge in interest in medical texts as well, including surgical treatises. Whilst the latter would become ever more elaborated and "rational" in the thirteenth century, evidence for some form of medical knowledge is already visible in the early laws.

Whilst there is considerable similarity to be drawn between the types of injury recorded in these later court cases, and the personal injury punished in the early medieval law codes, one crucial difference is apparent. Although many of the facial wounds recorded were likely to be disfiguring, at no point does the plaintiff refer to the shame or humiliation of her/his physical appearance. Either the wounds were serious enough to merit claiming permanent impairment—the "maimed" man (but not woman)—or they were dismissed because they had not caused any sensory damage. The close concern for visibility and humiliation set out in the earlier, prescriptive material is entirely lacking here. Several comments are possible: firstly, none of the cases discussed seem to involve injuries to elite males—none of the complainants uses any title signaling high status. Perhaps the issue at stake, then, was not the damage to appearance/reputation that their wounds had caused, but their economic enfeeblement due to being temporarily or permanently incapacitated. At any rate, we seem here to be dealing with a different constituency from the urban inhabitants studied by Demaitre, who were seeking cosmetic help with skin lesions in the same period.[116]

## CONCLUSIONS

The content of the laws on facial injury, the parameters of acceptable mutilation visible in the narrative texts, and the continued control of violence by the courts surely debunk once and for all the idea that medieval violence was unstructured and uncontrolled. Far from it. Violence to the face and head was the most serious of injuries, and as such, although it populates all our texts, it appears in highly specific contexts. Wrongful use of disfigurement was commented upon and condemned, and the horror of a facial injury is often talked up rhetorically to underline the wickedness or excess of the perpetrator.[117] At the same time, the power of a facial injury to convey social disgrace is expressed clearly in both early medieval laws and in personal attacks; none of the cases dealt with in this chapter was accidental. If there is any trend visible at all, it is perhaps a product of the multiplication of available sources rather than an upsurge in actual cases of disfigurement. If disfigurement becomes more visible, it must partly be due to the shift from summary execution for some crimes to a more "merciful" regime. Executed criminals did not linger in the same way, and did not have to be dealt with. Yet there is a barely perceptible shift toward shutting away victims of mutilation, rather than exhibiting them openly, and perhaps also toward less bloody forms of punishment. Later medieval court cases from England also highlight the fact that social class, and the type of text examined, shape accounts of how facial injury was represented and understood.

Of course, what we'd really like to have is a series of *early* medieval court cases that dealt with the types of personal injury outlined in the early laws—even better, along the lines of boundary-walking and other practices used in resolving land disputes, would be to see the rituals of throwing bits of extracted bone across roads and into shields, with the assembled witnesses agreeing that they did, indeed, make the requisite sound to proceed with the case. Such a performative element encoded in so many of the early medieval laws (as well as Lombard, Frisian and Welsh, similar clauses are found in Alemannic and Ripuarian codes) tempts speculation on their actual use. But in the absence of evidence, we can only imagine. How were people with acquired disfigurements, who mainly survived their ordeal, viewed by their peers? In the next chapter, the experience of disfigurement as stigma will be explored.

## NOTES

1. Epitomized by Valentin Groebner, *Defaced: the Visual Culture of Violence in the Later Middle Ages* (New York: Zone Books, 2004).
2. Michel Foucault, *Discipline and Punish: the Birth of the Prison*, tr. A. Sheridan (London: Allen Lane, 1977), 47–48 describes medieval punishment as a public, ritual display of the sovereign's "vengeance" on the criminal. Precursors: Johan Huizinga, *Waning of the Middle Ages* (Dutch first edition 1919, English translation published London: Edward Arnold, 1924), and Norbert Elias, *The Civilizing Process vol 1: The History of Manners, vol 2: State Formation and Civilization* (German first edition 1939, English translation Oxford: Blackwell, 1969 and 1982); Marc Bloch, *Feudal Society* (French first edition 1939, English translation London: Routledge, 1961). Piero Camporesi, *The Incorruptible Flesh: Body Mutation and Mortification in Religion and Folklore*, tr. T. Croft-Murray and H. Elsom (Cambridge: Cambridge University Press, 1988), 225, also characterizes the later middle ages as a "horrible, indescribable and sadistic age." On extreme bodily punishment in the later middle ages, Nathalie Gonthier, *Le châtiment du crime au moyen âge (xii-xiv siècles* (Rennes: Presses Universitaires de Rennes, 1998); Groebner, *Defaced*, 15–28.
3. E.g. Helen Carrel, "The ideology of punishment in late medieval English towns," *Social History*, 34 (2009): 301–320, at 307–8, disputes the supposed prevalence of mutilation. Foucault's depiction of imprisonment as a modern alternative to corporal punishment is also substantially undermined by the work of Guy Geltner, in particular *The Medieval Prison: a Social History* (Princeton: Princeton University Press, 2008), and earlier work such as "Medieval prisons: between myth and reality, hell and purgatory," *History Compass*, 4 (2006): 261–274.
4. William Ian Miller, *The Anatomy of Disgust* (Cambridge, MA: Harvard University Press, 1997), 151 and 170.
5. Sean McGlynn, *By Sword and Fire: Cruelty and Atrocity in Medieval Warfare* (London: Weidenfeld and Nicolson, 2008), 2. The essays

in *Violence in Medieval Society*, ed. R. W. Kaeuper (Woodbridge: Boydell, 2000) vary in their view of whether the period was any more violent than modern times. There also appears to be an associated taste for sensationalist titles for such volumes, e.g. Mitchell Merback, *The Thief, the Cross and the Wheel: Pain and the Spectacle of Punishment in Medieval and Renaissance Europe* (London: Reaktion Books, 1999); *Noble Ideals and Bloody Realities: Warfare in the Middle Ages*, ed. N. Christie and M. Yazigi (Leiden: Brill, 2006).

6. *Violence and Society in the Early Medieval West*, ed. Guy Halsall (Woodbridge: Boydell, 2002), 16.

7. Lucy Grig, "Torture and truth in late antique martyrology," *Early Medieval Europe*, 11.4 (2002): 321–336.

8. Randall Collins, "Three faces of cruelty: towards a comparative sociology of violence," *Theory and Society*, 1 (1974): 415–440.

9. Of particular relevance to this theme are Gerd Althoff, "Ira Regis: prolegomena to a history of royal anger," G. Bührer-Thierry, "'Just anger' or 'vengeful anger'? The punishment of blinding in the early medieval west," and W. Davies, "Anger and the Celtic saint," all in *Anger's Past: The Social Uses of an Emotion in the Middle Ages*, ed. B. H. Rosenwein (Ithaca and London: Cornell University Press, 1998), 59–74, 75–91 and 191–202 respectively.

10. William Ian Miller, *Eye for an Eye* (Cambridge: Cambridge University Press, 2006), 31–36 does, however, raise the question of how one *valued* (and how we still value) each of the body parts for financial compensation.

11. *Lex Frisionum* and its additions, ed. K. de Richthofen, in *MGH LL*, III, ed. G. Pertz (Hannover: Hahn, 1863), 673–700. The laws were even further elaborated in the rather confusingly-titled Old Frisian tariffs, which date from the later middle ages: Han Nijdam, "Compensating body and honor: the Old Frisian compensation tariffs," in *Medicine and the Law in the Middle Ages*, ed. Wendy Turner and Sara M. Butler (Leiden: Brill, 2014), 25–57.

12. Miller, *Eye for an Eye*, 118, picks up on this issue using the specific example of King Aethelberht of Kent's early (c. 600CE) lawcode. A new edition by Oliver, with slightly different numbering of clauses, is used in the following discussion and can be found at Aethelberht of Kent, *Laws*, ed. L. Oliver http://www.earlyenglish-laws.ac.uk/laws/texts/abt/ [Accessed 1 July 2015].

13. Pulling: *Pactus Legis Salicae*, ed. K. Eckhardt, in *MGH Leges Nat. Germ.*, IV.1 (Hannover: Hahn, 1962), III.104; *Leges*

*Burgundionum*, V.4–5, ed. L. R. de Salis, *MGH LL nat. Germ.*, II.1 (Hannover: Hahn, 1892); Laws of Aethelbeht, ed. Oliver, c. 33; *Leges Langobardorum*, Rothari c. 383, ed. F. Bluhme in *MGH LL*, IV, ed. G. H. Pertz (Hannover: Hahn, 1868); *Lex Frisionum* XXII.65; *Lex Frisionum Additiones Sapientium* III, 39–40; *The Laws of Hywel Dda (The Book of Blegywryd)*, tr. M. Richards (Liverpool: Liverpool University Press, 1954), 64. Cutting: *Pactus Legis Salicae* XXIV.2–3; *Leges Burgundionum*, XXXIII.1–5; *Leges Alamannorum*, Pactus, XVIII.1, ed. K. A. Eckhardt, *MGH LL nat. Germ.*, V.1 (Hannover: Hahn, 1966); *Lex Salica*, D,XXXV.1–2, and *Lex Salica Karolina*, XXXIII.2–3, ed. K. Eckhardt, *MGH LL nat. Germ.*, IV.2 (Hannover: Hahn, 1959); *Laws of Hywel Dda*, tr. Richards, 64. Shaving, tonsuring or scalping: *Leges Visigothorum*, VI.4.3, in *MGH LL. Nat. Germ.* I, ed. K. Zeumer (Hannover and Leipzig: Hahn, 1902); *Leges Alamannorum*, *Lex*, ALVII.28–29/BLXV.1–2, ed. Eckhardt; *Leges Langobardorum*, Liutprand 80 (dated 726) and 141 (734) and Aistulf 4 (dated 750).

14. Mustache: *Lex Frisionum* XXII.17, *Add. Sap.* III.17; eyebrows: *Lex Frisionum*. XXII.14, *Add. Sap.* III.15. Eyelashes feature in Welsh law: *Laws of Hywel Dda*, tr. Jenkins, 198.

15. *Pactus Legis Salicae*, XXIX.1 and 5, ed. Eckhardt; *Leges Burgundionum*, XXVI.1–5, ed. de Salis; Aethelberht of Kent, *Laws*, ed. Oliver, cc. 48–48.3 (canine teeth, teeth next to canines, back teeth); *Leges Langobardorum*, Rothari, cc. 51–2, 85–6, 109; *Bretha Déin Chécht*, 34 (six classes of teeth) in Fergus Kelly, *A Guide to Early Irish Law* (Dublin: Institute for Advanced Studies, 1988), 132; *Leges Alamannorum*, *Lex*, A, LVII.20–25, B, LXIII.3–8, ed. Eckhardt; *Lex Salica*, D, XLVIII.13 and *Lex Salica Karolina*, XVI.17, ed. Eckhardt; *Lex Frisionum*, XXII.19 (front teeth) and 21 (back teeth). That the appearance of teeth mattered is anecdotally indicated by the much later chronicler Ibn al-Athir, who notes in passing that the corpse of the king of Benares (d. 1193/4) was only recognized by the gold bridgework securing his teeth in his mouth: *The Chronicle of Ibn al-Athir for the Crusading Period from al-Kamil fi'l-Ta'rikh* Part 3: The Years 589–629, tr. D. S. Richards (Aldershot: Ashgate, 2008), 13.

16. E.g. *Lex Visigothorum*, VI.4.3, ed. Zeumer (*turpibus maculis*); Irish law punished anyone who verbally publicized a physical blemish in another: Kelly, *Guide*, 137.

17. E.g. *Leges Langobardorum*, Rothari c.74 states that the preceding list of penalties relates to injuries to a freeman, and clauses following it then repeat the injuries if inflicted on a semi-free or unfree victim.

18. *The Digest of Justinian*, Book 47.10, tr. and ed. A. Watson, 2 vols (Pennsylvania: Philadelphia University Press, 1985), II. Note however the written medium as a means to dishonor – the closest that medieval laws get to this is perhaps the defamatory – but still oral – poetry visible in early Irish law.

19. The Theodosian code, however, does punish those who self-mutilate their hands to avoid military service: Antonio Landi, Maria C. Facchini, Antonio Saracino and Giuseppe Caserta, "Historical aspects," in *Reconstructive Surgery in Hand Mutilation*, ed. Guy Foucher (London: Martin Dunitz, 1997), 3–12, at 5.

20. *Lex Frisionum Additio Sapientium*, III.16; *Laws of Hywel Dda*, tr. Richards, 64; *Laws of Hywel Dda*, tr. Jenkins, 196–197.

21. *Pactus Legis Salicae*, XVII.4, XXIX.14 and 16; *Lex Frisionum*, XXII.5 and 19.

22. Wound that cannot be staunched: *Pactus Legis Salicae*, XVII.7, ed. Eckhardt; *Lex Baiwariorum*, IV.4, ed. E. Liber, *MGH LL. Nat. Germ.*, V.2 (Hannover: Hahn, 1926); *Lex Salica Karolina*, XV.6, ed. Eckhardt.

23. Patrick Wormald, *The Making of English Law: King Alfred to the Twelfth Century*, vol 1 (Oxford: Blackwell, 1999), 476.

24. *Leges Alamannorum, Lex*, A LVII.13, B LXI.3, ed. K. A. Eckhardt, *MGH LL nat. Germ.*, V.1 (Hannover: Hahn, 1966), 119.

25. Aethelbehrt's laws, ed. Oliver, cc. 38 (deaf), 49 (speech damaged).

26. E. H. Freshfield, *A Manual of Later Roman Law: the Ecloga ad Procheiron Mutata* (Cambridge: Cambridge University Press, 1927), 1 and 138. On the difficulties of translating this particular clause, however, see above, Introduction, note 42.

27. *Gregorii Episcopi Turoniensis Libri Historiarum X*, VIII.29 (c.585 CE) and X.18 ("ad ridiculum laxaverunt"), ed. B. Krusch and W. Levison, *MGH SS Rer Merov.*, I (Hannover: Hahn, 1951), 393 and 509 [hereafter *GT*].

28. Above, Chap. 2.

29. *Leges Langobardorum*, Liutprand, 80.

30. E. H. Freshfield, *A Manual of Roman Law: The Ecloga published by the Emperors Leo III and Constantine V of Isauria at Constantinople*

*in 726 A.D.* (Cambridge: Cambridge University Press, 1926), cc. 17.2 (106, perjurer), 17.4 (106, thief) and 17.23–34 (109–111, sexual offences).

31. Freshfield, *Manual of Later Roman Law*, 1 and 33: chapter XXIII (XXXI), 139, reiterates the penalties of flogging, shaving and nose-slitting for sexual offences.

32. *II Cnut: Secular Laws*, 53 and 53.1, tr. D. Whitelock, *English Historical Documents I: 500–1042* (rev. ed., London, Routledge, 1979), 463.

33. The definition of "just" and "unjust" anger on the part of the ruler is discussed in Althoff, "Ira regis" and Bühler-Thierry, "'Just anger' or 'vengeful anger'?", both with numerous illustrative examples.

34. J. L. Nelson, "Peers in the early middle ages," in *Law, Laity and Solidarities: Essays in Honour of Susan Reynolds*, ed. P. Stafford, J. L. Nelson and J. Martindale (Manchester: Manchester University Press, 2001), 12–26 at 37; Paul Edward Dutton, "Keeping secrets in a dark age," in *Rhetoric and the Discourses of Power in Court Culture: China, Europe and Japan*, ed. D. R. Knechtges and E. Vance (Seattle: University of Washington Press, 2005), 169–198, at 175. The capitulary is edited as *MGH Capitularia Regum Francorum*, I, no. 44, ed. A. Boretius (Hannover: Hahn, 1883), 124.

35. Giorgio Agamben, *Homo Sacer: Sovereign Power and Bare Life*, tr. Daniel Heller-Roazen (Stanford: Stanford University Press, 1998) [Italian publication Torino: Einaudi, 1995], esp. 15 and 28.

36. Agamben, *Homo*, 47. It is when the exceptional becomes the norm that tyranny and atrocity result: Agamben cites Stalinist Russia and Nazi Germany as examples.

37. *GT*, V.18.

38. *Ibid.*; translation in Gregory of Tours, *History of the Franks*, tr. Lewis Thorpe (London: Penguin, 1974), 282–3.

39. Paul Fouracre, "Attitudes towards violence in seventh- and eighth-century Francia," and Janet Nelson, "Violence in the Carolingian world and the ritualization of ninth-century warfare," both in *Violence and Society in the Early Medieval West*, ed. Halsall, 60–75 and 90–107 respectively. On the rhetoric of peacekeeping see Paul Kershaw, *Peaceful Kings: Peace, Power and the Early Medieval Imagination* (Oxford: Oxford University Press, 2011).

40. Above, Chap. 2. The memory of Cnut's cruelty lingered on to resurface in William of Malmesbury: William of Malmesbury, *Gesta Regum Anglorum/The History of the English Kings*, II.179, ed.

R. A. B. Mynors, R. M. Thomson and M. Winterbottom, 2 vols, I (Oxford, Clarendon Press, 1998). On William's ambivalent portrayal of the king see Elaine Treharne, *Living through Conquest: the Politics of Early English* (Oxford: Oxford University Press, 2012), 38–40.

41. *MGH Epp. Karol. Aevi*, IV (Berlin: Weidmann, 1925), 595, LXXXVI: *Si fur vel latro deprehensus fuerit et negaverit quod ei impingitur, asseritis apud vos, quod iudex caput eius verberibus tundat et aliis stimulis ferries donec veritatem depromat, ipsius latera pungat. Quam rem nec divina lex nec humana prorsus admittit, cum non invita, sed spontanea debeat esse confessio, nec sit violenter elicienda...*

42. *Byzantine Defenders of Images: Eight Saints' Lives in English Translation*, ed. Alice-Mary Talbot (Washington: Dumbarton Oaks, 1998), 204.

43. *La vie d'Étienne le Jeune par Étienne le Diacre*, c.56, ed. M.-F. Auzépy (Ashgate: Variorum, 1997), 255–6.

44. Above, note 8.

45. "Three faces of cruelty," 419 and 421. He continues (421): "These cruelties are not only deliberate, they are ceremonially recurrent defenses of the structure of group domination."

46. Miller, *Eye for an Eye*, 52.

47. *Making of English Law*, 361; Mary P. Richards, "I-II Cnut: Wulfstan's *Summa?*", in *English Law before Magna Carta*, ed. Stefan Jurasinski, Lisi Oliver and Andrew Rabin (Leiden: Brill, 2010), 137–156, comments that the adultery laws in II.50–55 "have no identified source."

48. G. R. Evans, *Law and Theology in the Middle Ages* (London and New York: Routledge, 2002), vii, quote at 53; Wormald, *Making of English Law*, 122. L. K. Little, "Anger in monastic curses," in *Anger's Past*, ed. Rosenwein, 9–35, comments, 27, on early medieval society's "decidedly Old Testament stamp." Kelly, *Guide*, 125 comments that Irish laws relating to killing and injury had as their starting point Exodus 21:24, demanding a life for a life, etc.

49. Patricia Skinner, "The gendered nose and its lack: 'medieval' nose-cutting and its modern manifestations," *Journal of Women's History*, 26.1 (2014), 45–67, and Chap. 5 below explore these in more detail.

50. "Three faces of cruelty," 427.

51. J. A. Lokin, "The significance of law and legislation in the lawbooks of the ninth to eleventh centuries," in *Law and Society in Byzantium: Ninth-Twelfth Centuries*, ed. Angeliki Laiou and Dieter Simon (Washington: Dumbarton Oaks, 1994), 71–91, at 77.

52. Reported in *The Chronicle of Theophanes Confessor: Byzantine and Near Eastern History, AD 284–813*, tr. C. Mango and R. Scott with G. Greatrex (Oxford: Clarendon Press, 1997) under the years AM6101 (608/9CE), 6133 (640/1CE), 6161 (668/9CE), 6187 (694/5CE), 6190 (697/8CE), 6198 (705/6CE – blinding of the patriarch Kallinikos), 6205 (712/13CE), 6210 (717/18CE), 6211 (718/19CE), 6235 (742/3CE), 6257 (764/5CE), 6263 (770/1CE), 6284 (791/2CE), 6285 (792/3CE), 6289 (796/7CE – the notorious blinding of Constantine by his mother Irene), 6291 (798/9CE), 6296 (803/4CE) and 6303 (810/11CE). The infamous cases of mutilated popes expressed the continuing purchase of this biblical injunction: see below, 00. The blemished were also excluded from rule in early Ireland: Kelly, *Guide*, 19–20.

53. *Chronicle of Theophanes Confessor*, AM 6187 (694/5CE). Justinian's life is reconstructed, with a certain amount of apologetic licence to compensate for the hostile sources, in Constance Head, *Justinian II of Byzantium* (Madison: University of Wisconsin Press, 1972). See also Bogdan-Petru Maleon, "La role de la mutilation dans la lutte politique a Byzance," in *Le corps et ses hypostases en Europe et dans la société roumaine du Moyen Âge à l'époque contemporaine*, ed. Constanţa Vintilă-Ghiţulescu et Alexandru-Florin Platon (Bucharest: New Europe College, 2010), 125–146 and *id.*, "The impossible return: about the status of deposed and mutilated emperors," *Medieval and Early Modern Studies for Central and Eastern Europe*, 3 (2011): 31–49.

54. *Pauli Historia Langobardorum*, VI.31, ed. L. Bethmann and G. Waitz, *MGH SSRLI*, ed. G. Waitz (Hannover: Hahn, 1878), 175: *qui post iterum adsumpto imperio, quotiens defluentem gutta reumatis manum detersit, pene totiens aliquem ex his qui contra eum fuerant iugulari praecepit.*

55. *Agnelli Liber Pontificalis Ecclesiae Ravennatis*, c.137, ed. O. Holder-Egger, *MGH SSRLI*, 367: *et potitus imperio, nares sibi et aures ex obrizo fecit.*

56. Judith Herrin, "Blinding in Byzantium," in *Polypleuros nous: Miscellanea für Peter Schreiner zu seinem 60 Geburtstag* (München: Saur, 2000), 56–68.

57. J. Lascaratos and S. Marketos, "The penalty of blinding during Byzantine times: medical remarks," *Documenta Opthalmologica*, 81.1 (1992), 133–144, outlines the ways in which deliberate blinding could be accomplished, including by hot vinegar.
58. Michael Psellos, *Chronographia: Fourteen Byzantine Rulers*, tr. E. R. A. Sewter (London: Penguin, 1966), IV.49 (115). Greek: καὶ συλλαβὼν αθρόου της τε ρινὸς καὶ των οφθαλμών αφαίρεται, μαγειρική σφαγίδι άμφω συνεξέλων: Michele Psello, *Imperatori di Bisanzio (Cronografia)*, ed . and tr. Salvatore Impellizari, Ugo Criscuolo and Siliva Ronchey, 2 vols (Milan: Fondazione Lorenzo Valla/Mondadori, 1984), 174.
59. Psellos, *Chronographia*, II.2–3, tr. Sewter, 53–54.
60. Psellos, V.14 (Orphanotrophos); VI.15 (Skleros); VI.123 (Tornikios and Vatatzes). "Nobly": γενναίως.
61. His purpose in highlighting the flaws of individual emperors is discussed in detail by Anthony Kaldellis, *The Argument of Psellos's Chronographia* (Leiden: Brill, 1999), especially 41–47.
62. See below, Chap. 6.
63. A. Kazhdan, "Some observations on the Byzantine concept of law: three authors of the ninth through twelfth centuries," in *Law and Society in Byzantium*, 199–216, at 215.
64. Bührer-Thierry, "'Just anger' or 'vengeful anger'?"
65. *vanissima Hellade in suis sedibus exsuperata*: Notker, *Gesta Karoli*, II.6, *MGH SS rer. Ger. n.s.* XII, ed. H. Haefele (Berlin: Weidmann, 1959), 55.
66. *Thietmar*, II.15.
67. Mutilation: *Rodulfi Glabri Historiarum Libri Quinque / Rodulfus Glaber The Five Books of the Histories*, ed. and tr. John France (Oxford: Clarendon Press, 1989), Book I.12, 24–25.
68. *Iohannis Diaconi Chronicon Venetum et Gradense*, s.a. 998, in *MGH SS* VII, ed. G. H. Pertz (Hannover: Hahn, 1846), 31.
69. Discussion in Gerd Althoff, *Otto III* (University Park: Pennsylvania State Press, 2003), 72–81, at 73.
70. *Einhardi Vita Karoli Magni*, ed. O. Holder-Egger, *MGH SS rerum. Germ.* XXV (Hanover: Hahn, 1911), III.28; Notker, *Gesta Karoli, MGH SS rer. Ger. n.s.* XII, ed. H. Haefele (Berlin: Weidmann, 1959), I.26: *in signum virtutis illius pulcherrima cicatrix in modum fili tenuissimi turturinas acies niveo candore decorabat*; translation in Einhard and Notker the Stammerer, *Two Lives of Charlemagne*, tr. L. Thorpe (London, Penguin, 1969), 122–124.

71. Iconodules: St George Limnaiotes (nose slit, c. 730) and Paul of Kaioumas (nose cut off, c. 750): *Dumbarton Oaks Hagiography Database*, directed by A. Kazhdan and A.-M. Talbot, http://www.doaks.org/document/hagiointro. pdf [accessed 15 January 2012]; the life of St Stephen the Younger (c. 715–767) also highlights widespread mutilations including nose-cutting among his contemporary iconodule monks: *Vie d'Étienne le jeune*, ed. Auzépy, 157 and 161. I am grateful to Dr Stavroula Constantinou for bringing these references to my attention. Milan: *Andrea da Strumi, Arioaldo: passione del santo martire milanese*, tr. M. Navoni (Milan: Jaca Book, 1994), 144.

72. E.g. the restoration of the sight of Ailward, discussed above.

73. Cited in Wormald, *Making of English Law*, 125–6.

74. *Leges Langobardorum*, Rothari c.180; *Laws of Hywel Dda*, 78.

75. *Leges Langobardorum*, Rothari c.377 – a freeman so blinded was paid two-thirds of the price payable for his murder, whilst the same injury to a semi-free or unfree man was payable as if they had been killed.

76. *The Annals of St Bertin: ninth-century histories vol I*, tr. J. L. Nelson (Manchester, Manchester University Press, 1991), 181n; Michael McCormick, *Eternal Victory: Triumphal Rulership in Late Antiquity, Byzantium and the Early Medieval West* (Cambridge: Cambridge University Press, 1986), 334. The ultimate source for this information is Gregory of Tours.

77. K. van Eickels, "Gendered violence: castration and blinding as punishment for treason in Normandy and Anglo-Norman England," *Gender and History* 16 (2003): 588–602.

78. *GT*, V.14.

79. van Eickels, "Gendered violence," 588.

80. Edward Wheatley, *Stumbling Blocks before the Blind: Medieval Constructions of a Disability* (Ann Arbor: University of Michigan Press, 2010), 60.

81. *Ibid.*, 33, with numerous examples.

82. *Ibid.*, 34–5.

83. *Erchemperti Historia Langobardorum Beneventanorum*, c.39 (s.a. 877), ed. G. Waitz, in *MGH SSRLI*, 249: Sergius, the *magister militum* of Naples, is blinded and sent to Rome, where he "ended his life miserably (*ibique miserabiliter vitam finivit*)."

84. Kelly, *Guide*, 221.

85. Patricia Skinner, "The Political uses of the body in Norman texts," paper read at *People, Texts and Artefacts: Cultural Transmission in the Norman Worlds of the Eleventh and Twelfth Centuries*, Ariano Irpino, Italy, 20–22 September 2013 [publication forthcoming].
86. This episode is reported in *Orderic*, III.ii.15.
87. William of Malmesbury, *Gesta Regum*, II.137 (attempt to blind King Athelstan); II.145 (blinding of Riulf in prison by William Longsword); II.165 (Aethelred's blinding of Aelfric's son); II.188 (blinding of Alfred son of Aethelred).
88. The episode is extensively discussed by Wheatley, *Stumbling Blocks*, 175–179 and van Eickels, "Gendered violence," 595.
89. John Hudson, "Violence, theft and the making of the English common law," in *Crime and Punishment in the Middle Ages*, ed. T. H. Haskett (Victoria, BC: Humanities Centre of the University of Victoria, 1998), 19–35, at 31. As we shall see, Chap. 6 below, blindings were difficult and risked killing the victim.
90. The count was accused of treachery, fought and lost, leading to his blinding and castration: *The Anglo-Saxon Chronicle: a revised translation*, ed. Dorothy Whitelock (London: Eyre and Spottiswoode, 1961), version E (Peterborough) s.a. 1095; *Orderic* VIII.iii.23.411; William of Malmesbury, *Gesta Regum*, IV.319. See also Jane Martindale, "Between law and politics: the judicial duel under the Angevin kings (mid-twelfth century to 1204," in *Law, Laity and Solidarities*, 116–149.
91. *Bernardi Cremifanensis Historiae*, s.a.1251, in *MGH SS*, XXV, ed. G. H. Pertz (Munich: MGH, 1880), 658.
92. The three volumes of *I Placiti del "Regnum Italiae,"* ed. C. Manaresi (Rome: Tipografia del Senato, 1955, 1957 and 1960), for example, only feature violence in the form of judicial duels to settle disputes over property, and even these are rare: II, nos 170 (Verona, 972), 236 (Rome, 998), 250 (Gaeta, 999, highly exceptional) and 274 (Cesa, 1010). Earlier land disputes, featured in volume I, do use the term "altercatio" to describe the dispute much more frequently than later cases, and whilst this may represent a simple change in notarial practice, it does suggest some violence was involved, even if it did not form the grounds for the court case.
93. On violence as a strategy, see the discussion in Chris Wickham, *Courts and Conflict in Twelfth-Century Tuscany* (Oxford: Oxford University Press, 2003), 219–222.

94. *Select Pleas of the Crown, volume I: AD 1200–1225*, no. 4, ed. F. W. Maitland (Selden Society Publications, 1, London: Bernard Quaritch, 1888), 2. The case is also included in *Pleas before the Kings or his Justices, 1198–1202, volume II: Rolls or Fragments of Rolls from the Years 1198, 1201 and 1202*, no. 288, ed. D. M. Stenton (Selden Society Publications, 68, London: Bernard Quaritch, 1949), 61–2.

95. *Select Pleas of the Crown, volume I: AD 1200–1225*, no. 9, 4. Also included in *Pleas before the Kings or his Justices, II*, ed. Stenton, no. 350, 79.

96. E.g. Peter v. Anketill for four wounds in the head; *Pleas before the Kings or his Justices, II*, ed. Stenton, nos 386, 89–90 (female victim, accusing the same man who had assaulted her husband) and 389, 90–91.

97. *Pleas before the Kings or his Justices, II*, ed. Stenton, nos 289, 62 (4 bones extracted); 348, 78–9 (number of bones not stated, additional wound on the nose); 357, 81–2 (number of bones not stated); 382, 88 (victim Edith of St Teath, 16 bones extracted).

98. Archaeological studies of earlier and contemporary skull lesions show that some healing might take place, but that complete closure was rare: e.g. cases reported in M. Rubini and P. Zaio, "Warriors from the East: skeletal evidence of warfare from a Lombard-Avar cemetery in central Italy (Campochiaro, Molise, sixth to eighth century AD)," *Journal of Archaeological Science*, 38 (2011): 1551–1559; and N. Powers, "Cranial trauma and treatment: a case study from the medieval cemetery of St Mary Spital, London", *International Journal of Osteoarchaeology*, 15 (2005): 1–14. Modern examples assist in visualizing the effects of missing pieces of the skull, e.g. the case of builder Elvis Romeo Lingurar, whose skull was rebuilt when he shattered it falling from scaffolding: *Daily Telegraph*, 31 July 2014, at http://www.telegraph.co.uk/news/worldnews/europe/romania/11001905/Builder-has-crushed-skull-rebuilt-thanks-to-donations-from-public.html    [accessed 31/7/14]. On medieval industrial injuries of this type, none resulting in head wounds, see Metzler, *Disability in Medieval Europe*, 150–151.

99. *Bald's Leechbook*, I, 25, ii, quoted in S. Rubin, *Medieval English Medicine* (London, David and Charles, 1974), 131.

100. I should like to thank former colleagues and the service users at Headway (Portsmouth and SE Hampshire) for educating me first-hand in the often debilitating after-effects of traumatic brain injury.

101. William of Brienon's complaint of a knife wound in the jaw from William Torell, heard at Essex in 1202, seems just such a case, for the bulk of the record contains Torell's counterclaim that Brienon had been caught in Torell's bedroom "plotting his [Torell's] shame in respect of his wife": *Select Pleas of the Crown, I*, ed. Maitland, no. 87, 44. Wendy Davies and Paul Fouracre, "Conclusion," in *The Settlement of Disputes in Early Medieval Europe*, ed. Wendy Davies and Paul Fouracre (Cambridge: Cambridge University Press, 1986), 233: "Some disputes may well have been undertaken for reasons other than those which were the immediate object of the dispute..."

102. *Rolls of the Justices in Eyre for Gloucestershire, Warwickshire and Staffordshire, 1221, 1222*, ed. D. M. Stenton (Selden Society Publications, 59, London: Bernard Quaritch, 1940), no. 939, 402.

103. *The Roll of the Shropshire Eyre of 1256*, ed. A. Harding (Selden Society Publications, 96, London: Selden Society, 1980), Crown pleas, nos 494, 501, 518, 520, 543, 562, 587, 593, 595, 628, 657, 675, 678, 687 and 757. [Hereafter cited as *Shropshire Eyre Roll*.] I have excluded from my count one case where Harding has translated "percussit" as "hit on the head" but where the Latin omits the location of the wound: no. 582, 221.

104. Thus although another boy, Gregory, was named in the report of the accidental, self-inflicted fatal injury of one Nicholas of Willey, he was exonerated of all culpability. Nicholas had been beating him with a staff [*virga*] when the accident happened: *Shropshire Eyre Roll*, no. 658, 239.

105. *Ibid.*, no. 541, 209.

106. *Ibid.*, no. 596, 224.

107. *Rolls of the Justices in Eyre for Yorkshire in 3 Henry III (1218–1219)*, ed. D. M. Stenton (Selden Society Publications, 56, London: Bernard Quaritch, 1937), no. 553, 218–9

108. *Pleas before the Kings or his Justices, II*, ed. Stenton, no. 344, 76–7.

109. *Shropshire Eyre Roll*, nos 747–8, 261–3.

110. *Ibid.*, no. 794, 274–5.

111. *The Roll and Writ File of the Berkshire Eyre of 1248*, ed. M. T. Clanchy (Selden Society Publications, 90, London: The Selden Society, 1973), no. 896, 353–4.
112. *Select Pleas of the Crown, I*, ed. Maitland, no. 41, 18.
113. *Ibid.*, no. 24, 10.
114. See below, Chap. 7, and Appendix 2 for detail.
115. Pollock, F., and F. W. Maitland, *The History of English Law before the Time of Edward I*, 2 vols (Cambridge: Cambridge University Press, 1895), I, 66. The fate of the law in England after 1066 was, of course, signaled as the subject of the never-written second volume of Wormald, *Making of English Law*.
116. Luke Demaitre, "Skin and the city: cosmetic medicine as an urban concern," in *Between Text and Patient: The Medical Enterprise in Medieval and Early Modern Europe*, ed. Florence Eliza Glaze and Brian K. Nance (Florence: SISMEL-Edizioni del Galluzzo, 2011), 97–120.
117. E.g. an episode from *Thietmar*, IV.21, in which a certain Margrave Henry seized and blinded one of Bishop Bernward of Würzburg's men – this usurpation of the king's right to punish in this way led to the margrave's exile.

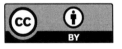

# CHAPTER 4

# Stigma and Disfigurement: Putting on a Brave Face?

This chapter will ask whether acquired (as opposed to congenital) facial disfigurement marked a person as stigmatized in medieval Europe, or whether "abnormal" faces were so commonplace—through disease, infection, birth defects, accidental and deliberate violence—that a disfigured person was effectively invisible. Jacques Le Goff certainly thought so, opining that medieval Europe teemed with the impaired, the blind, the sick and the mutilated.[1] This may well be true, although the visibility of such groups is undoubtedly exaggerated by their appearance in hagiographic texts: medieval Europe was teeming with would-be saints as well, and the most common context for extended descriptions of people with disabilities is in accounts of miraculous alleviation of their condition. More will be said on "cures" to the face in Chapter 7. This chapter, however, largely bypasses the hagiography to explore examples of different types of disfigurement reported in chronicles and legal material, considering not only the nature of the disfigurement, but also the nature and context of the report itself. Do the writers stigmatize their subjects simply through drawing attention to them, and do they make clear how contemporaries viewed those subjects? Did ubiquity of visible difference in fact mute its potential to cause surprise, shock or disgust? The chapter will ask whether responses to facial disfigurement were conditioned by class or circumstances, and will present some case studies supporting my contention that facial impairment, whether accompanied or not by side effects such as brain injury or loss of senses, was treated differently from maiming of limbs or disease of

© The Author(s) 2017
P. Skinner, *Living with Disfigurement in Early Medieval Europe*,
DOI 10.1057/978-1-137-54439-1_4

the body, in that very little could be done either to mitigate its effects or disguise its appearance.

The notion of "stigma" of course immediately brings to mind the distinction made in the social sciences between in-groups and out-groups in any given society.[2] Medieval historians have long found it useful to consider the work of social scientists, particularly in the fields of anthropology and sociology, to provide insights into less well-documented societies and groups of the early Middle Ages.[3] Such studies, however, have only recently begun to focus on the margins of medieval society, exploring the socially-excluded, the poor, dissidents and criminality.[4] I have already suggested that it is difficult to posit disfigured people as a recognizable group in medieval society: certainly they were not conceptualized as such. They therefore seem to have escaped the fate of other groups, highlighted in studies following the seminal work of Bob Moore, but adapting, as well as adopting, his notion of a "persecuting society,"[5] such as the blind, lepers, the poor, Jews or even women, all of whom were and still are discussed with little sense of differentiation or recognition that individuals within these groups might be experiencing their perceived "difficulties" in different ways. This is a point made by Edward Wheatley in his ground-breaking study of visually impaired people in medieval Europe: visual impairment not being understood as a range of abilities, the partially-sighted, in particular, faced a dilemma as to whether to reveal their ability to see a little, and thus be accused of faking their "blindness."[6] Wheatley's work is highly relevant to the history of disfigurement, given that a significant number of the visually impaired may have been deliberately blinded, rather than lacking or losing their sight through natural causes. Those who lost their eyes, in particular, would have looked rather different to those whose blinding was through non-invasive methods.

Medieval sources, as we have seen, had no stable term to describe disfigurement, nor were those so afflicted identified as a group. "The disfigured," linguistically at least, do not exist. That is not to say that acquired disfigurement affected only individuals—group disfigurement of defeated enemies is often reported. Thietmar of Merseberg's early eleventh-century history, for example, refers to the shaving and flogging of six men.[7] Reports of such group mutilation seem to increase sharply from the thirteenth century onwards. Some of the most notorious examples are clustered in accounts of the Albigensian crusade, in which both sides were condemned or excused by chroniclers for tit-for-tat acts of cruelty. In 1210 a local lord, Gerard de Pepieux, abandoned the crusade and mutilated two of its knights whom he had captured at Puisserguier by blinding them and cutting off their ears, noses, and upper lips, then sent them back to Simon de Montfort. Later, in retaliation, de Montfort blinded over a hundred defenders of Bram and cut off their noses, leaving one man with a single eye to lead the rest to Cabaret, another fortress resisting the Crusade. The *Canso de la Crozada* reports another, similar attack by Count Ramon Roger of Foix against a group of German and Frisian crusaders. In 1228, Roger of Wendover reports, Count Raymond of Toulouse captured and mutilated some 2000 French prisoners and sent them back to their homes "shamefully mutilated, a deformed spectacle to their own people."[8] The strong message running through these and earlier sources relating to the wounded faces of warriors, or the legal codes discussed in Chapter 3 dealing with personal injury, is that disfigurement inflicted on another was unsightly or shameful—*turpis*—and invited ridicule. The sheer impact of a whole group of mutilated bodies in the thirteenth-century cases ensured they were recorded. With the apparent exception of Old Norse society, facial scarring (and, for that matter, congenital deformity) was not seen as a sign of prowess, but instead was read more often as a sign of defeat and disgrace.[9]

Yet the picture we have is made more complex by medieval reflections on the relationship between bodily imperfection and the health of the soul, and the prioritizing of the latter. Writing in the early eleventh century, Thietmar commented:

> In me, however, you will see a tiny little man whose jaw and left side of the face are deformed by an ulcer which erupted there and continues to swell. The nose, broken in childhood, gives me a laughable appearance. Of all that I would regret nothing, if only my inner character were bright.[10]

Whilst Thietmar's self-reflection about his appearance is a rarity, the sentiment it expresses is commonplace in medieval texts. A century after Thietmar, Abbot Guibert of Nogent (d.1125) echoed a similar sentiment about physical appearance: "If their internal models are beautiful and good, those who manifest their image, especially if they do not depart from their measure, are beautiful, and hence they are good."[11] We shall return to the subject of beauty presently.

Medieval authors in fact had a highly sophisticated sense of the difference between the material and the figurative, illustrated most frequently by the differentiation between literal and spiritual sight and blindness.

The tenth-century Old English version of the *Deeds of Andrew and Matthew among the Cannibals*, for example, reports that when his eyes were gouged out with a sword, Matthew prayed to God for inner light.[12] Guibert comments that those who elected him to the abbacy of Nogent were "blind or short-sighted," asking, "what would they have said if they had seen my inner self?"[13] In his account of the martyrdom of the missionary Bruno in 1009, Bruno's companion Wipert recounts how, despite accepting baptism, the Russian king "Nethimer" ordered the execution of Bruno and four of his chaplains. Wipert, the only survivor, then reports matter-of-factly: "he had my eyes taken out [*meos oculos eruere fecit*]." From that time, he says, he had wandered as a pilgrim of God through many provinces, invoking the aid of the saints to help the Christians, and asking the charitable help of all Christians for the defense of his life and the remedy of their sins.[14] Wipert hints at the material reality of his situation, but nevertheless sees in his peregrinations the opportunity for others to acquire spiritual rewards by helping him. Such distinctions, despite being didactic in nature, caution against uncritically applying modern assumptions about the misfortune of disfigurement to the medieval cases under review.

So the disfigured were perhaps not a conventionally identified "out-group" linguistically. But there are different degrees of difference/strangeness, both figurative and literal. Wipert was permanently impaired, but Thietmar's disfigurement placed him on the relatively mild end of the spectrum. Broken noses must have been a common occurrence, after all. More importantly, the major cause of disfigurement to his face, the *fistula* or ulcer, was a natural phenomenon rather than being inflicted by a third party. But his protest—indeed the fact he raises the issue of his appearance at all—does suggest the potential for others to respond negatively to his facial deformities, and as the number of examples drawn from his text suggests, Thietmar may have had a specific interest in physical difference that has not hitherto attracted much attention from historians.

Disfigured faces were "read" and commented on in medieval texts, it seems, only if their visual impact was obvious and immediate. A late example, but fulfilling a similar didactic function, comes in the thirteenth-century chronicle of Salimbene. Describing a certain brother Aldevrandus, he says "He had a deformed head in the shape of a helmet of the ancients, with copious hair on his forehead." Although he suffered laughter from the brothers when his turn came to start the antiphon (so all eyes would have been on him?), Aldevrandus's case is used by Salimbene to highlight the lessons of Christ's humility before his persecutors.[15] We might note here the appearance of excessive hair as one element in Aldevrandus's "strange" appearance: Miller comments that this is often the focus for feelings of disgust in modern studies.[16]

Modern studies of facial disfigurement and facial perception focus on the psychological impact on the self and others of "normal" and disrupted appearance. This "first impression" might—or might not—be reinforced by other body language such as speech or gestures, and could be severely disrupted by facial difference. But as sociologists of stigma have pointed out, damaged physical appearance is not only a key factor in shaping the perception of others, but also reinforces the behavior of the stigmatized individual in that s/he may withdraw more and more from potentially "embarrassing" situations.[17] Was a disfigured person a stranger to themselves, abject in the Kristevan sense that "the skin, a fragile container, no longer guaranteed the integrity of one's 'own and clean self' but ... gave way before the dejection of its contents?"[18] Aldevrandus, in Salimbene's report, was certainly "disturbed and made to blush" by the ridicule of the other brothers.[19] Did acquired disfigurement throw up issues of recognition and social exclusion among family or community, especially if the damage had occurred away from home, for instance in warfare? And might it lead to a need for physical relocation—spatially "outside" the community—if the disfigurement were read in the wrong way?

Sociologists have extensively explored the concept of stigma since the pioneering work of Erving Goffman in 1963. Goffman's work has also constituted a useful point of reference for medieval historians, although the editors of a volume on stigma published in 1986 commented on historians' rather belated adoption of the concept as an interpretative filter.[20] His model of difference, relegating the person to a tainted, discounted member of the community,[21] however, has not been without its critics. Colin Barnes suggests that applying stigma theory to the physically-impaired, and viewing their impairment as a personal tragedy, not only denies the impaired their own voices, but also "over-emphasizes subjective physiological and cognitive limitations through the professionally-determined authenticity of those determinations."[22] The modern advent of professional care and segregation of the impaired, in other words, has increased and reinforced dependency and isolation. Barnes contrasts this situation with the Middle Ages and early modern periods when the impaired may have been viewed as "abnormal in the purely statistical sense of belonging to a minority group," but were not separated from the mainstream.[23] The disfigured, of course, might or might not fall into the category of the "abnormal." As Sally Crawford and Christina Lee have observed in their discussion of health and sickness, such categories are highly fluid: "it is only when normal health becomes 'abnormal' that it becomes unhealthy, when people move from the normative—in behavior, appearance or emotional or physical well-being—to the boundaries."[24] Yet the concept of stigma can be useful for drilling down into medieval texts that did not, for the most part, explicitly consider the wider implications of a damaged face. A useful study by social psychologist Edward Jones and his colleagues offered "six dimensions of stigma:" concealability; course; disruptiveness; aesthetics; origin and peril.[25] How useful are these in understanding the medieval experience of damaged appearance?

## CONCEALABILITY: CAN THE STIGMA BE HIDDEN?

According to sociologist Shlomo Shoham, visible difference automatically stigmatizes and sets the individual outside the group, as "these individuals and the groups are manifestly different. Their apartness is inherent in their physical attributes."[26] All modern commentators agree that the solution to stigma is to learn to "pass," to conceal or disguise the physical difference sufficiently so as not to be noticed.[27] In the Middle Ages, the possibilities for concealing facial disfigurement were limited: women, more than men, might be able to cover their heads and faces and look relatively "normal," since a married woman, in particular, was expected to cover her hair (and lawcodes often include penalties for dishonoring women by removing or touching their scarves and hair, as we have already seen).[28] A striking depiction of head and face covering on a woman is incorporated in the Becket windows at Canterbury cathedral: here the mother of the leprous boy is, somewhat ironically, all wrapped up, presumably to prevent contagion, whilst his disease is indicated with a few generic dots on the face and not concealed at all. Whether male lepers went about with their heads and faces partly covered or not is hard to judge: the few and late depictions we have clearly show them concealing themselves.[29] But having an extensive head wrapping might, in fact, have become an *indicator* of leprosy: for men the choice of headgear was perhaps more highly charged.

A visible scar, on the other hand, might also have functioned as a memory device, recalling the circumstances in which it was acquired. For example the Flemish count William, involved in a violent confrontation at Avesnes (c.1147), received a sword wound on the head, whilst climbing down a ladder from the church tower which left him scarred for life.[30]

The almost contemporary Gerald of Wales develops this idea further, uti-lizing a scar acquired in battle as a device to discuss legitimacy: the knight Erchembald, he reports, bore exactly the same scar at his birth as his father had acquired in battle when nicked on the top lip by a spear, thereby sav-ing his mother from suspicion of adultery.[31]

Three cases of missing ears demonstrate that the visibility of, and level of stigma attached to, a mutilated person could very much vary with the circumstances in which the mutilation had been suffered. The sixth-century history of Bishop Gregory of Tours provides the first example, a character assassination of Count Leudast of Tours, whom he portrays as the son of a slave. Sent to work in the royal kitchens as a child, Leudast ran away, and was punished by having one of his ears slit. "As there was no possibility of concealing this mark on his body," the young Leudast fled to Queen Marcovefa, who took pity on him and gave him a job in her stables. From here on, Gregory relates, Leudast essentially worked his way up to his comital position, and was appointed as a punishment to the people of Tours for their immense sins.[32] It is easy to dismiss Gregory's jaundiced view of the count as nothing more than a series of rhetorical flourishes—assigning low birth to a prominent figure was, throughout this period, a well-known tool for attacking them.[33] But clearly Leudast's ear was "wrong," and by drawing attention to it Gregory was able to construct the image of a man without much honor, in his eyes. Similar processes are at work in a case reported by the ninth-century Byzantine chronicler Theophanes. He reproduces a story relating to the fifth-century patrician Illos, whose right ear was cut off in an assassination attempt:

> When he was cured of the wound, he used to wear a cap. He asked the emperor to send him to the East so that he could enjoy a change of air because he was weak from the wound.[34]

This story is told as a prelude to a later rebellion—from the very eastern provinces to which Illos had retired—by the same man. It seems pretty clear that Illos is being set up by Theophanes as in some way dishonored by his wound (possibly by the circumstances in which it was acquired—he clearly was not popular), hinting that his withdrawal was not for health reasons but to render his lack of ear, which he also tried to hide with a cap, even less visible. Examining Byzantine iconography, it is in fact quite difficult to find evidence of male headgear except in the case of imperial crowns and head-dresses, so in highlighting the cap Theophanes may well have been drawing further attention to Illos's misfortune and status as "outside" the norms of the court once he withdrew.

Contrast these cases, in which the missing or damaged ear functioned as a negative element, with Thietmar of Merseberg's account of Bishop Michael of Regensburg (d. 972). He comments that Michael had lost an ear in battle, but "his mutilation was not to his shame but more to his honor."[35] The bishop's lack of an ear would have been apparent, but since he had acquired the injury in battle against the pagan Hungarians, the possible shame inherent in the injury was countered by the heroic way in which it had been acquired. In fact, Irina Metzler makes the important point that if a mutilation occurred *after* a priest had entered holy orders, he was permitted to maintain his position. Hence, Thietmar took the time to tell Michael's story.[36] For Leudast, Illos and Michael the visible injury was the same, but the stigma attached to it by those reporting the cases differed greatly, according to the back-story of its acquisition. (And the story mattered: Theophanes features an earlier, mutilated priest in the figure of Maximus, who became patriarch of Jerusalem in the early fourth century despite his lack of one eye. Theophanes attributes this to Maximus having "endured many tortures ($\pi o \lambda \lambda \acute{\alpha}\varsigma \ \beta \alpha \sigma \acute{\alpha} v o v \varsigma \ v \pi o \sigma \tau \alpha \varsigma$), implying that he had been caught up in the last great persecutions of Christians before toleration was decreed by Constantine, and thus, like Michael, could be presented as a hero for his faith.)[37] Was Thietmar in fact inclined to be more sympathetic to those who, like him, looked different? Or was his account shaped purely by his terms of reference, in this case the need to defend a deformed bishop from the accusation that his loss of an ear compromised his suitability to serve as a priest (and, by extension, reinforce his own legitimacy as a bishop despite *his* deformity)?

There is another dimension to the loss of ears, since the most famous case, which all of our protagonists would have been well aware of, was the attack by Simon Peter on Malchus, servant of the high priest, as Christ was arrested in the Garden of Gethsemane (John, 18:10). The Biblical account does not say whether this is whom Simon Peter was *aiming* at, but he succeeded in cutting off Malchus's ear with his sword. John's account shows Christ rebuking Peter for his action, and later artists would use this scene to show him miraculously re-attaching the missing ear. Either way, the episode with Malchus is adopted by medieval authors such as Orderic Vitalis to express violence, significantly in defense of the pope in 1106.[38]

Of course, what links all these cases is the fact that most of the men concerned were all expected to be highly visible in public—whether attending court as elite men (Illos at the imperial court, for example), or officiating in public offices (Patriarch Maximus, Bishops Michael and Thietmar). In early Irish laws, the *Bretha Déin Chécht* took account of the long-term effects of disfigurement when it awarded the victim one *cumal* (the price of a slave-girl) for every occasion on which he had to attend the public assembly with his visible scars.[39] The issue of visibility recurs in many other early lawcodes, including the Welsh laws of Hywel Dda as transmitted in the *Book of Blegywryd*.[40] As we have already explored in Chapter 2, the requirement to live a life in public, particularly for men of high status, meant that their appearance mattered.

## COURSE: COULD THE STIGMATIZING CONDITION BE CHANGED OVER TIME?

There are two aspects to the question of change over time: the possibility of changing one's physical appearance, and the possibility of changing the meaning of, and response to, the disfigurement. For medieval people, facial disfigurement was not easy to remedy or improve. The loss of ears, for instance, was permanent, and probably brought with it some auditory impairment as well. In the case of wounds acquired in warfare, however, the care received at the time might radically affect how bad the subsequent disfigurement might be: the work of Piers Mitchell has demonstrated that care on the battlefield, or immediately afterwards, was available to crusaders in the Holy Land.[41] Depending on time and place, therefore, there was a slight possibility of modifying, if not totally changing, the disfiguring condition.

Medieval case studies of such care are still very rare, but the potential difference it could make to subsequent appearance has been startlingly illustrated by an example drawn from antiquity: the reconstruction of King Philip of Macedon's face (based on his archaeological remains) by John Prag and Richard Neave and their team at Manchester. Philip had been hit diagonally across his face by an arrow shot from above, shattering his eye socket and depriving him of an eye. The reconstruction team, aided by make-up artists from the local television station, was able to produce a highly realistic wax effigy, complete with the devastating wound. However, just as this model was being completed it was learnt that Philip, as reported in Pliny's *Natural History*, had in fact received care from one of the most skilled surgeons of his era (the late fourth century BC), Kritoboulos, and so the team also reconstructed the face to reflect the possibility of this intervention. In place of a raw, open chasm in his face there is a neat line indicating suturing, complete with closed eye socket. These full-color "before" and "after" images, however, were thought too disturbing to go on display, and a bronze rendition was eventually made for Manchester Museum.[42]

Whilst Philip's may be a special case, it is important not to assume that wounded medieval warriors lacked any kind of care. Arrow wounds were ubiquitous, reflecting the fact that the face was the most vulnerable part of a warrior's body.[43] An illustration from Peter of Eboli's *Liber ad Honorem Augusti*, produced at the end of the twelfth century, suggests that immediate care was sometimes available. Depicting in one scene Count Richard of Acerra's face being horizontally pierced by an arrow at the siege of Naples (1191), the narrative then continues with another illustration depicting Richard being attended to by a man labeled "medicus" and two female assistants.[44] We know that Richard survived his wound (only to be executed for treachery some years afterwards): the detailed pictures suggest that the arrow hit Richard's cheeks, narrowly missing his jawbone, but he must nevertheless have had two major scars on his face thereafter. Arrow wounds to the head and face, in fact, are one of the most common disfiguring (but often also fatal) injuries reported by chroniclers.[45]

The only evidence we have of potential change in the form of a facial prosthesis in the early Middle Ages, however, is the highly-suspect western account by the ninth-century author Agnellus of Ravenna of the Byzantine Emperor Justinian II's golden nose and ears.[46] The basic problem with Agnellus's account, besides its geographical and chronological distance from the events it describes, is that it is our only evidence for the prosthetic nose and ears. Byzantine sources in the east report the mutilation, but the idea of a golden nose may well derive from Agnellus's proximity to the richly decorated mosaic portrayals of Justinian's earlier namesake still extant at Ravenna. A recent report of a gold *solidus* of Justinian II, on which both the emperor's and Christ's faces have been disfigured by a blow to the nose, opens the intriguing possibility that the power of images was understood and in this case used to undermine the emperor further.[47]

For most, however, a facial disfigurement was unlikely to improve, and would become worse with age as the facial muscles lost their tension. As Irina Metzler has rightly highlighted, referring to acquired impairment, the stage in a person's life when disfigurement occurred, as well as its severity, could also have a greater or lesser effect on their future.[48]

## Disruptiveness: Does the Stigmatizing Condition Disturb Social Interactions?

Here, the circumstances in which the disfigurement had been acquired had direct implications. Medieval life was played out far more publicly and communally than life today. The study of medieval *fama*, the common knowledge within a community spread by gossip and rumor, has revealed how important gaining and maintaining a reputation could be.[49] We have also already seen how quickly news of misfortune could spread, as illustrated by Thietmar's account of the pirate attacks of 994 and capture of hostages.[50] If a person had a terrible accident or disease that left them scarred, the knowledge of that event would spread and then remain in the memory of her/his family, friends and neighbors, and whilst the victim remained in the locality, that knowledge might have formed a protection of sorts.[51] The recorded use of nicknames indicating disability or facial difference, whilst apparently highlighting a person's misfortune, might actually indicate that they were still accepted as part of the community.[52] Conversely, mutilation inflicted as a penalty, or suffering mutilation at the hands of the enemy in a military defeat, would also be remembered, and whether the victim's social interactions continued in the same vein as before would depend very much upon the opinion of the community regarding their crime or the damage to their honor inflicted by defeat.[53] This was contingent upon the circumstances in which the disfigurement was acquired, and a further distinction affecting the reception of the injury might have been whether it was accidental or deliberate. Our sources, however, are almost entirely concerned with the latter, and in some cases the disfigurement (or threat of disfigurement) follows on from illegitimate acts, that is, the person has already jeopardized their communal ties by their behavior, whether treasonous, criminal or adulterous. We have already met, and will continue to meet, guilty men and women who were disfigured and either paraded as a lesson to others *or* shut away and deprived of their normal social interactions. Here, the disfigurement simply marks that person out, and links the stigma to the assumed deviance of the person concerned.

Even rare cases of reports of "accidental" facial injury turn out to be loaded with significance for future social interactions. An apparently trivial aside in the Anglo-Saxon "Fonthill Letter" turns out to be anything but. The subject of the letter, dated between 899 and 924, is Helmstan, whose repeated thefts of property caused confiscations of land to which he does not appear to have had full title. The author of the letter is essentially defending his own right to the estates at issue. In passing, however, the writer recounts that Helmstan had stolen some oxen and driven them to Cricklade where he was apprehended by a man who recognized the cattle. "When he fled, *a bramble scratched him in the face and when he wished to deny it, that was brought as evidence against him* [my emphasis]."[54] Without suggesting that Helmstan was seriously or permanently disfigured by the bramble scratches, they were clearly sufficiently visible and serious to function as proof of his flight; moreover, in marking him out as a thief they had generated a memory of his actions that was now being rehearsed again and committed to writing even after his face had—presumably—healed up. Helmstan may or may not have been scarred or disfigured by the theft, but his reputation surely was.

As a thief, Helmstan was fortunate to escape further physical punishment. Other crimes, such as treason, attracted more severe penalties: the would-be assassins of King Childebert II of Francia, as we have seen, were deprived of their ears and noses then "let out as a subject of ridicule," according to Gregory of Tours.[55] Wheatley comments that blinded criminals "would have been shunned as long as they remained in locations where their criminal past was known."[56] This brings to mind the comment of sociologists Mark Stafford and Richard Scott, who point out that the process of stigma depends very much on the "power weight" of the person stigmatizing:[57] these mutilations—and their permanent, exclusionary effect on the victims' lives—were legitimized by the fact that they were inflicted by royal or religious authorities. As we have seen in Chapter 3, however, such acts could only be justified, in our authors' accounts, in very specific circumstances. Inflicting such injuries without the authority to do so was a sign of another type of social disruption.

## Aesthetics: Is the Condition Viewed as Repellent or Ugly?

This question raises interesting issues as to what was considered beautiful or ugly in the early Middle Ages. As Umberto Eco has pointed out, beauty can be contemplated dispassionately, the perfection of form being appreciated but not necessarily desired. Ugliness, by contrast, frequently evokes an emotive response, and this might be one of disgust, if the ugliness was caused by a severe disfigurement. We have already met William Ian Miller's framing of the disgust response, but the notion of "disgust" is still also employed in modern studies of disfigurement perception.[58] Given that early medieval artists were not concerned to produce a faithful depiction of facial features (as will be explored in Chapter 6), we are reliant on medieval authors describing beauty for us, rather than visual evidence. Texts were no less generic, of course, but they do reveal for us something of the ideals of physical appearance. Anna Komnena, for example, reflects on the Norman leader Robert Guiscard's ruddy complexion, fair hair and broad shoulders, further noting that "In a well-built man, one looks for breadth here and slimness there; in him all was admirably well-proportioned and elegant."[59] Anna also provides a description of her mother as a young woman: "her body absolutely symmetrical...her face... slightly oval in shape. There were rose blossoms in her cheeks...Her light blue eyes were both gay and stern... For the most part her lips were closed and when thus silent she resembled a veritable statue of Beauty, a breathing monument of Harmony."[60] In Anna, proportion and symmetry are at the heart of her ideals, reflecting her classical education, and as we have seen, symmetry lies at the heart of human cognitive processing of faces.[61] Abbot Guibert of Nogent (d. 1121) also presents us with an idealized portrait of his own mother's beauty, but uses it to reflect on moral quality: however fleeting physical beauty might be, he opines, it symbolizes goodness. Yet it could only fulfill that function when allied with chastity, as in his mother's case.

The destruction of beauty, then, could be read as a sign of moral failure—Guibert suggests that "a blemished exterior is rightly a matter for sorrow."[62] As we have seen, several sets of laws threatened women (and some men, in the Byzantine laws) who committed sexual misdemeanors such as adultery, prostitution or pimping, with the loss or mutilation of their noses.[63] Mutilation prevailed in the laws of mid-thirteenth-century Cyprus, themselves based on earlier provisions in the Kingdom of Jerusalem (and not only for sexual transgression), but in the absence of earlier evidence it is unclear whether such penalties arrived with the crusaders.[64] Furthermore, just as the laws threatened mutilation after the sexual acts (and implied in doing so that the offenders would be rendered repellent to future sexual partners), so hagiographers presented self-disfigurement as an effective deterrent (for female saints, at least) to unwanted sexual attention. Thus the ninth-century abbess Ebba of Coldingham and her nuns are famously reported as self-mutilating in order to avoid rape by Viking attackers in England.[65] The self-humiliation that such a mutilation would cause was taken up by hagiographers of the twelfth and thirteenth centuries, who revived this early medieval motif in the *vitae* of three holy women, Oda of Brabant (d. 1158), who succeeded in cutting her nose; St Margaret of Hungary (d. 1270), who threatened to do so in order to avoid unwanted marriage, but also as a deterrent to the invading Mongols—an echo of the earlier example of fear of rape by pagans—and St Margaret of Cortona (d.1297), whose regret at her earlier life of promiscuity included a plea to be allowed to destroy her (notably) beautiful face, a request turned down by her confessor.[66] What is striking here is the fact that whilst the holy women all *wanted* to self-mutilate, only one (Oda) succeeded, and she was never in fact canonized, suggesting at least some ambivalence regarding her "heroic" gesture. In essence, by taking matters into her own hands she stigmatized herself in the eyes of a Church that valued and promoted obedience and abhorred the shedding of blood.[67]

Extreme examples of ugliness in fictional works can also offer further insight into ideals of good looks. Salimbene's tale of brother Aldevrandus, mentioned earlier, simply repeats tropes found in other tales of hirsute people, such as those in early Irish myths. These often combine disfigurement with other conditions to describe unfortunate individuals, but their descriptions seem to verge on the non-human in their bestial qualities: "if his snout were thrown against a branch it would stick there... if her snout were thrown against a branch, the branch would support it, while her lower lip extended to her knee."[68] The fantasy of facial change is also embedded in stories such as Marie de France's *Bisclavret*: the treacherous wife, deprived of her nose by her angry, werewolf husband, subsequently gives birth to similarly disfigured, noseless daughters, a permanent reminder of her betrayal.[69] Guibert of Nogent, too, equates ugliness with evil in his portrayal of Thiégaud, servant of Enguerrand of Coucy, responsible for collecting bridge tolls. Abusing this position, Thiégaud would rob and even murder travellers: "the unrestrained wickedness of his heart," Guibert comments, "was displayed in his hideous face."[70]

## ORIGIN: CAN THE STIGMATIZING CONDITION BE BLAMED ON THE PERSON HIMSELF OR HERSELF?

This element of the discussion engages with one of the enduring tensions surrounding medieval disease and impairment, whether it was attributable to some flaw of character or behavior in the person her/himself (thus interpreted as a punishment of sorts), or whether external forces working through the body's humors resulted in the condition. Acquired disfigurement falls between these two stools, in that it was usually the work of a third party rather than God, yet could sometimes be attributed to the behavior of the person disfigured (Bisclavret's wife's daughters carried the sign of their mother's transgression, for example.) Helmstan's guilt, as we have seen, was writ large in the bramble scratches on his face. As Sander Gilman comments, sight has the power to create a moral indictment.[71] The framework of assigning blame for disfigurement has of course a particularly rich applicability for analyzing medieval texts, since many of the stories considered so far were clearly included to impart moral lessons to the reader. In some instances, the same incident was recorded by different authors, such as the pirate attacks in Thietmar and Adam of Bremen, but opinions might vary as to what the reader was supposed to conclude from the inclusion of such stories.

A case in point is the tale of Young Charles, the son of the Carolingian Emperor Charles the Bald, severely wounded in the face with a sword during a bout of play-fighting. The Annals of St Bertin record for the year 864:

> Young Charles ... while he only meant to enjoy some horseplay with other young men of his own age ... by the work of the devil was struck in the head with a sword by a youth named Albuin. The blow penetrated almost as far as the brain, reaching from his left temple to his right cheekbone and jaw...[72]

Here, the major injury Charles received was presented as accidental—there was no hint in the source that his assailant intended to injure him (and thus no reference in the annals to compensation by, or punishment of, Albuin being demanded). Following from this, secondly, Charles appears not to have been dishonored by his injury—in fact, continued in the honorable position as sub-king of Aquitaine for the two remaining years of his life. The annals do report, however, that he suffered epileptic fits thereafter, and it is doubtful whether he escaped other impairments given the severity of the injury.[73] Yet the chroniclers disagreed on the circumstances of the injury: whilst the St Bertin annals present it as accidental and remain silent on the issue of honor, Ado of Vienne (d. 870) reports that Charles was *"molestatus et dehonestatus"* by his injury.[74] Moreover, Regino of Prum (d. 915) tells a rather different story of the incident, saying that Charles provoked Albuin's attack "out of the levity of youth" and that his assailant struck him on the head with his sword, leaving him half-dead with a "deformed face [*vultu deformatus*]."[75] For Regino, therefore, the disfigurement was Charles's own fault, a condition that his irresponsible behavior had brought upon himself.

Thietmar also recounts an example hinting at moral opprobrium: his nephew Henry's blinding of a soldier. As we have seen, the soldier is described as "distinguished but over proud (*egregium set nimis superbum*)." Moreover, Henry is also described as having suffered (unspecified) injuries which, as we now know, might have consisted of either physical or verbal abuse. Despite the fact that Henry was exiled for his extreme response, Thietmar is careful to point out that he and the king were soon reconciled. It is hard to avoid the conclusion that he is doing everything he can to suggest to the reader that, in some way, the unnamed soldier was partly responsible for his own fate through his pride and his provocation, and Henry's guilt is further ameliorated by Thietmar's addition that his exile ended and he was eventually reconciled with the king.[76] A detail in Peter of Eboli's account of Richard of Acerra also hints that the count's non-fatal but marking arrow injury was his own fault, for climbing up to the walls of Naples he "makes a mockery of men whose skill lay in the bow" below and gets his just reward: "The arrow flashed as it shot through the middle of his cheek."[77]

## PERIL: DOES THE STIGMA REPRESENT DANGER TO OTHER INDIVIDUALS OR THE COMMUNITY?

Facial deformity might be taken as a signal of disease, specifically referring to leprosy, but the isolation of lepers does not appear to have been as straightforwardly stigmatizing as might be assumed. Disfigurement, arguably, did not in and of itself represent peril to the community, but if the message of mutilated noses and ears was of criminality and deviance, then a person might find himself or herself treated as a threat. Still more worrying would be the arrival of the disfigured stranger in a town or village community, but their unfamiliarity, rather than their facial difference, would mark them out straightaway.[78] It is hard, therefore, to see facial disfigurement as an actual sign of "peril" in medieval society. Moreover, on occasion facial modification is presented as an (ill-conceived) attempt at self-protection: Theophanes reports the story of a group of Turks, captured and sent to Constantinople in 588/9, who had "the symbol of the cross tattooed [literally 'embroidered' in black (τον τύπον του σταυρού δια μέλανος κεντητου]" on their foreheads. When asked why they had this sign, they responded that they had been advised by Christians to get the tattoos to protect themselves from plague.[79]

Yet, discussions of stigma often include the notion of taboo: the stigmatized individual carrying with them so much ill fortune that their fate can have wider repercussions. One specific society, early Ireland, seems to have had a much stronger sense of the potential threat posed by a damaged face, especially if it was the face of a leader. Fergus Kelly points out that the *lóg n'enech* or honor price in Irish laws (a concept mirrored in most early medieval lawcodes—*wergild* in England and on the continent, *sarhaed* and *wynebwerth* in Wales—to express the status of the person and the compensation to be paid in the event of injuring or killing them) had the literal meaning of the "price of her/his face." An Irish king's body, however, needed to be perfect—any mutilation or injury was a taboo or *geis*, requiring his removal from power and threatening the well-being of the community if he stayed. Kelly cites the case of Congal Cáech, ruler of Ulster and Tara, who was blinded in one eye by a bee sting and who was thus "put from the kingship of Tara" (though not Ulster, which he ruled until 637—such is the fluidity of taboos).[80]

## Messages in a Marked Face

It has proven a useful exercise to combine six modern categories of stigma with the evidence of medieval texts, but this rather skirts round the original question as to whether the medieval disfigured were stigmatized in their communities. So let us return to one of those categories, disruptiveness, and expand a little more on whether disfigurement damaged or broke an individual's ties with her or his community. A well-known law of King Cnut seems to suggest, in fact, that disfigurement might be the *expression* of social marginalization. In clause 30 of his secular laws it is stated:

30. And if any man is so regarded with suspicion by the hundred and so frequently accused, and three men together then accuse him, there is then to be nothing for it but that he is to go to the three-fold ordeal...
30.3b And if he is then convicted, on the first occasion he is to pay two-fold compensation...
30.4 And on the second occasion there is to be no other compensation...but that his hands, or feet, or both, in proportion to the deed, are to be cut off.
30.5 And if, however, he has committed still further crimes, his eyes are to be put out and his nose and ears and upper lip cut off, or his scalp removed, whichever of these is then decreed by those with whom the decision rests; thus one can punish *and at the same time preserve the soul* [my emphasis].[81]

Now whilst this series of increasingly severe penalties relies upon serious recidivism to reach the stage of selective or wholesale disfigurement (slaves, it might be noted, were branded on their first offence), nevertheless the path toward becoming disfigured starts here with the man being "regarded with suspicion."[82] So again we see reputation as a key element—and disfigurement as the sign that there had been a real social breakdown. Although the king was keen to "preserve the soul," death might well have been preferable to the punishment meted out here.

Another key question is how to quantify disfigured people: were maimed and damaged faces so commonplace as to resist stigmatization? In fact, reports of disfigurement in narrative sources, whilst surprisingly frequent, seem to counter Le Goff's view, emphasizing more often than not the exceptionality, and often the *illegitimacy* of facial mutilation. They also share a generic language to express this. In many examples, in fact, extending from the reports of Gregory of Tours to Orderic Vitalis's portrayals of Robert of Bellême and William Talvas,[83] to the chronicles of thirteenth-century conflicts, facial disfigurement functions as an act of retaliation or extreme anger (*furor*), and is used to indict the lack of control (*demens*, literally madness) or cruelty on the part of the person mutilating.[84] A classic example is Amatus of Montecassino's extended description of Prince Gisulf II of Salerno's cruelty to his Amalfitan hostages in the eleventh century: "Besides being deprived of a limb, or sometimes half a limb, they lost an eye, a hand or a foot. If someone could not ransom himself, they would gouge out both his eyes."[85] Slightly later, Emperor Frederick II's treatment of Genoese archers, "manu et oculo mutilati" after his capture of Milan in 1245, would just be another atrocity of war, had not the report by Bartholomew *Scriba* also included the detail that the mutilated men received a pension when they returned to their home city.[86] This underlines the contingency of mutilation and disfigurement: to Frederick, the Genoese were traitors, but to their co-citizens (and Bartholomew) they were heroes, worthy of economic support now that they were deprived of their livelihood. As in so many cases, however, this report is exceptional: it does not permit us to claim that all war-wounded men were treated with such sympathy and practical help.

Taken together with the numerous and extraordinarily detailed clauses in almost every early medieval lawcode condemning injuries to head, face and body parts (see Chapter 3 and Appendix 2), such reports caution against the assumption that a person with a disfiguring injury would automatically be stigmatized, still less evoke disgust in the viewer. It does seem, however, that individuals with acquired disfigurements had to have a special story in order to be recorded in narrative and other sources—the account of Helmstan's scratched face is a case in point. Whether these exceptional cases prove Le Goff's point about the ubiquity of disfigurement and disease among the larger population is a moot point. It is also worth noting that those whose stories were recorded in the chronicle evidence cited in this chapter were exclusively drawn from the social elite. Arguably, these men (I will revisit the women in Chapter 5, when the gendering of disfigurement will be explored in greater detail) were secure enough in their status to be able to override any doubts about the facial damage they suffered or were willing to suffer. We cannot discount the possibility that the writing-up of their cases was itself a carefully managed operation—it is striking that later accounts of Young Charles's injury, for example, take a progressively less sympathetic line.[87]

At the same time, the strong sense that the earthly body was less important than inner cleanliness, expressed by Thietmar, seems to have given license to reporters to explore facial disfigurement in more imaginative ways. Such a case is the extended treatment, in Orderic Vitalis's *Ecclesiastical History*, of Walchelin the priest's vision of the walking dead, including being attacked and dragged along the ground by an evil knight with burning hands. Fifteen years later, he recounted his tale to Orderic, who believed his informant on the basis that "I saw the scar on his face caused by the touch of the terrible knight."[88] Clearly Walchelin had a visibly-scarred face, possibly from a rather more mundane accident with fire, but his story, it seems, was designed to deflect the attention of viewers, providing a supernatural explanation worthy of recording and gaining him belated attention. If Walchelin was able to turn his scar into something positive, it is striking too that whilst political maiming, as seen in the case of Justinian II, was intended to disbar him from rule, he was able to overcome his stigmatizing condition through sheer determination and the acquisition of allies from outside the court (if not, more's the pity, through sporting a matching set of gold nose and ears).

Returning then to the questions with which this chapter opened, it does not appear that early medieval authors automatically wrote stigma into their accounts of people with disfigurements. Class does seem to have been a major factor both in the generation of records and in how they were viewed. The damaged faces of the elite might provoke questions, and on occasion were attributed negatively to the fault of the disfigured person. The early medieval laws attributed more compensation to the well-born victim of disfigurement than the peasant or the unfree, recognizing that shame—or, to use the sources' own term, ridicule—might result from attending public events with a mutilated face. Much more frequently, however, disfigurement as a result of interpersonal violence indicted the *perpetrator* in the narrative texts, rather than the victim: if disgust was present as a response to the victim, it is not manifested in the written accounts, and this absence is telling. And whilst there might have been a clear, biblical framework for assessing the parameters of acceptable violence, there is no clear or uniform scheme framing reports of disfigurement. An exception to this statement may have been a heightened awareness, among clerical writers, of the Levitical disbarring of priests with deformities, but this does not, as a rule, seem to have prevented such men from serving the Church, if Thietmar's text or Orderic's story of Walchelin are any indication. Indeed, it is possible to suggest, in light of several of the stories discussed in this and the previous chapter, that the Christian values underpinning most of our authors' accounts provided *space* for those with disfigurements, albeit space conditioned by pity for the victim's condition, or the opportunity to draw moral lessons from that condition or the behavior of the person who had inflicted their terrible injuries. Pope Leo's shining scar, discussed above, bore witness to the miracle of his sight being returned to him, Wipert turned the adversity of his blinding to a triumph of patient humility and a tool for others' salvation, and Walchelin won an ally in Orderic by presenting his burns in the entirely orthodox language of a vision. Unfortunately, Thietmar does not elaborate on why Duke Henry of Bavaria ordered the blinding of the archbishop of Salzburg and the castration of the patriarch of Aquileia (note again the contiguity of the two mutilations), simply branding this act "impious," but his resultant land grab for his vassals provides us with a clue.[89]

Disfigurement in and of itself was not sufficient to generate a written record, however, nor did it alone generate social marginalization. The Irish evidence highlights the other main issue raised at the start of the chapter: whether geographical region conditioned written or recorded responses to disfigured people. It does appear there was some distinction between different parts of Europe. It has been suggested that Old Norse society valued, rather than abhorred, the battle-scarred face; Celtic societies, on the other hand, seem to have had a heightened sensitivity to facial difference, and linked honor linguistically to the face and nose, as evidenced by Welsh and Irish laws, and myths from the latter region. Between these two poles lay the vast majority of cases, whose presentation and interpretation in written narratives was heavily contingent upon the circumstances of the acquisition of the disfigurement, and do not offer a universalizing, stigmatized view of disfigured people.

## NOTES

1. J. Le Goff, *Medieval Civilization, 400–1500*, tr. J. Barrow (Oxford: Blackwell, 1988), 240.
2. An idea made popular by Henri Tajfel: see his "Intergroup relations, social myths and social justice in social psychology," in *The Social Dimension*, ed. H. Tajfel, II (Cambridge: Cambridge University Press, 1984), 695–716.
3. Starting with J. M. Wallace-Hadrill's work on the Franks, *The Long-Haired Kings and other Studies on Frankish History* (New York: Barnes and Noble, 1962), utilizing classic anthropological studies such as Marcel Mauss, *The Gift: the Form and Reason for Exchange in Archaic Societies* (London: Cohen and West, 1954) and Max Gluckmann, "The peace in the feud," *Past and Present*, 8 (1955): 1–14; *The Settlement of Disputes in Early Medieval Europe*, ed. Wendy Davies and Paul Fouracre (Cambridge: Cambridge University Press, 1986); *Property and Power in the Early Middle Ages*, ed. Wendy Davies and Paul Fouracre (Cambridge: Cambridge University Press, 1995); *The Languages of Gift in the Early Middle Ages*, ed. Wendy Davies and Paul Fouracre (Cambridge: Cambridge University Press, 2014).
4. E.g. Bronislaw Geremek, *The Margins of Society in Late Medieval Paris* (Cambridge: Cambridge University Press, 1987); Michael Goodich, *Other Middle Ages: Witnesses at the Margins of Medieval Society* (Philadelphia: University of Pennsylvania Press, 1998); *Monks and Nuns, Saints and Outcasts*, ed. Lester K. Little, Sharon H. Farmer and Barbara H. Rosenwein (Ithaca, NY: Cornell University Press, 2000); Andrew McCall, *The Medieval Underworld* (Stroud: Sutton, 2004).
5. R. I. Moore, *The Formation of a Persecuting Society* (Oxford: Blackwell, 1987, 2nd ed. 2007).
6. Edward Wheatley, *Stumbling Blocks before the Blind: Medieval Constructions of a Disability* (Ann Arbor: University of Michigan Press, 2010).

7. *Thietmar*, VIII.22: *Namque homines sex flagellati ac depilati cum edificiis turpiter mutilatis approbant, qualiter tanti seniores ab aliis precaveri debeant.* Note the use of "shamefully" here.

8. Puisserguier: *The History of the Albigensian Crusade: Peter of Les-Vaux-de-Cernay's Historia Albigensis*, tr. W. A. Sibly and M. D. Sibly (Woodbridge: Boydell, 1998), I.142. I am grateful to Daniel Power for reminding me of this notorious case, on which see also Megan Cassidy-Welch, "Images of blood in the *Historia Albigensis* of Peter des Vaux-de-Cernay," *Journal of Religious History*, 35 (2011): 478–491, especially 487. Karen Sullivan, "The good, the bad and the beautiful: violence in the *Canso de la Crozada*," in *Violence and the Writing of History in the Medieval Francophone World*, ed. Noah D. Guynn and Zrinka Stahuljak (Cambridge: D. S. Brewer, 2013), 99–114; *Rogeri de Wendover, Chronica*, ed. H. Coxe (London: Sumptis Societatis, 1842), IV.170: *sic turpiter mutilatos ad propria remittens deforme spectaculum Francigenis...*

9. Patricia Skinner, "Visible prowess? Reading men's head and face wounds in early medieval Europe to 1000CE," in *Wounds and Wound Repair in Medieval Culture*, ed. Larissa Tracy and Kelly de Vries (Leiden: Brill, 2015), 81–101. The ambiguity of attitudes toward disfigurement in the saga literature is explored by Lois Bragg, "Disfigurement, disability and dis-integration in *Sturlunga saga*," *alvíssimál*, 4 (1994[1995]): 15–32.

10. *Thietmar*, IV.75 (51): *...videbis in me parvum homuncionem, maxillum deformem leva et latere eodem, quia hinc olim erupit semper turgescens fistula. Nasus in puericia fractus de me ridiculum facit. Idque totum nil questus essem, si interius aliquid splendescerem.* English translation in *Ottonian Germany: the* Chronicon *of Thietmar of Merseburg*, tr. David A. Warner (Manchester: Manchester University Press, 2001), 203–4.

11. *Self and Society in Medieval France: The Memoirs of Abbot Guibert of Nogent*, ed. and tr. John Benton (New York: Harper and Row, 1970), I.2, 39.

12. Cited in Paul Beekman Taylor, "Wounds, wit and words," in *Fleshly Things and Spiritual Matters: Studies on the Medieval Body in Honour of Margaret Bridges*, ed. Nicole Nyffenegger and Katrin Rupp (Newcastle: Cambridge Scholars Press, 2011), 125–139, at 126.

13. *Self and Society*, I.19, 100.

14. *Ex illo tempore pro Deo peregrinando circuivi plurimas provincias, invocans sanctos sanctasque in christianorum auxilia...Omnium christianorum in karitate Dei deposco auxilium, quod mee vite fiat patrocinium, vestrorum peccatorum eternum remedium*: Wipert's account is reproduced in the preliminary matter to the *Vita S. Adalberti Episcopi*, in *MGH SS*, IV, ed. G. H. Pertz (Hannover: Hahn, 1841), 579–580.

15. *Habebat enim caput deforme et factum ad modum gálee antiquorum, et pilos multos in fronte*: *Chronica Fratris Salimbene Ordinis Minorum. Liber de Praelatio*, ed. O. Holder-Egger, in *MGH SS*, XXXII, ed. G. H. Pertz (Hannover: Hahn, 1913), 137.

16. William Ian Miller, *The Anatomy of Disgust* (Cambridge, MA: Harvard University Press, 1997), 54.

17. Erving Goffman, *Stigma: Notes on the Management of Spoiled Identity* (Englewood Cliffs, NJ: Prentice-Hall/London: Penguin, 1963). See also James Partridge, *Changing Faces* (London: Penguin, 1990). Partridge, the survivor of major burns in a car crash, notes how reading Goffman helped him to rationalize his own situation.

18. Julia Kristeva, *Powers of Horror: an Essay on Abjection*, tr. Leon S. Roudiez (New York: Columbia University Press, 1982), 53. Cf. Miller, *Anatomy* and Chap. 2, above, on the skin as a container.

19. *Ipse turbabatur et erubescebat*: the imperfect tense here indicates that Aldevrandus's distress was repeated or continuous: *Chronica Fratris Salimbene Ordinis Minorum*, 137.

20. E.g. William Ian Miller, *Bloodtaking and Peacemaking: Feud, Law and Society in Early Saga Iceland* (Chicago: Chicago University Press, 1990), 4–5, comments that "the saga writers of the thirteenth century anticipated the perspicacity of Erving Goffman" in their presentation and analysis of social interactions. Criticism: "Introduction: stigma reconsidered," in *The Dilemma of Difference: a Multidisciplinary View of Stigma*, ed. Stephen C. Ainlay, Gaylene Becker and Lerita M. Coleman (New York and London: Plenum Press, 1986), 1–13, at 8.

21. Goffman, *Stigma*, 12.

22. Colin Barnes, *"Cabbage Syndrome": the Social Construction of Dependence* (London/New York: The Falmer Press, 1990), 8–9.

23. *Ibid.*, 18–19. Irina Metzler, *A Social History of Disability in the Middle Ages: Cultural Considerations of Physical Impairment*

(London/New York: Routledge, 2013), 174, makes much the same point – provision for the medieval poor and sick did not encompass caring for the impaired if they were capable of working or begging.

24. Sally Crawford and Christina Lee, "Introduction," in *Bodies of Knowledge: Cultural Interpretations of Illness and Medicine in Medieval Europe*, ed. S. Crawford and C. Lee (Studies in Early Medicine 1/BAR International Series 2170, Oxford: Archaeopress, 2010), 2.

25. E. E. Jones, A. Farina, A. Hastorf, H. Markus, D. Miller and R. A. Scott, *Social Stigma: the Psychology of Marked Relationships* (New York: Freeman, 1984).

26. S. Shoham, *The Mark of Cain: the Stigma Theory of Crime and Social Deviation* (Jerusalem: Israel Universities Press, 1970), 1. Shoham thus summarily dismissed the physically-different from his subsequent discussion of stigma.

27. "...almost all persons who are in a position to pass will do so on some occasion by intent": Goffman, *Stigma*, 95; Sander Gilman, *Making the Body Beautiful: a Cultural History of Aesthetic Surgery* (Princeton/Oxford: Princeton University Press, 1999), 22.

28. See above, Chap. 3.

29. Luke Demaitre, *pers. comm.* July 2015, notes however that hats and hoods remain the exception in the sample of 25 or so pre-1200 depictions of lepers he has found. He is currently preparing a study on medieval disease and disfigurement.

30. *Cuius vulneris cicatrix quamdiu vixit apparuit*: *Chronicon Laetiense*, c.12, ed. I. Heller, in *MGH SS*, XIV, ed. G. H. Pertz (Hannover: Hahn, 1883), 500.

31. Gerald of Wales, *The Journey Through Wales*, II.7, tr. L. Thorpe (London: Penguin, 1978), 190–1. Gerald adds that he himself had seen the same scar on Erchembald's son Stephen.

32. *GT*, V.48.

33. Cf. the case of Conrad vs. Henry discussed above.

34. *The Chronicle of Theophanes Confessor: Byzantine and Near Eastern History, AD284–813*, ed. and tr. C. Mango and R. Scott with the assistance of R. Greatrex (Oxford: Clarendon Press, 1997), AM5972 (479/80CE). Greek: ιαθείς δε την πληγήν εφόρει καμελαυκιον. και ητήσατο τον βασιλέα επί την ανατολήν απελθεῖν δια τὸ τους αερας αλλάξαι, ότι ηοθένει εκ τηξ πληγής: *Theophanis*

*Chronographia*, ed. C. de Boor, 2 vols (Hildesheim: Georg Olms, 1963), I, 128.

35. *Thietmar*, II.27: *...et fuit eiusdem mutilatio non ad dedecus, sed ad honorem magis*; translated in *Ottonian Germany*, 112.

36. Levitical ban: Ruth Mellinkoff, *Outcasts: Signs of Otherness in Northern European Art of the Late Middle Ages*, 2 vols (Berkeley: University of California Press, 1993), I, 113–114; Irina Metzler, *Disability in Medieval Europe* (London: Routledge, 2006), 40.

37. *Chronicle of Theophanes*, AM5817 (324/5CE), 42; *Theophanis*, ed. De Boor, 27.

38. A knight "struck the pope's assailant more powerfully and fatally than Peter struck Malchus": *Orderic*, X.1 (V, 196–7).

39. *Bretha Déin Chécht*, clause 31, cited in Fergus Kelly, *A Guide to Early Irish Law* (Dublin: Dublin Institute of Advanced Studies, 1988), 132.

40. *The Laws of Hywel Dda (The Book of Blegywryd)*, tr. Melville Richards (Liverpool: Liverpool University Press, 1954), 65.

41. Piers Mitchell, *Medicine in the Crusades: Warfare, Wounds and the Medieval Surgeon* (Cambridge: Cambridge University Press, 2004); *id.*, Y. Nagar and R. Ellenbaum, "Weapon injuries in the twelfth century crusader garrison of Vadum Iacob castle, Galilee," *International Journal of Osteoarchaeology*, 16.2 (2006): 145–155.

42. J. Prag and R. Neave, *Making Faces: Using Forensic and Archaeological Evidence* (London: British Museum Press, 1997). Images of the two effigies, kindly provided by Professor Prag and courtesy of the museum, can be viewed on my project blog: http://medievaldisfigurement.wordpress.com

43. Cf. Gerald of Wales' somewhat hazardous reports of Hugh, Earl of Shrewsbury ("the arrow struck his right eye and penetrated his brain"), who died, and Harold, king of the English, who allegedly survived ("wounded in many places, losing his left eye through an arrow which penetrated it but, although beaten, he escaped to these parts"): *The Journey Through Wales*, II.7 and 11, tr. L. Thorpe (London: Penguin, 1978), 188 and 198–9 respectively. And see below, Chap. 7.

44. *Liber ad Honorem Augusti di Pietro da Eboli*, XV, ed. G. B. Siragusa (Rome: Istituto Storico Italiano, 1906), 34. On the limited possibilities of surgery in early medieval Italy, see Clare Pilsworth,

*Healthcare in Early Medieval Northern Italy* (Turnhout: Brepols, 2014), 104–111.

45. The present study went to press just as *Wounds and Wound Repair*, ed. DeVries and Tracy, was published. The collected essays in this volume represent a significant leap forward in the study of wound care, including that of injuries received on the battlefield.

46. Above, Chap. 3. Agnellus is our only source for this: Joaquín Martinez Pizarro, *Writing Ravenna: The* Liber Pontificalis *of Andrea Agnellus* (Ann Arbor: University of Michigan Press, 1995), 183.

47. Pers. comm. Dr Mark Bradley, 4 March 2014. Compare the gold nose commissioned by Emperor Otto III for the slightly crumbling corpse of Charlemagne when the latter's tomb was opened in the year 1000: *Chronicon Novaliciense*, III.32, ed. G. H. Pertz, *MGH SS rer. Germ.*, XXI (Hannover: Hahn, 1846), 55. This, too, has misled subsequent scholars into thinking that it was *Otto* who wore it: Julie Singer, *Blindness and Therapy in Late Medieval French and Italian Poetry* (Woodbridge: Boydell and Brewer, 2011), 149. See also Antony Eastmond, "Between icon and idol: the uncertainty of imperial images," in *Icon and Word: the Power of Images in Byzantium*, ed. A. Eastmond and L. James (Aldershot: Ashgate, 2005), 73–85.

48. Metzler, *Disability in Medieval Europe*, 31.

49. On the power of gossip and reputation, Ronald S. Burt, *Brokerage and Closure: an Introduction to Social Capital* (Oxford: Oxford University Press, 2005), and on words as violent acts, William Ian Miller, *Humiliation and Other Essays on Honor, Social Discomfort and Violence* (Ithaca/London: Cornell University Press, 1998), 83. On the middle ages specifically: Susan E. Phillips, *Transforming Talk: the Problem with Gossip in Late Medieval England* (University Park: Penn State University Press, 2007); *Fama: the Politics of Talk and Reputation in Medieval Europe*, ed. Thelma Fenster and Daniel Lord Smail (Ithaca, NY: Cornell University Press, 2003); Chris Wickham, "Gossip and resistance among the medieval peasantry," *Past and Present*, 160 (1998): 3–24.

50. Above, Chap. 1.

51. As modern examples illustrate, however, the level of stigmatization experienced by an individual might increase sharply if they moved to an area where the circumstances of their disfigurement were unknown: Gaylene Becker and Regina Arnold, "Stigma as a social

and cultural construct," in *Dilemma of Difference*, ed. Ainlay, Becker and Coleman, 39–57, at 49, highlight the case of a disfigured World War II freedom fighter's experiences when moving from Europe to the United States.

52. See the discussion in Stephen Wilson, *The Means of Naming: a Social History* (London: UCL Press, 1998), especially 118–123 and 280–289. Nicknames referring to appearance are noted by Bragg, "Disfigurement, disability and dis-integration," and by Metzler, *A Social History of Disability*, 37; Patricia Skinner, "'And her name was?' Gender and naming in medieval southern Italy," *Medieval Prosopography*, 20 (1999), 23–49. Gerald of Wales, *Journey through Wales*, II.8, mentions Iorwerth Drwyndwn "which is the Welsh for Fat-Nosed"; in fact the term suggests a nose that is broken, and thus appears wider.

53. On this issue: Skinner, "Visible prowess?"

54. Mechthild Gretsch, "The language of the 'Fonthill letter'," *Anglo-Saxon England*, 23 (1994): 57–102, at 99: *Ða he fleah, ða torypte hine an breber ofer ðæt nebb; ða he ætsacan wolde, ða sæde him mon ðæt to tacne*. English translation cited from *ibid.*, 101. I am grateful to Charles Insley for introducing me to this fascinating text.

55. *GT*, VIII.29 (c. 585 CE) (393) and X.18 (509: "ad ridiculum laxaverunt").

56. Wheatley, *Stumbling Blocks*, 21.

57. Mark C. Stafford and Richard R. Scott, "Stigma, deviance and social control: some conceptual issues," in *Dilemma of Difference*, ed. Ainlay, Becker and Coleman, 77–91, at 86. Stafford and Scott comment that at the time of writing this dynamic of power had not been fully explored within stigma studies.

58. Umberto Eco, *On Beauty*, tr. A. McEwan (London: Secker and Warburg, 2004), 8; U. Eco, *On Ugliness* (London: Harvill Secker, 2007), 19.

59. *Alexiad*, I.x. All English quotations from *The Alexiad of Anna Comnena*, tr. E. R. A. Sewter (London: Penguin, 1969).

60. *Alexiad*, III.iii.

61. For the most part, however, according to Eco, "medieval man did not apply a mathematics of proportions to the appraisal or reproduction of the human body": *On Beauty*, 77.

62. *Self and Society*, I.2, 38 (mother) and 40 (quote).

63. For a full discussion see Skinner, "Gendered nose and its lack."

64. In Codex 1 of *The Assizes of the Lusignan Kingdom of Cyprus*, tr. Nicholas Coureas (Nicosia: Cyprus Research Centre, 2002), corporal punishments include cutting the tongue of a slave who dares to summon his master to court (I.16), or someone who wrongly challenges a judgment in court and cannot pay compensation (I.253); loss of a hand for an assault leaving an open wound, including to the head (I.118 and 254) and for forging documents (I.273); loss of the penis for ravishing a virgin if no settlement can be reached (I.127); and branding on the palms of the hands of a person offering testimony for gain (I.131). In addition, a first-time thief could be beaten, paraded publicly and branded (the clause does not specify where: I.281). Specific mutilation of the *face*, however, does not figure in this collection.

65. The relevant report is reproduced and discussed in Philip Pulsiano, "Blessed bodies: the *vitae* of Anglo-Saxon female saints," *Parergon* 16.2 (1999): 1–42.

66. *Acta Sanctorum*, vol. XI, 20 April, *Vita Ven. Oda Praemonstratensis*; *Acta Sanctorum*, vol III, 28 January, *B. Margaritae Hungariae Virginis*; *Acta Sanctorum*, vol. VI, 22 February, *De B. Margarita Poenit. Tertii Ord. S. Francisci Cortonae in Etruria* respectively.

67. For a fuller discussion of these three saints, see Patricia Skinner, "Marking the face, curing the soul? Reading the disfigurement of women in the later middle ages," in *Medicine, Religion and Gender in Medieval Culture*, ed. Naoë Kukita Yoshikawa (Woodbridge: Boydell, 2015), 287–318.

68. *The Destruction of Da Derga's Hostel*, in *Early Irish Myths and Sagas*, tr. Jeffrey Gantz (London: Penguin, 1981), 71.

69. The tale is discussed in Tory Vandeventer Pearman, *Women and Disability in Medieval Literature* (New York: Palgrave Macmillan, 2011), 74–83.

70. *Self and Society*, III.8 (176).

71. Gilman, *Making the Body Beautiful*, xix.

72. *Annales Bertiniani* s.a. 864, ed. G. Waitz, *MGH SS rer. Germ.*, V (Hannover: Hahn, 1883), 67: *Carolus iuvenis... noctu rediens de venatione in silva Cotia iocari cum aliis iuvenibus et coaevis suis putans, operante diabolo ab Albuino iuvene in capite spatha percutitur pene usque ad cerebrum; quae plaga a timpore sinistro usque ad malam dextrae maxillae pervenit.* English translation: *The Annals*

*of St Bertin: Ninth-Century Histories vol I*, tr. J. L. Nelson (Manchester: Manchester University Press, 1991), 111–112.

73. Janet L. Nelson, *pers. comm.*, comments that Charles seems not to have *done* anything as sub-king thereafter, implying that he was effectively incapacitated.

74. *Ex Adonis Archiepiscopi Viennensis Chronico*, ed. I. de Arx, *MGH SS*, II (Hannover: Hahn, 1829), 323. "*Dehonestatus*" implies loss of dignity *and* looks, since the adjective *honestus* could be used to describe a handsome man as well as an honest or honorable one.

75. *Reginonis Abbatis Prumiensis Chronicon*, s.a. 870, ed. F. Kurze, *MGH SS rer. Germ.*, L (Hannover: Hahn, 1890), 101.

76. *Thietmar*, IV.21 and see above, Chap. 2.

77. *Liber ad Honorem Augusti*, ed. Siragusa, XV, 34: *Illudensque viris ars quibus arcus erat... Lapsaque per medias arsit arundo genas.* Translation from *The Book in Honour of the Emperor*, tr. G. A. Loud, I. Moxon and P. Oldfield (2006), online at http://www.leeds.ac.uk/arts/info/125040/medieval_studies_research_group/1102/medieval_history_texts_in_translation [accessed 15 May 2015].

78. On this topic (for a later period) see the collected essays in *The Stranger in Medieval Society*, ed. F. R. P. Akehurst and Stephanie Cain Van d'Elden (Minneapolis: Minnesota University Press, 1997).

79. *Chronicle of Theophanes*, AM6081 (588/9CE), 389; *Theophanis*, ed. de Boor, 266.

80. Kelly, *Guide*, 8 (face price) and 19 (kingship).

81. II Cnut, in *English Historical Documents*, I, tr. D. Whitelock (2nd edition, London: Routledge, 1979), 458–9.

82. Slave: II Cnut, 32, in *ibid.*, 459.

83. Gregory: above, Chap. 3, note 33; Orderic: above, Chap. 3, note 71.

84. See above, Introduction, discussion of Ezzelino da Romano. The use of extreme violence towards corpses is another common marker of the evil of the perpetrators, as for example in Walter's extended description of the killing and mutilation of Charles the Good of Flanders in 1127. Having killed the count, the murderers continued to wound his head and cut off his right arm: *Walteri Vita Karoli Comitis Flandriae*, in *MGH SS*, XII, ed. G. H. Pertz (Hannover: Hahn, 1856), 549.

85. Amatus of Montecassino, *The History of the Normans*, tr. Prescott N. Dunbar with introduction by G. A. Loud (Woodbridge: Boydell, 2004), VIII.2, 188, and see also VIII.3 (189–90) and VIII.11 (192).

86. *Bartholomaei Scribae Annales* s.a. 1245, in *MGH SS*, XVIII, ed. G. H. Pertz (Hannover: Hahn, 1863), 219.

87. Gaylene Becker and Regina Arnold, "Stigma as a social and cultural construct," in *Dilemma of Difference*, ed. Ainlay, Becker and Coleman, 39–57, at 46, also make the point that stigma can be mitigated by social class – the individual can literally rise above her or his condition.

88. *faciem eius horrendi militis tactu lesam perspexi*: Orderic, VIII.17 (IV, 248–9).

89. *Thietmar*, II.40.

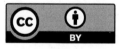

# CHAPTER 5

# Defacing Women: The Gendering
# of Disfigurement

The discussion of disfigurement in early medieval Europe has so far mostly explored cases of men becoming disfigured. This reflects one of the clear findings to emerge from the sample of over 400 instances found in the legal and narrative sources before 1200: that men make up the vast majority of cases documented, whether as victims or perpetrators of the disfiguring injuries. The minority sample of women, however, is itself interesting in that the *type* or form of the disfigurement they suffer as victims frequently differs from that experienced by men. For a start, almost all the cases of female disfigurement center around some perceived sexual betrayal. This may—in the written reports at least—reflect the concerns of the biblical stories that, I have suggested, underpin the ways in which medieval clerics, the authors of almost all our written material, made sense of and presented their accounts of disfigurements. Women were, in this epistemological framework, the second and secondary sex. They were not—in theory at least—permitted to have authority over men, to teach, to stray beyond their allotted role of obedient daughters, wives and mothers. In some legal codes, they had no separate legal personality from their male relatives, but were under the latters' protection. Their bodies, whether viewed through a religious or a medical lens, were weaker, colder, impaired versions of the male ideal.[1] Eve's betrayal of Adam had left women with an insuperable

---

This chapter further develops points made at the conference *European Perspectives on Cultures of Violence*, held at Leicester University in June 2013.

© The Author(s) 2017
P. Skinner, *Living with Disfigurement in Early Medieval Europe*,
DOI 10.1057/978-1-137-54439-1_5

burden to carry, perceived always as prone to curiosity, lust and deceit, unable to control themselves and yet at the same time blamed for their power to tempt men into transgression.[2] Women also rarely make it into the record as writers in this early period, and when they do it seems that they draw their authority to write from pre-existing rank or religious status, trumping their gender.[3] Their writing might not mirror exactly that of their male, clerical counterparts, but nor does it appear to challenge significantly the norms visible in that output.

It is important to rehearse these issues, for all that they will be familiar to anyone who has studied medieval women's or gender history, because the ideological structures shaping the medieval record become highly visible when exploring representations of the twin subjects of women as victims *and* as instigators of disfigurement. Women's bodies, as numerous legal frameworks reveal, were off-limits in ways that men's were not. Violence by men against women, however, has a long history. Often (and crudely) explained as the outcome of men's superior physical strength over women, and their need to control women's productive and reproductive capacity for their own benefit, discussions of gendered violence have tended to focus on specific issues such as rape, sexual assault and/or domestic abuse.[4] But men were also expected to protect "their" women from such violence: hence rape (from *raptus*—seizure/abduction) was literally the "theft" of the woman from her menfolk (fathers, brothers, husband). An injury to a woman—as we have begun to see with the case of Theodoric's daughter, discussed in Chapter 2—was considered an insult to the honor of her menfolk, rather than to her, a principle mirrored in Lombard law on the subject.[5] This reflects the world of mutilation-by-proxy introduced above, and girls and women could function equally effectively as the proxies. Nowhere is this more apparent than in a tale told by Orderic Vitalis. Eustace of Breteuil, son-in-law of King Henry I of England and husband of the latter's daughter Juliana, was in dispute with Ralph Harenc over the castle of Ivry, and the two men exchanged hostages whilst the king considered Eustace's demand that the castle be returned to him. Henry sent Eustace Ralph Harenc's son, whilst Eustace sent his two (unnamed) daughters, the king's granddaughters. On the malevolent advice of Amaury of Montfort, however, Eustace took out the boy's eyes (*oculos eruit*) and sent him back to Ralph. Henry, in an act of breathtaking callousness, then handed over his granddaughters to Ralph so that he could take his revenge "with the permission of the angry king." Ralph not only took out their eyes, but also cut off the tips of their noses (*nariumque summitates truncavit*). The incident is used by Orderic as a prelude to Eustace and Juliana's rebellion against her father, Henry, their distress a catalyst for their actions.[6] Juliana ended up being enclosed in the nunnery at Fontevrault, but we hear nothing more of the two girls. In this political tit-for-tat, however, no comment is made about Ralph's excessive revenge—going beyond blinding to literally deface Eustace's daughters. Unpacking the episode further, however, Eustace's initial mutilation of Ralph's son, while the king himself was overseeing negotiations, represents an act of defiance, betraying the trust established between the two parties by the exchange of hostages. Children, even royal children, were mere tokens in this dangerous game—recall the fact that in 994, Thietmar of Merseberg's mother had been willing to trade him to the Saxon pirates in exchange for her brother's safety. Were two girls worth less than one boy in such exchanges? Or was Ralph's total destruction of their faces, the tipping point for Eustace to go into open rebellion, recognition of their high potential worth as marriage partners? Either way, whilst Orderic recorded the sorry tale, the fact that he did not even name the girls themselves effectively effaces them from the narrative.[7]

## WOMEN "PROTECTED"

As Chapter 3 outlined, early medieval law codes punished injuries inflicted upon the face and body. William Ian Miller suggests that violence is largely coded male, with female violence less imaginable.[8] Since the Latin in many of the legal clauses takes the gender-neutral (or, more precisely, gender-inclusive masculine) formula "Si quis...alii"/"If anyone [injures the body part] of someone else," it would be reasonable to assume in fact that the detailed injury clauses were intended to apply to men and women. Indeed, Jinty Nelson and Alice Rio have addressed precisely this issue, hypothesizing that early medieval laws did not differentiate by gender except in clauses where the injury concerned—whether shaming or physically painful or both—specifically identified the victim as female.[9] Yet the genitive "alii" in the "si quis" clauses (and its more direct accusative, *alium*) is a grammatically different element from *quis*, since it implies the injury done to some other *male* person's body, unless we assume the gender-inclusive masculine to stand for male and female victims. The careful and gendered distinction between terms for male and female slaves in the same sets of laws, however, suggests that if female victims were envisaged, they might have been indicated by *"aut aliae/aliam"* or similar additions to the text. Only the Visigothic lawcode makes it clear that the provisions are intended to apply to both men and women: "tam in viris quam in feminis observande sunt."[10] This suggests that the matter was anything but clear, and that the world of interpersonal early medieval violence was conceived predominantly as one of men.

Nelson and Rio's study outlines in some detail the ways in which violence and injury against women is presented in the medieval laws, so what follows will be a brief restatement. Exploring the early legal texts, all of which date before 1000 CE, it becomes apparent in fact that women appear in very specific contexts of violent acts. Penalties are exacted for causing abortions by potions or blows,[11] free women are beaten for marrying or copulating with slaves,[12] rape is punished,[13] and a husband was permitted to do as he wished with an adulterous wife in Visigothic law, some of the earliest extant material.[14] Ripuarian and Salic laws in Francia punished grabbing a woman's hand, arm, finger or grabbing or exposing her breasts, and Lombard law in Italy extended the prohibition of touching and grabbing to "any shameful place."[15] Blocking a woman or girl's way also attracted a penalty in Frankish and Lombard laws.[16] Medics were forbidden to bleed women in the absence of her close family.[17] The latter three categories underline the unauthorized nature of strangers approaching and touching women's bodies, expressed also in numerous clauses about uncovering or cutting a woman's hair, particularly within her own home.[18] These provisions essentially establish a no-go zone around a woman's body, reinforced and defended by the protection or *mund* of her male relatives. (This probably explains Adam of Bremen's detail that the pirates in 994 came ashore and stole women's *earrings*—a symbolic mutilation to correspond with the physical harming of the men, rather than—or in addition to—plundering the jewelry for its intrinsic value.) Invading that space, whether through unauthorized approaches and proximity (say, into a woman's house, or blocking her way) were as threatening to the woman's own reputation as to that of her family. Touching, whether sexual in nature or not, represented an unwelcome penetration, since *all* touching represented a sexual approach transgressing the *mund* in these provisions (Rosi Braidotti's image of the body as an interface again comes to mind here).[19]

Work on medieval violence between men, and on knightly culture in particular, emphasizes the need for an injured man to reciprocate, often equally violently, unless bought off with considerable compensation, or risk losing his honor in the eyes of others. How this honor code worked in cases of disfigurement among men has already been discussed in detail in previous chapters, especially Chapter 2. Women, however, were not expected to participate in this reciprocal contest of physical prowess: female honor and reputation might well be at stake, but violence was not, it seems, part of the process of defending it (the exception being the fierce women—often mothers and wives—depicted in Norse sagas and Irish legends, who goad their menfolk into violent acts and, in some cases, undertake the violence themselves).[20] Exploring the early medieval law-codes with a gendered eye reinforces the idea that women's place was con-structed largely as passive victims of violence, if they are mentioned at all. As Ross Balzaretti has pointed out for Lombard Italy, the laws had a prob-lem with even conceptualizing women defending their honor with vio-lence in the same way as men.[21] Irish laws, too, are particularly dismissive of fights between women. Indeed, injuries inflicted in such fights were not considered actionable. The laws go on to allow a first wife to inflict inju-ries on a second wife, and the latter's retaliation could take the form only of scratching, pulling hair or speaking abusively about her rival.[22] Whilst scratches to the face might well leave marks, it is clear that the actual disfigurement of another woman was not being envisaged or encouraged here. In the Burgundian laws, if a woman dishonored by having her hair cut in her own home tried to reciprocate in any way, she lost the right to claim for injury.[23] Much later on, the belief that women's violence did not amount to much is expressed in the thirteenth-century Assizes of the kingdom of Cyprus: here, a woman beating a man paid half the fine a male assailant would.[24] The key issue here was where the violence might take place—within the Irish home, cat-fights were not thought particu-larly actionable—but if a woman or group of women crossed outside the boundary of their men's protection to pursue a grievance, then they were effectively rejecting the privileges that such protection brought.

The theme of female passivity in the face of violence is also represented in narrative sources. Writing a letter of advice, the eleventh-century car-dinal, and later saint, Peter Damian (1007–1072) relates a story which he says was told to him by Pope Alexander II. It involves a certain Ardericus of Milan, who got into an argument with his mother at his own wedding feast when it was reported to him by one of the servants that the food was not seasoned properly. Matters came to a head when, in his fury, he struck her about the face "as only a stepson would have." Almost immediately he was afflicted with alternating pain and numbness, swelling and putrefac-tion in his own face, the jaw becoming deformed as pus and poison oozed from an abscess. It became so bad that he feared he would lose his wife (recall here that they are newlyweds). His mother, far from rejoicing in this divine punishment, in fact prayed to St Nazarius to release her son from the torment, and her wish was granted. Although Ardericus lost a chunk of bone and flesh, and was permanently disfigured, he was healed and freed from pain.[25] (We do not actually learn whether his wife stayed with him, but the assumption is that she probably did.)

What is striking about Peter's account is the detail with which he packs this story of a son who was ultimately disfigured for having treated his mother so badly—a moral tale from Peter to his correspondent not to treat his mother disrespectfully. Ardericus is punished—and permanently disfigured, the most visible of punishments—for treating his apparently blameless mother with a lack of respect (*inreverenter*). As her face was the target of his violence, so his face becomes the site of redress. Of course, the serving of bland, unseasoned food at his wedding feast might have been construed as bringing him into disrepute as co-host of the feast, as might his mother's indignant (and presumably fairly public) response to his accusation that she was to blame. Nevertheless, the message is one of excessive violence here. Having broken the commandment to "honor thy mother and thy father," Ardericus is punished by divine justice (*divina iustitia*), and loses his honor both as a son and a husband. His permanently deformed face, the passage continues, acted as a sign of his human fault, albeit cured by divine mercy. But why did Ardericus think he was going to lose his wife? Was his public loss of self-control, and consequent punishment, a threat to his "face"? And were his mother's selfless prayers intended to try to "save face" by saving his physical face? Peter's suggestion that this was an issue may ultimately hark back once again to the biblical idea of male authority diminished by deformity, but the new marriage might also have been put at risk if Ardericus' bride was so disgusted by his appearance that it affected their ability to consummate the union. Earlier Lombard law, after all, had also permitted that an engagement could be broken off if the *bride* became leprous (*lebrosa*), possessed (*demoniaca*) or was blind in both eyes (*excecata*).[26] Either way, this tale introduces a number of the themes to be discussed in this chapter: violence against women, the dynamics of patriarchy in male-female relationships and masculinity expressed through violence, and the participation of women (or not) in that language of violence. On the surface, Peter Damian's tale adheres to and reinforces the normative framework of male activity and female passivity: the response of the unnamed mother is not to retaliate in any way to the blow at the time, and because she is such a good mother (Peter draws a relatively early contrast between her actions and those of a wicked stepmother), she prays to the saint to stop the divine punishment being meted out on her son. This she achieves, underlining the idea that the correct response for women in difficulties was to turn to prayer, rather than reciprocal violence.

Relatively little academic work has been done on the female face as a site of violence in medieval Europe. This is surprising given that ideals of beauty in European culture have most often been represented using women's features (with the possible exception of the perfect young men in classical Greek statuary). Recall again the quote from Peter Damian's letter—the human fault in his story was to be shown up in a facial sign (*humanae culpae signaculum retinetur*). Now, whilst medieval philosophers, in Umberto Eco's words, "had few reasons to deal with female beauty, given that they were all men of the Church and medieval moralism caused them to mistrust the pleasures of the flesh...", they nevertheless understood the power of the body as a symbol. For Thomas Aquinas, beauty emanated from integrity.[27] A flawed or mutilated body, or face, was therefore a sign of some other deficiency. This has implications for how we understand women's faces as sites of violence. Visible facial injury or its aftermath, indeed any sign of having been beaten, was understood and described as shameful, a sign of weakness in a man, rather than a source of pride—the "battle-scarred hero" did not exist in real life. Early medieval lawcodes make this visual aspect of honor and shame explicit, fining injuries which could be perceived from a certain distance away, or those which left a permanent scar.[28] Yet women's injuries do not appear to have been read in the same way.

Several of the injuries to women outlined in early laws, however, seem again to be symbolic rather than permanently disfiguring. Hair cutting is a case in point. Discussing corporal punishments, Guy Geltner comments that a punishment did not necessarily have to incorporate pain to be classified as "corporal," and that "penal shaving... was broadly perceived not merely as humiliating but as an outright form of mutilation."[29] We have already met cases of men being shaved and tonsured as punishment, but did the removal of a women's hair signal even greater shame? Read in the light of multiple lawcodes throwing up a virtual fence around female bodies and heads, it seems that hair cutting could have as profound a symbolism as a more permanent marker of shame. This is apparent in accounts of the downfall of Byzantine empresses. Michael Psellos reports the exile of

Empress Zoe (d. 1050) at the hands of Michael V, which included a party being sent to cut off her hair. Psellos' language here is interesting, since the disgrace of Zoe's hair being cut is equated with her death: "She was to be offered up, so to speak, as a whole burnt-offering (αλοκαρπωμα)... whether to appease God or the wrath of the emperor who gave this order, I do not know."[30] Other empresses, too, whether consorts or rulers in their own right, are also recorded as having been exiled, but what is striking is that, unlike their male counterparts, prominent Byzantine women do not appear to have been blinded or otherwise mutilated permanently as part of the process of their downfall.[31] This was despite some having acquired notoriety for their multiple sexual liaisons (for example, the tenth-century empress Theophano, not to be confused with the western empress Theophanu, wife of Otto III) and/or their cruelty whilst in power. Empress Zoe, for example, is presented by Psellos as having inherited a tendency to blind indiscriminately from her father, Constantine VIII.[32] Why then were these powerful women left unharmed? Again we meet gendered, ideological parameters that dictated that women, although they might rule, were exceptions to the norm. Their very femaleness, which might briefly be trumped by imperial birth (Zoe and her sister Theodora were, after all, both Purple-Born), contingency (in particular a temporary lack of viable adult male to take the imperial throne, necessitating a regency such as Empress Irene's in the late eighth century) or the sexual partners they were able to ally with (Theophano is a case in point here, marrying two successive emperors and nearly securing a third), meant that they were tolerated only as long as they were able to secure strong, male allies. When the latter abandoned them, their vulnerability as women was sufficient to disbar them from future rule: confinement to a female space such as a nunnery might be considered, but usually retirement or exile was accepted as marking the end of their ambitions. It was not necessary to mutilate them, as their claim to authority was compromised already by their sex.

## Women Defaced

I suggested earlier that female sexuality underpins presentations of women and punishment; laws on adultery specifically threatened to mutilate female faces of perpetrators in an apparent move away from the death of both parties.[33] The female head and face, however, also feature here in an entirely different category of legal provisions. In Visigothic Spain, if a slave prostituted herself she was publicly beaten, shaved ( *decalvata* ) and returned to her master (a free woman was simply beaten).[34] Considerable uncertainty surrounds the meaning of *decalvata*, however, for it could also indicate that the slave girl was scalped, a rather more violent head injury which, assuming she survived the procedure and that the injury healed, would have left a visible, permanent, bald patch of scar tissue on her head.[35] Visigothic law also punished with disfigurement any Jewish woman participating in or allowing a circumcision to take place: she was to lose her nose (men doing this were castrated). Although the latter provision was part of a wider program targeted against the expansion of the Jewish community through proselytism, both of the Visigothic clauses fall into the broad category of associating women with sexuality, and punishing them accordingly.[36]

Yet even if the offence was not of a sexual nature, some clerical writers still saw in their female protagonists the opportunity to present all women as Jezebels. A case in point is a story of double disfigurement, recounted by Gregory of Tours, suggesting that punitive violence could be gendered. In Book IX of his history, Gregory tells the rather unlikely story of Septimina, nurse to King Childebert's children, who was implicated in a plot to persuade the king to banish his mother, Queen Brunhild, and his consort, Faileuba, from court, or to kill him by witchcraft (*maleficiis*). Arrested and tortured alongside one Droctulf, who had been deputed to assist her with the children, Septimina admitted that she had killed her husband with witchcraft and then become Droctulf's lover. The pair confessed to the plot and named two further accomplices (who in fact successfully denied their involvement).[37] They were both severely beaten, Septimina's faced was disfigured with red-hot irons (*cauteriis accensis in faciae vulnerata*—note the lack of a specific Latin term), and Droctulf lost his ears and hair. Both were then sent to royal estates to do manual labor, she grinding corn for the women in the spinning and weaving room, he working in the king's vineyards.[38]

This case, as reported by Gregory, needs considerable unpacking to get at why Septimina and Droctulf suffered differentiated punishments. Droctulf's mutilation partly equates him with the (unnamed) conspirators against Childebert mentioned above in Chapter 4, but unlike them, he did not lose his nose, and was not let off to be an example to others. Instead, he was confined to work on the king's estate, from where he absconded once but was recaptured. His confinement here appears to be as much of a punishment as the mutilation meted out to him; his hair would, after all, grow back, and he might be able to conceal his missing ears.

So why was the same punishment not inflicted upon Septimina? Why target her face? Remembering that the case is being reported by a clerical author, Septimina's guilt was on three counts: first, she plotted against the king (as Droctulf had), but in addition she confessed to killing her husband *and* taking another sexual partner *and* contemplating and using witchcraft. Note the emphasis on magic to get what she wants—at no point is Septimina presented as a violent woman, just a scheming witch. Gregory's language is blunt: "[she acted] out of love for Droctulf and to join with him like a prostitute/*ob amorem Droctulfi ipsumque secum scorto miscere.*"[39] Here Septimina as woman trumps Septimina as traitor, and her main asset, her face, is targeted for punishment. Thereafter she was sent to work in penal servitude in an all-female space, the *genitio* or *gynaeceo*, where cloth was made, but her role was even more menial, grinding the corn for the workers' food. Why she was not simply executed for her many crimes is open to question: perhaps her former position as a trusted nurse earned her some mercy. It remains to ask, however, why this high-profile couple was packed off (*deducitur*) to rural estates to work, rather than being exhibited for public ridicule, as other plotters were. The answer may simply lie in their former positions: advertising that members of the royal household could be disloyal might not have been wise. These are named figures, whereas those who had been let out "to be ridiculed" are not even named by Gregory—they were, literally, nonentities.

## DEFACING WOMEN

Miller notes that women are barely present in Norbert Elias's account of the progress from medieval barbarism to a civilized society, "except as early guardians of the civilized style."[40] This would seem to set up women as a separate group, detached from, and possibly immune to, the violence exchanged between men. Early medieval narrative sources, in particular the work of Gregory of Tours in the sixth century and Einhard in the ninth, rapidly disprove that idea. For example, Gregory reports the attempted rape of an unnamed girl by Duke Amato, in which her face is punched and slapped so hard by his servants and himself that his bed is covered in her blood. As the duke falls asleep (Gregory suggests that this happens without him carrying out the rape), the girl attempts to kill him, and is only saved from the penalty for this attempted murder by his admission that he was at fault, at which point he promptly dies.[41] Here, a woman slapped and punched around the face fights back, and ultimately wins out, but most women participating in violent acts are written up doing so indirectly. Gregory, for instance, reports the punishment of the would-be assassins of Childbert II, two clerics with poisoned daggers, sent by Queen Fredegund. Confessing to their crime, their hands, ears and noses were cut off and they were put to death, but she emerges unscathed from the episode.[42] A little later, Einhard reports that a group of conspirators against Charlemagne were exiled, some having their eyes put out first. Einhard attributes the plots against the king, if not the punishments, which after all could be entirely justified by contemporary standards, to "the cruelty of Queen Fastrada," rather than to the king himself.[43] The Bible provided plenty of examples of cruel or scheming women as models for medieval writers, and undue female influence on rulers was a common *topos* of the chronicles. Blinding as a punishment and political tool was certainly not unheard-of in Carolingian Francia, but a woman's hold over him was squarely blamed for Charles deviating from his usual "kindness and gentleness." Of course Fastrada had a hard act to follow in Charlemagne's deceased wife Hildegard, and what Einhard sees as cruelty might actually simply be the reality of being part of a large and complex family in which she was the stepmother to his existing children, as well as mother to two daughters by Charles.

Peter Damian drew a contrast, in his story of Ardericus, between the kindness of a natural mother and the hard-heartedness of a stepmother. As Pauline Stafford reminds us, early medieval mothers, particularly royal ones, fought to ensure their own children succeeded to power, and in fact the dynamics visible in Gregory's story of Septimina adhere to this model.[44] Septimina was, after all, nurse to the king's existing children, and her accuser in the treason case was Faileuba, the king's concubine, who had recently given birth. Faileuba's new baby was thus a direct competitor to Septimina's charges. Disrupting their upbringing, however temporarily, was at least one way for Faileuba to create space for her own child at court, and ultimately secure her own position.

When a mother did not live up to this early medieval maternal ideal, she might be the object of particular disapproval. Such was the case of Empress Irene of Byzantium, who acted as regent for her son Constantine from 780 until he came of age c. 790, but ruled alone after removing him from power and having him blinded in 797. Steven Runciman's rather picturesque assessment of her conveys the ambivalence of modern scholars to her actions: "In these days of Women's Liberation... whether she was, in her methods and her achievements, an ornament to the movement, is a matter of opinion." Linda Garland states that Irene had "manipulated events and personalities to this conclusion."[45] Even the contemporary chronicler Theophanes, understood as something of an apologist for the empress because of her support for icon-worship, describes the blinding as "cruel and grievous" and intended (unlike other political blindings) to kill the young emperor. Whether it succeeded is unclear.[46] Either way, Irene's blinding of her son actually differs from some other instances not because she was his mother, but because her actions could not be justified: Constantine was not a usurper, after all, even if his attempt to rule alone could be interpreted as disrespectful to his mother. Yet Theophanes, in an earlier passage, sets Constantine up as an equally cruel ruler who, in putting down a plot by the Caesar Nicephoros (whom he blinded), also had the tongues of his four paternal uncles cut out. "God avenged this unjust deed" when Irene blinded Constantine in turn.[47] Irene managed to stay in power for a further five years before being deposed in 802 and exiled to Lesbos. Notably, as in the cases of other empresses already discussed, she was neither mutilated nor blinded: despite having been called *basileus/emperor* on at least one coin issue, it was unnecessary to incapacitate her further.

Irene's actions expressed her power at its height. Much later, Abbot Guibert of Nogent interprets another apparently unjust action by a woman as an "exhibition of power" as well, when he discusses (but does not name) Alais, the mother of Count John of Soissons. She is reported as having ordered the tongue and eyes of a certain deacon to be cut out, but suffered divine punishment with paralysis and the loss of her own ability to speak. More horribly, the treatment that she received involved the cutting of her own tongue, which in fact hastened her death. This story needs to be set in context: Guibert, as Anna Sapir Abulafia has demonstrated, considered John and his family heretics, particularly close to the Jews of Soissons, and so his portrayal of Alais effectively martyring a servant of the church represents an [un]edifying tale.[48] It is notable, however, that he credits the dowager countess with the ability to exhibit her power—perhaps this, too, was the sign of a family out of control. Yet we have relatively few examples of female "cruelty" to set alongside the innumerable episodes that involve men giving the orders.

## WOMEN, HONOR AND FACE

Despite the occurrence of women apparently fighting back or inflicting disfiguring injuries on others, it is difficult to categorize their actions as engaging fully with the "honor culture" of medieval society. To characterize it as such ignores the fact that women did not, as a general rule, enjoy the "rough equality" (a striking echo of Eileen Power's famous statement) characteristic of honor-based social relationships.[49] Rather, they formed part of the group that Miller has termed "those not deemed good enough to play" the honor game.[50] Although he more likely was thinking in class rather than gender terms, Miller's comment is suggestive—women did not in general participate in the reciprocal rituals of defending honor through direct or indirect violence. As we have seen, female violence was regarded as aberrant, absurd. If women sought redress at all, it was in the courts, and even there they might not achieve their goals. Battered Welsh wives, for example, if their husbands had not drawn blood, might find themselves condemned for bringing the case; they were expected to be submissive, particularly to their husbands, and to know their place in the hierarchy, and challenging their husband in public disrupted this framework.[51] The vulnerability of women, as we have already seen, came from the fact that their faces were, to a certain extent, symbolic of their bodily integrity. A woman or girl with a damaged face was immediately suspect, and her shame reflected upon her family and community. In targeting the physical face of a woman, whose beauty has already been noted as a cause for concern, those carrying out assaults were well aware that the resultant bruises, scars or permanent disfigurement would be interpreted by viewers as having a deeper, more damaging meaning for the victim's social status *and* for the standing of her menfolk.

Women's position, therefore, is much more explicable if we instead conceptualize their medieval society as governed by a "face culture," concerned with preserving the dignity of fathers, brothers, husbands *and* sons within their social class, and careful not to demean themselves or their families by having sexual relationships outside of marriage or with lower-status men. Motherhood afforded them some authority, as Peter Damian's letter and numerous studies on medieval mothering illustrate,[52] but only over their children, and when sons were grown men they might assume the role of their mother's protector after the death of her husband. This, as Constantine and Irene found, was a relationship fraught with problems.

Licit and illicit sexual relations are central to this scheme of female agency, since it is a focus not only of legislation that prescribes the dreadful mutilation of a guilty woman's face, but also of legislation, such as that in Wales, about when a husband was permitted to beat his wife (adultery being one instance). Earlier, continental laws permitted a husband to kill his adulterous wife and her partner. Such provisions persisted into the later Middle Ages: a cuckolded husband in the kingdom of Cyprus could kill his adulterous wife and her lover with impunity, but was forbidden to kill one and spare the other (the law here cites an earlier ruling of King Aimery, ruler of Cyprus from 1194 and Jerusalem from 1197 till his death in 1205).[53] Either way, the legal material assumes that knowledge of the adulterous relationship will become public, and this is where the mutilation of the physical face (of the woman) intersects with the preservation of the metaphorical face (of the man).

Medieval marriages, like their ancient precursors, were highly hierarchical: the husband had total dominion over his wife, and she was expected to show him submission and obedience. The influence of the Church mitigated this somewhat by demanding mutual respect. Hence an admonition issued in Charlemagne's name after 801 reinforces the wife's duty to obey: she should be "subject to her husband in all honesty and chastity, keeping herself away from fornication, favors and selfishness, as those who [indulge in] these are repugnant to God." Husbands, in return, were ordered to love their wives, and not speak dishonorably to them.[54] The hierarchy of marriage demanded that the wife obey her husband and care for *his* reputation—his "face"—as studiously as her own (recall the Welsh law about a wife who disrespected her husband's "beard" and could be legitimately beaten for doing so).[55] This explains why legal texts often condemn marriages between socially unequal partners where the woman is of higher social status than her husband (but not vice versa), for such marriages challenged the norm of male domination. If a wife showed a lack of deference, or betrayed her husband, or was even suspected of doing so, she committed a face-threatening act. Let us remind ourselves again of Cnut's law: an adulterous woman, he says, shall become "a public disgrace" and lose her nose and ears.[56] But the publicity of the case, and the supposed intervention of royal justice and/or the local bishop who was to "judge sternly" if her attempt at exculpation failed, clearly had the potential not only to disgrace the woman herself, but also her husband, whose position as cuckold would have been exposed by any proceedings. The fact that he was to receive all that his wife owned seems to be related to the compensation culture that accompanied other laws. There is, predictably enough, a double-standard at work here, for previous clauses of the code, dealing with male adulterers, fornicators, rapists and men committing incest, are punished by compensation and fines (in contrast to earlier Byzantine law on the same topics).[57] Not only did she lose her own reputation and status, but she damaged her husband's reputation and standing as well (although we have to wait till the later Middle Ages to engage with the figure of the "cuckold", so prominent and so targeted in early modern culture).[58] And this, I suggest, is why her own, physical, face was seen as a legitimate target for punishment.

What responses might a facially-mutilated woman expect from her community? The association between women's sexual transgression and punishment targeted at the face had a long history. I have noted above how mutilation of the nose, or even its complete removal, was an Old Testament penalty against loose women that found its way into multiple legal codes. In Byzantium, we should note, it was threatened for sexual misdemeanors by women and men, and for incestuous as well as adulterous relationships, and in Sicily it was targeted at women who pimped their daughters. In Spain, the penalty occurs in Jewish rabbinic responsa on the adulterous wife, where the purpose of such a mutilation was set out plainly—it was to deprive the woman of the beauty with which she had wooed her lover.[59] So beauty here was a threat, and needed to be made ugly to neutralize its danger. Thus Septimina's punishment—as reported above by Gregory—addressed not (or not just) her treasonous act but also her sexual history. It therefore went beyond the penalty imposed upon Droctulf (who is not, we might note, ever referred to as a fornicator). Similarly, although Cnut's laws demand that an adulterous wife be deprived of her property—a financial compensation for her husband's loss of face—they also demand the physical mutilation of the woman herself. William Ian Miller comments that here "the idea of compensation has lost out completely to ideas of punition... The point is to render her so physically repulsive that she will have sexual virtue foisted upon her and leave her so poor that no one will be inclined to overlook the disfigurement for the benefits of her property."[60] Returning to Eustace's two daughters, the unevenness of Ralph's retaliation signaled the complete closing-off of their futures as wives, but the nose-cutting was also calculated as an insult to their father, who had failed to protect them. Here, then, there *is* a sense that destroyed beauty might well elicit disgust from a potential sexual partner, magnifying the value of taking a gendered approach to disfigurement.

Early legislators clearly had no problem with including facial mutilation of women in their laws dealing with sexual transgression. The mere threat of such extreme treatment was intended to terrify women into submission. What about other types of crime? The case of Septimina, ostensibly a traitor to her king but written up as a witch and a whore by Gregory, confuses the issue by inserting her infidelity to (and murder of) her husband into the plot. A much later case, however, suggests that women taken for other crimes might expect to be treated in the same way as men. An infamous, and to my knowledge unique, case features in the court records in England in the thirteenth century. In the Shropshire Eyre of 1203 we find the following case:

> [Following the death of a woman slain at Lilleshall, Alice Crithecreche and others were taken for her death]. And Alice, at once after the death, fled to the county of Stafford with some of the chattels of the slain, so it is said, and was taken in that county and brought back into Shropshire and there, as the king's serjeant and many knights and lawful men of the county testify, in their presence she said, that at night she heard a tumult in the house of the slain; whereupon she came to the door and looked in, and saw through the middle of the doorway four men in the house, and they came out and caught her, and threatened to kill her unless she would conceal them; and so they gave her half the pelf that she had. And when she came before the justices in Eyre she denied all this. Therefore she has deserved death, but by way of dispensation let her eyes be torn out. The others are not suspected, therefore let them be under pledges.[61]

This case, which to my mind ranks as one of the most spectacular miscarriages of justice in the medieval record,[62] seems to indicate that once convicted of criminality, gender had little bearing on the punishment meted out. Alice's crime, it seems, was the fact that she had fled and recanted her "confession" to being involved, and we should note that none of the four men she mentions appear to have been apprehended, nor are they named. Alice's eyes, therefore, were symbolic of much more than her apparently involuntary (if we believe her original account) entanglement with this case. They were to be taken as a means of enforcing the authority of the court, whose real targets, the violent thieves, had evaded its reach. In effect, this is yet another mutilation-by-proxy: she is the only "hostage" the court has, and so she is condemned to punishment for the much more serious actions of others. Her permanent blindness would stigmatize her for the remainder of her life, assuming she survived the procedure, but perhaps the written record (which after all took the trouble to include her account), and associated oral narratives, would elicit sympathy from her community rather than disapprobation.

Cases such as this (and the Eyre cases explored above in Chapter 3) underline the fact that in later medieval Europe, the incidence of records of extreme bodily and facial mutilations appears to have increased exponentially. Note here I that focus on the record—Valentin Groebner, too, highlights the increase in documentation of violence, but attributes it to a change in culture in the fourteenth-sixteenth centuries, with more monitoring and recording of behavior.[63] At the same time, however, he demonstrates that the association of damaged face with loss of status maintained its hold on medieval writers such as Albertus Magnus, and cites reports of attacks on women's faces, often targeting the nose.[64]

## BEHIND CLOSED DOORS

All of the cases used thus far have featured violence done to women's faces in public arenas, whether as judicial punishments or as incidents of interpersonal violence recorded to make a moral or other point. But some of the early medieval lawcodes we have considered assumed that women remained within, or at least close to, their homes. Thus anyone entering a woman's home to injure her also challenged the authority of her menfolk: a law of King Liutprand of the Lombards addresses deliberately setting fire to another man's house in the same clause as penalizing rape.[65] Lombard society, of course, was one where the *mundium*, the legal protection of women by men, held sway more strongly than perhaps any other region of Europe. Thus her menfolk might demand compensation, but she was forbidden from taking direct action. The home, though, was not always a safe haven. Houses were accidentally or deliberately set alight in times of war (as the graphic detail on the Bayeux Tapestry of a woman fleeing her burning house with her child, complete with caption "Here a house is burnt," illustrates). Accidents with fire or sharp implements could happen within and out of doors. Such incidents do not make it into the early medieval record, although the evidence of later coroners' rolls underlines what a dangerous place a home could be for women and their children.

And the home was also the setting for domestic violence, the likely ubiquity of which is largely concealed from view unless it reached an extreme whereby the woman herself, or members of her wider family, took action through the courts. Citing work by Sara Butler, Lizabeth Johnson argues that in later medieval England, at least, spousal violence barely registered in the plentiful court records and coroners' rolls, and that even if it did, two-thirds of the cases were actually homicides.[66] As Hannah Skoda has pointed out, using French examples, "domestic violence operates at the interface of the public and the private."[67] Of course the face, unless covered with a veil or other wrapping (and clearly covering of the head and hair was pretty ubiquitous among married women), was itself the most public site of injury: one could attempt to conceal the violence done, but this was rather more difficult than covering up wounds or bruises to the torso. Yet the disfigurement of women by their own family members, so ubiquitous among modern cases in the media, hardly figures in the medieval evidence. Medieval authors, after all, had a stake in upholding the ideal of the male protector: this is why Peter Damian's story of transgression by an ungrateful son has such value, in demonstrating where the limits lay. Hitting one's mother in the face was unacceptable behavior, a shameful act. In fact hitting any woman in the face—even the unnamed target of Duke Amato's rape—seems to cross a line that is rarely explicitly mentioned. Was the sustained attack on this girl meant to reduce her to a state similar to a whore, or does Gregory (who as we have seen does not flinch from describing the mutilation of guilty women) include this detail to indicate just how wrong Amato's act was from start to finish? Would we even have had the story if the duke himself had not dropped dead at the end of it?

## CONCLUSIONS

Gender history draws much of its energy from the analysis of the historically unequal relationships between men and women, and certainly the cases of actual disfigurement discussed here seem to argue for a double-standard at work, not only in the ways in which sexual activity was regulated, but in the way that women's faces were targeted as a means of marginalizing them and taking them out of the social arena. There is unevenness in the apparent "extra" element in the way that the appearance of women's faces is altered as well as or instead of the penalties and disfigurements meted out to men. Septimina's is burnt, Eustace's daughters lose their noses *as well as* their eyes, exceeding the blinding handed down to Ralph's son. Theodoric's daughter is mutilated on mere suspicion. In all three cases, the women and girls are marked visibly, whether or not also impaired physically. I have argued elsewhere, and continue to maintain, that the key to understanding women's faces as sites of violence is to be found in the honor networks in which their menfolk participate. As Jurgen Frembgen has pointed out in the case of nose-cutting in modern Pakistan and Afghanistan, "'honor' and 'shame' are encoded in body morphology."[68] Discussing modern cases in Pakistan, Frembgen describes the men's mutilation of wives or daughters as a reciprocal act within the code of honor. Yet the women in these cases are not "rough equals" either, despite Islamic law offering more protection of wives than westerners might in fact imagine; the honor being satisfied here is male honor, restoring the man's place within the male community by "imprint[ing] his power on the surface of her body."[69] This is a useful way of understanding medieval violence against women's faces too: it is striking that the law of King Cnut on adulterous wives, threatening their mutilation, does nothing to penalize the male partner in the adultery. Instead, II Cnut 50 simply orders that anyone committing adultery is to pay compensation for it in proportion to the deed.[70] Men, then, enjoyed a right to a "proportional" punishment: the punishment threatened for female adulterers, on the other hand, as almost all the cases of violence against women's faces in the evidence, was an entirely disproportionate response born out of the need to maintain "face" and masculinity.

## NOTES

1. Monica Green, "Bodily essences: bodies as categories of difference," in *A Cultural History of the Human Body in the Medieval Age*, ed. Linda Kalof (London: Bloomsbury, 2010), 149–172, explores sexual differentiation as well as other markers of difference such as disease and disability.
2. See, e.g., John Flood, *Representations of Eve in Antiquity and the English Middle Ages* (New York: Routledge, 2011).
3. Although the literature is vast on this topic, one of the best single-volume works in terms of its relevance to the early Middle Ages remains *Women Writers of the Middle Ages: a Critical Study of Texts from Perpetua to Marguerite Porete*, ed. Peter Dronke (Cambridge: Cambridge University Press, 1984). Surprisingly, the otherwise excellent *Oxford Handbook of Women and Gender in Medieval Europe*, ed. Judith Bennett and Ruth Mazo Karras (Oxford: Oxford University Press, 2013) does not have a section addressing female writers, perhaps a deliberate response to their celebration in earlier work as "women" rather than "writers"?

4. Rape: A. Musson, "Crossing boundaries: attitudes to rape in late medieval England," in *Boundaries of the Law: Geography, Gender and Jurisdiction in Medieval and Early Modern Europe*, ed. A. Musson (Aldershot: Ashgate, 2005), 84–101.

5. *Leges Langobardorum*, Rothari, c.186, ed. F. Bluhme, in *MGH LL*, IV, ed. G. H. Pertz (Hannover: Hahn, 1868), 44.

6. *Orderic*, XII.10 (VI, 210–213). On Orderic's treatment of Juliana, see Susan Johns, *Noblewomen, Aristocracy and Power in the Twelfth-Century Anglo-Norman Realm* (Manchester: Manchester University Press, 2003), 17–18.

7. Adam J. Kosto, *Hostages in the Middle Ages* (Oxford: Oxford University Press, 2012), 85 notes a rise in the number of female hostages recorded after c.1000, but comments that "gender does not seem to have been a pressing issue." I disagree: damaging elite marital plans through the retention and/or mutilation of female family members was surely a gendered strategy? See Katherine Weikert, "The princesses who might have been hostages: Margaret and Isabella of Scotland," and Gwen Seabourne, "Female hostages: definition and distinctions," both in *Hostage-Taking and Hostage Situations: the Medieval Precursors of a Modern Phenomenon*, ed. Matthew Bennett and Katherine Weikert (Routledge, forthcoming). Seabourne, in particular, takes issue with Kosto's claim.

8. William Ian Miller, *Humiliation and other essays on Honor, Social Discomfort and Violence* (Ithaca, NY: Cornell University Press, 1998), 62.

9. Janet L. Nelson and Alice Rio, "Women and laws in early medieval Europe," in *Oxford Handbook of Women and Gender*, 103–117, at 105.

10. *Leges Visigothorum*, VI.3.3, in *MGH LL. Nat. Germ.* I, ed. K. Zeumer (Hannover and Leipzig: Hahn, 1902), 266.

11. *Leges Visigothorum*, VI.3.1 and 2 (260–1); *Leges Alamannorum*, LXXXVIII.1, ed. K. A. Eckhardt, *MGH LL nat. Germ.*, V.1 (Hannover: Hahn, 1966), 150; *Lex Baiwariorum*, XVIII, ed. E. Liber, *MGH LL. nat. Germ.*, V.2 (Hannover: Hahn, 1926), 361.

12. *Leges Visigothorum*, III.2.3, 135.

13. *Leges Visigothorum*, III.3.1–12; *Leges Burgundionum (Gundobada)*, XXX and XXXV, ed. L. R. de Salis, *MGH LL nat. Germ.*, II.1 (Hannover: Hahn, 1892), 66 and 68; *Leges Burgundionum (Romana)*, XIX, ed. de Salis, 142–3; *Lex Ribvaria*, 38.1, ed.

F. Beyerle and R. Buchner, *MGH LL nat. Germ.*, III.2 (Hannover: Hahn, 1954), 90; *Pactus Legis Salicae*, XIII (gang rape by three men), ed. K. Eckhardt, *MGH LL nat. Germ.*, IV.1 (Hannover: Hahn, 1962) 58 ; *Lex Salica*, XIV, ed. K. Eckhardt, *MGH LL nat. Germ.*, IV.2 (Hannover: Hahn, 1959), 52; *Leges Langobardorum*, Liutprand 72, ed. F. Bluhme in *MGH LL*, IV, ed. G. H. Pertz (Hannover: Hahn, 1868), 136.

14. *Leges Visigothorum*, III.4.1 (147), III.4.3 (148).

15. *Lex Ribvaria*, XLIII, 96; *Pactus Legis Salicae*, XX.1, 83; *Lex Salica*, XXVI.1, 66 and XXVI.4, 68; *Leges Langobardorum*, Liutprand 121 [*alium locum unde turpe esse potest*], 158. See also *ibid.*, Liutprand 125, 160.

16. *Pactus Legis Salicae*, XXXI.2, 121; *Lex Salica*, XXXVIII.2, 215; *Leges Langobardorum*, Rothari 26 and 371, 17 and 86. For more on the implications of way-blocking, see below, Chap. 5.

17. *Leges Visigothorum*, XI.1.1, 400.

18. *Leges Burgundionum (Gundobada)*, XXXIII.1–4, 67. *Pactus Legis Salicae*, XXIV.3 forbade the cutting of girls' hair without the consent of her parents, 90. *ibid.*, Addition CIV, 260, brackets cutting a woman's hair with other injuries such as causing miscarriage and death.

19. William Ian Miller, *Eye for an Eye* (Cambridge: Cambridge University Press, 2006), 135–139, discusses this "holy" space at length, comparing *mund* with the Icelandic *helgi*. Braidotti: above, Chap. 2.

20. For example, Hallgerda encouraging Brynjolf to kill Atli in Njallsaga, c.38; and see Miller, *Eye for an Eye*, 69.

21. Ross Balzaretti, "'These are things men do, not women': the social regulation of female violence in Langobard Italy," in *Violence and Society in the Medieval West*, ed. G. Halsall (Woodbridge: Boydell, 1998), 175–192, citing *Leges Langobardorum*, Rothari 278 (67): *absurdum videtur esse, ut mulier libera, aut ancilla, quasi vir cum armis vim facere possit*, and 378 (88), denying women getting injured in such fights among men any compensation for their injuries. *Leges Langobardorum*, Liutprand 141 (170) reiterated the prohibition of using women in fights.

22. Fergus Kelly, *A Guide to Early Irish Law* (Dublin: Dublin Institute for Advanced Studies, 1988), 79.

23. *Leges Burgundionum (Gundobada)*, XXXIII.5, elaborated in XCII.1–6.

24. *The Assizes of the Lusignan Kingdom of Cyprus*, tr. Nicholas Coureas (Nicosia: Cyprus Research Centre, 2002), Codex I, clause 280.

25. *MGH Die Briefe in der deutschen Kaiserzeit, IV.2: Die Briefe des Petrus Damiani II*, no 85, ed. K. Reindel (Munich: MGH, 1988), 458. Translation in *The Letters of Peter Damian 61–90*, tr. Owen J. Blum (Washington DC: Catholic University of America Press, 1998), 250–4.

26. *Leges Langobardorum*, Rothari 180, 42.

27. U. Eco, *On Beauty*, tr. A. McEwan (London: Secker and Warburg, 2004), 154 (quote). Thomas Aquinas, *Summa*, I, 39.8, quoted in U. Eco, *On Ugliness* (London: Harvill Secker, 2007), 15.

28. See above, Chap. 3.

29. Guy Geltner, *Flogging Others: Corporal Punishment and Cultural Identity from Antiquity to the Present* (Amsterdam: AUP, 2014), 25.

30. Michael Psellos, *Chronographia*, V.23: Michele Psello, *Imperatori di Bisanzio (Cronografia)*, ed . and tr. Salvatore Impellizari, Ugo Criscuolo and Siliva Ronchey, 2 vols (Milan: Fondazione Lorenzo Valla/Mondadori, 1984), I, 136.

31. An early exception, reported by Theophanes, is that of Martina, mother of Heraklonas, deposed in 640/1, but whilst his nose was cut off, she lost her tongue, perhaps signalling the end of her motherly advice and guidance: *Theophanis Chronographia*, ed. C. de Boor, 2 vols (Hildesheim: Georg Olms, 1963), AM 6133/640–1 CE. English translation: *The Chronicle of Theophanes Confessor: Byzantine and Near Eastern History, AD284–813*, ed. and tr. C. Mango and R. Scott with the assistance of R. Greatrex (Oxford: Clarendon Press, 1997), 475.

32. Psellos, *Chronographia*, VI.157.

33. Despite passages explicitly repealing the eighth-century laws of the "heretic emperors" Leo III and Constantine V in subsequent codes issued by Basil I (d. 886) and Leo VI (d. 912), the nasal mutilation of both parties in an adulterous relationship was reiterated in Leo's Novels: *Les Novelles de Léon VI Le Sage*, ed. and tr. P. Noailles and A. Dain (Paris: Les Belles Lettres, 1944), Novel 32, 127–129.

34. *Leges Visigothorum*, III.4.17, 157.

35. Head-shaving of women for perceived and actual sexual misconduct has persisted across the centuries, from the treatment of convicts to the shaving of "horizontal collaborators" in post-World

War II France: Shani d'Cruze and Louise A. Jackson, *Women, Crime and Justice in England since 1660* (London: Palgrave Macmillan, 2009), 129; Alison M. Moore, "History, memory and trauma in photography of the *tondues*: visuality of the Vichy past through the silent image of women," *Gender and History*, 17 (2005), 657–681.

36. *Leges Visigothorum*, XII.3.4, 433. On the specific context of Visigothic relations with the Jews, Norman Roth, *Jews, Visigoths and Muslims in Medieval Spain: Cooperation and Conflict* (Leiden: Brill, 1994), especially 7–38. Note here the apparent reciprocation of damage to a penis (circumcision) by damage to a nose, and see above, Chap. 2.

37. One was the count of the stables, Sunnigisil, who would later be involved in another plot against Childebert: *GT*, X.19.

38. *GT*, IX.38.

39. Thorpe's translation, in Gregory of Tours, *History of the Franks*, tr. Lewis Thorpe (London: Penguin, 1974) 524–5, "whose mistress she had then become," does not do justice to Gregory's invective here.

40. William Ian Miller, *The Anatomy of Disgust* (Cambridge, MA: Harvard University Press, 1997), 174.

41. *GT*, IX.27.

42. *GT*, VIII.29.

43. *Einhardi Vita Karoli Magni*, III.20, ed. O. Holder-Egger, *MGH SS rerum. Germ.* XXV (Hannover: Hahn, 1911), 26.

44. Pauline Stafford, "Sons and mothers: family politics in the Middle Ages," in *Medieval Women: Essays presented to Professor Rosalind M. T. Hill*, ed. Derek Baker (Oxford: Blackwell, 1978), 79–100.

45. Steven Runciman, "The Empress Irene the Athenian," in *Medieval Women*, ed. Baker, 101–118, at 101; Linda Garland, *Byzantine Empresses: Women and Power in Byzantium, AD527–1204* (London: Routledge, 1999), 86.

46. Theophanes, *Chronographia*, AM6285, tr. Mango, 649.

47. *Ibid.*, AM6284, 642.

48. *Self and Society in Medieval France: The Memoirs of Abbot Guibert of Nogent*, III.16, ed. and tr. John Benton (New York: Harper and Row, 1970), 209; Anna Sapir Abulafia, "Theology and the

commercial revolution: Guibert of Nogent, St Anselm and the Jews of northern France," in *Church and City, 1000–1500: Essays in Honour of Christopher Brooke*, ed. D. Abulafia, M. Franklin and M. Rubin (Cambridge: Cambridge University Press, 1992), 23–40, at 28.

49. Angela K.-Y. Leung and Dov Cohen, "Within- and between-culture variation: individual differences and the cultural logics of honor, face and dignity cultures," *Journal of Personality and Social Psychology*, 100.3 (2011): 507–526; Eileen Power, *Medieval Women* (Cambridge: Cambridge University Press, 1975), 34.

50. *Eye for an Eye*, xi.

51. L. Johnson, "Attitudes towards spousal violence in medieval Wales," *Welsh History Review*, 24 (2009): 81–115.

52. E.g. *Motherhood, Religion and Society in Medieval Europe*, ed. Conrad Leyser and Lesley Smith (Farnham: Ashgate, 2011); Pauline Stafford, *Gender, Family and the Legitimation of Power* (Aldershot: Ashgate, 2006); Mary Dockray-Miller, *Motherhood and Mothering in Anglo-Saxon England* (New York: Palgrave, 2000); Patricia Skinner, "'The light of my eyes': medieval motherhood in the Mediterranean", *Women's History Review*, 6.3 (1997): 391–410; *Medieval Mothering*, ed. J. Carmi Parsons and Bonnie Wheeler (New York: Garland, 1996).

53. *Assizes of the Lusignan Kingdom*, Codex I, 271. A striking parallel here is Chapter XXI (XIX).8 of the almost contemporary rendering of Byzantine law for the Greek subjects of the Norman kingdom of Italy, which also forbade killing one and not the other of the adulterous couple: E. H. Freshfield, *A Manual of Later Roman Law: the Ecloga ad Procheiron Mutata* (Cambridge: Cambridge University Press, 1927), 139.

54. *Mulier sint subiecti viri sui in omni bonitate et pudicitia, custodiant se a fornicatione et beneficiis et abaritiis, quoniam qui hec facit Deo repugnant.... Vir diligant uxorem suam et inhonesta verba non dicat ei...*: Additamenta ad Pippini et Karoli M. Capitularia, no 121, "Missi cuiusdam admonitio," in *MGH Capitularia Regum Francorum I*, ed. A. Boretius (Hanover: Hahn, 1883), 238–240, at 240.

55. See above, Chap. 2, note 54.

56. Above, Chap. 3.
57. *II Cnut: Secular Laws*, 50–52, tr. D. Whitelock, *English Historical Documents I: 500–1042* (rev. ed., London, Routledge, 1979), 462–3. Byzantine law: above, Chap. 3.
58. On this figure see *Cuckolds, Clerics and Countrymen: Medieval French Fabliaux*, ed. and tr. John DuVal and Raymond Eichmann (Fayetteville: University of Arkansas Press, 1982); Louise Mirrer, "The 'unfaithful wife' in medieval Spanish literature and law," in *Medieval Crime and Social Control*, ed. Barbara Hanawalt and David Wallace (Minneapolis: University of Minnesota Press, 1999), 143–155; Elizabeth Foyster, *Manhood in Early Modern England: Honour, Sex and Marriage* (London: Longman, 1999, repr. Oxford: Routledge, 2014), esp. 103–147 on "lost manhood."
59. Patricia Skinner, "The gendered nose and its lack: 'medieval' nose-cutting and its modern manifestations," *Journal of Women's History*, 26.1 (2014): 45–67.
60. Miller, *Eye for an Eye*, 36. Miller suggests that some may have taken pleasure in such cruelty.
61. *Select Pleas of the Crown, I: AD 1200–1225*, ed. F. W. Maitland (London: Bernard Quaritch for the Selden Society, 1888), 33–34.
62. It is mentioned without comment by Edward Wheatley, *Stumbling Blocks before the Blind: Medieval Constructions of a Disability* (Ann Arbor: University of Michigan Press, 2010), 36–7.
63. Valentin Groebner, *Defaced: the Visual Culture of Violence in the Late Middle Ages* (New York: Zone, 2004), 15.
64. *Ibid.*, 75–6.
65. *Leges Langobardorum*, Liutprand 72.
66. Johnson, "Attitudes towards spousal violence," 86, citing S. M. Butler, *The Language of Abuse: Marital Violence in Later Medieval England* (Leiden and Boston: Brill, 2007).
67. Hannah Skoda, *Medieval Violence: Physical Brutality in Northern France, 1270–1330* (Oxford: Oxford University Press, 2013), 194. Her magisterial study of domestic violence, *ibid.*, 193–230, draws a stark contrast between the unambivalent punishment of women who beat their husbands and the reluctance of the authorities to intervene when it was the husband beating his wife.

68. J. W. Frembgen, "Honour, shame and bodily mutilation: cutting off the nose among tribal societies in Pakistan," *Journal of the Royal Asiatic Society* 16.3 (2006): 243–60, at 243.

69. *Ibid.*, 252.

70. II Cnut 50, in Whitelock, *English Historical Documents* I, 462.

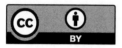

# CHAPTER 6

# Ways of Seeing: Staring at and Representing Disfigurement

Vision lies at the heart of all medieval responses to disfigurement and difference: modern campaigners for facial equality argue that whilst the *visual impact* of a different face might be unavoidable, a *negative response* is almost always conditioned by socialization, that is, prejudice is learned, not inborn. A child growing up with visibly-different parents may realize that difference quite early in life, but will not make value judgments until it witnesses the responses of peers and/or *their* parents. In medieval culture, the assumption that a disfigured or scarred face might be seen and cause shame underpins the compensation demanded of the perpetrator of the injury (payments which, as we have seen, might continue long after the actual injury itself). The flipside, the exhibition of the judicially-marked, did not work without an audience to understand the meaning of such marking. Yet the potential for sympathy, rather than derision, from onlookers suggests that the meaning of such marking was far from stable. It clearly motivated some rulers, for example, to disfigure and then seclude their "treacherous" subjects. The visible bramble scratch on the face singled out Helmstan as a cattle rustler, a branded face marked the repeat Lombard thief, noseless hostages were a sign of Cnut's ruthlessness. But difference might also attract attention because of attempts to conceal it: Notker the Stammerer tells the strange tale of a young man who, ashamed of his red hair and lacking a cap to cover it, attended Mass balancing one of his boots on top of his head. The bishop, annoyed at the lack of respect inherent in not removing headgear in church (and this is Notker's point

© The Author(s) 2017

P. Skinner, *Living with Disfigurement in Early Medieval Europe*, DOI 10.1057/978-1-137-54439-1_6 in telling the bizarre story, it seems), seized the boot and cried "Lo and behold all you people, this fool is red-headed!"[1].

"Vision forces us to face the ugly and horrific," according to Miller.[2] He continues, "In a harsher age there would be little or no guilt on the observer's part for the emotions [of disgust] that the stigmatized elicit; in ours there is."[3] And Notker's story does seem to bear him out on this: the bishop had no qualms whatsoever in singling out and ridiculing a member of his congregation whose only offence seems to have been his poverty. "Ridicule" is the word that most often stalks examples of disfigurement: a beaten-up man in the Lombard laws was rendered open to it, conspirators in Gregory of Tours were freed in order to be exposed to it, and Aldevrandus, discussed in Chapter 4, was also laughed at for his appearance. In this chapter, however, I want to explore in more detail the broader assumption inherent in Miller's statement—that seeing a disfigured person evoked disgust in medieval viewers *and* that they felt no shame in being disgusted. I will use the work of Rosemarie Garland-Thomson on staring to broaden out the possibilities for visual contacts between those with disfigured faces and those without. "Staring," she says, "is an ocular response to what we don't expect to see...[it] is an interrogative gesture that asks what's going on and demands the story."[4] Although Garland-Thomson, like Miller, draws a contrast between premodern village societies, in which a person "knew everyone they saw," and the sprawling, impersonal world in which most are strangers, she nevertheless opens up interesting analytical possibilities for the medievalist by restoring to the "staree"—the object of stares—a voice and opinion based on the testimonies of modern people with visible differences.[5] Another point that she makes is that "We don't usually stare at people we know, but instead when unfamiliar people take us by surprise."[6] Herein lies the first quandary for a person with a disfigurement: if the stranger was an object of curiosity, how much more would a stranger with facial difference be the object of questions, suspicion or even downright hostility? Although we do not have such spectacular cases of misrecognition as exist in early modern archives, the very fact of a face being changed by disfigurement potentially limited mobility, physical and social.[7] At the same time, we have already met the perceived shame inherent in a disfigurement being noticed. Miller weaves the subject of the stare into his description of medieval honor culture: honor, he comments, "governed... how long you could look at someone or even dare to look at him at all."[8] The male pronoun is suggestive here.

The subject of looking and staring has engaged theorists of visual culture for some decades, and their work on viewers of pictures and film has been influential in the burgeoning field of disability studies. In this chapter, however, we shall leave the pictorial till later, and firstly explore written accounts. Garland-Thomson's work provides a rich range of possibilities for interrogating medieval texts. As many medieval narratives of disfigurement, and indeed the legal material, often highlight the unexpected in their accounts or additions, and often demand a story be told to justify the inclusion of that material, they may indeed reveal the gaze of authors or protagonists stunned into staring—physical or textual—by what *they* did not expect to see.

What, though, is "textual staring"? Alongside narratives of actual, eyewitness accounts by the author, two of which are included at some length in the present chapter, I define "textual" staring as a broader spectrum of accounts, where the writer might not be present as an eyewitness, but where the narrative is sufficiently extended to suggest that the author, or reader, or both, are expected to share some pleasure in consuming the scene being described. A possible analogy to this is the modern French literary device of *chosisme*, the detailed, almost tortured description of events, people and particularly the objects they owned as if through a camera lens. The major difference between this and the textual staring I propose, however, is that *chosisme* detached these objects and made them tell the story, whilst the scrutiny visible in the medieval texts is packed with details to heighten emotional response to the actors. As we read extended accounts, whether shocked or curiously fascinated, our focus on the text is itself a stare that verges on the uncontrolled.[9] The account might verge on the prurient (lengthy accounts of the torture of saints have been accused of this), or display an apparent relish in the gory detail that might not be expected of the author.[10] These are textual prostheses—additions, enhancements, unnecessary to the basic account but deployed all the same. Most of our reporters were, after all, highly-skilled rhetoricians. Gregory of Tours is a master of textual staring, sharing extended and detailed passages of gruesome injuries and murders with his readers, such as the death of Duke Rauching who, having fallen over the threshold of a doorway, is set upon by his assailants who "cut and sliced his head this way and that so that it all looked like a brain (*ita minutatim caput eius conliserunt ut simile totum cerebro puteretur*)."[11] Thietmar, as we have seen, actually *invites* his readers to consider his "ridiculous" face, in a passage that is as out of place in his text as his broken nose is on his countenance. And all writers have a purpose to their texts beyond the simple report: to draw a lesson about bodily vanity compared with cleanliness of soul. Accounts in lawcodes of the extraction of bone shards from a wounded head, with highly-ritualized means for measuring their size, also generate a vivid, performative scene: the reader is invited to look at the bone, to imagine the test in metal receptacles, to judge the outcome themselves, but also to *remember*. But we do not *see* these injuries directly. Like all the other cases in this study, they are mediated for us, and earlier readers, by their presentation, repeated for a secondary visual consumption in the written record. But what is the reader to make of such accounts? Are they designed to give pleasure even as they shock or horrify us? As William Ian Miller has commented, "Pain and pleasure have such an unseemly relationship, each never quite knowing how to keep neatly to itself."[12]

The stare, however, that visual engagement with something that has captured attention for its unexpected qualities, is differentiated by Garland-Thomson from the gaze. The latter—that "oppressive act of disciplinary looking that subordinates its victim"—has been used to explore the increasingly unequal relationship between doctors and their patients (Foucault's "clinical gaze") and has also been posited as a gendered phenomenon, with the female body its object and the male viewer in the position of power.[13] Gender theory, however, is not simply confined to the oppositional categories of male and female, but also encompasses other situations of unequal power relations. According to Miller, "Deformity and ugliness... are disordering... they force us to look and notice."[14] This somewhat complicates the binary between viewer/powerful and viewed/powerless, as the glance turns to full-on stare that is difficult to resist. James Partridge, in his personal account of becoming and being disfigured, states bluntly, "Staring can simply be accepted as part of the disfigurement package: changing faces is partly to do with getting used to being an object of scrutiny wherever you go."[15] In fact, once we start to look, we find a lot of staring going on in medieval texts. Gerald of Wales, for example, reflecting on the scar below the nose just above the upper lip with which a certain Erchembald was born, supports this unlikely story of a "miracle of nature" by saying, "I myself saw Erchembald's son, whose name was Stephen, *and there is no doubt that he had the same mark*. A chance accident had become a natural defect."[16] Gerald's report, and that of Orderic Vitalis about Walchelin, discussed earlier, suggest not so much disgust as wonder, a phenomenon that Rosemarie Garland-Thomson posits as the reason for the uncontrolled staring which, she suggests, "opens up toward new knowledge."[17]

In a stimulating article utilizing evidence from medical texts, in particular Henri de Mondeville's surgical manual of the thirteenth century, Luke Demaitre proposes that facial difference became a real issue for medical practitioners from this period onwards, when they were faced with "a sharper perception of superficial features, which was no doubt enhanced by the proximity of town life," and concomitantly a demand from urban elites (aristocratic and mercantile) for assistance in remedying conditions that would not have concerned country folk: red or pale skin, sun- or windburn, dark or ugly complexion, an excess or lack of hair or beard.[18] The next chapter will expand on the earlier types of treatment that might have been available for rather more serious disfigurements, but Demaitre's study centers on two issues. The first was the widening-out of a wealthy class able to pay doctors for cosmetic and other enhancements to their appearance, previously the preserve of a very narrow elite. The second, and pertinent to the current discussion, is the idea that town life, with its crowds, public spaces and frequent need to interact with others, led to "changes in sensitivity" about personal appearance. Clearly the conditions that are described here are some way along the spectrum from the disfigurements and injuries that have attracted our attention so far. Whilst largely accepting the economic factor Demaitre posits—there is little doubt that the link between material prosperity and "worried well" is not simply a modern phenomenon—I am troubled by the chronology he proposes.[19] After all, as we have seen, appearances in public assemblies, and proximity to observers, had been features of early medieval legislation regarding facial appearance, and translating Apuleius's *Herbarium* into Anglo-Saxon surely suggests that curing "uncouth blisters that sit on a man's *neb*" was not simply an intellectual exercise.[20] The change he identifies, however, relates as much to the increasing intensity of texts dealing with the surface of the body, as the rising and concentrated populations of towns. Moreover, the apparent triviality of some of the conditions he discusses suggests that people were scrutinizing *themselves* a lot more closely, a point that we shall return to.

## CASE STUDY: BYZANTINE STARING

This raises the question of how much staring was going on. Can we access the stare or the gaze in the medieval evidence? I want to use two Byzantine authors, Michael Psellos (d. c. 1078) and Anna Komnena (d. 1153), whose texts contain multiple examples of blindings and mutilation, to explore how their descriptions evoke a visual image in the reader's mind, and whether it is possible that any of the episodes were reported by eyewitnesses. Psellos is in fact a useful barometer, reflecting on the right and wrong times to use blinding and disfigurement, and his extended description of nose-cutting as a practice of the "Scythians," not of cultured, Byzantine society, reflects the theme of facial violence as done by Others.[21] Many of the examples he describes, however, evoke sympathy for the victims, most apparently in an extended episode in which he is a direct eyewitness.[22] The scene is the downfall of Emperor Michael V and the *nobilissimos* Constantine (brother of John Orphanotrophos), who sought refuge from the mob in the Studite monastery. Following them in, along with a baying mob, Psellos is greeted by the sight of the two fugitives hanging on for dear life to the altar, and he comments at length on how this pitiable sight moved him to tears rather than the anger he had felt at the men. At the same time, the threat from the mob outside remained, and Psellos builds the tension by adding: "I was fascinated by the drama of the thing."[23] The standoff in the church continues until a new officer comes with orders to remove the fugitives, promising that they will not be harmed. When they refuse, the sanctuary of the church is breached (illegally, as Psellos notes), and the crowd and officers drag the two fugitives outside "like wild beasts," heedless of their cries of anguish. Having set the story up as a drama, Psellos now switches the action back to the palace, where the fate of Michael and Constantine is being discussed. Finally, it is agreed that they present too much of a danger to be allowed to remain unscathed, but that killing them would be equally risky. A party of men is therefore sent to the monastery with orders to put out the fugitives' eyes, provided that this is done outside the church. Back at the church, of course, the victims are already outside and awaiting their fate, so the newcomers sharpen the branding-iron and prepare to do the deed. At this point "The emperor [Michael]... moaned and wailed aloud and... begged for help. He humbly called on God, raised hands in supplication to Heaven, to the Church, to anything he could think of." By contrast, his uncle remained silent,

> braced himself for the trial and... faced suffering bravely....Seeing the executioners all ready for their work, he at once offered himself as the first victim and calmly approached them. They waited with hands athirst for his blood. As there was no clear space between himself and the mob... the Nobilissimus quietly looked round for the man to whom the miserable job had been

entrusted. "You there," he said, "please make the people stand back. Then you will see how bravely I bear my calamity!"

When the executioner tried to tie him down, to prevent movement at the time of blinding, he said, "Look here, if you see me budge, *nail* me down!" With these words he lay flat on his back on the ground... His eyes were then gouged, one after the other.[24] Meanwhile the emperor, seeing in the other's torment the fate that was about to overtake him, too, lived through Constantine's anguish in himself, beating his hands together, smiting his face, and bellowing in agony. The Nobilissimus, his eyes gouged out, stood up from the ground and leaned for support on one of his most intimate friends... With Michael it was different, for when the executioner saw him flinch away and lower himself to base entreaty, he bound him securely. He held him down with considerable force, to stop the violent twitching when he was undergoing his punishment. After his eyes, too, had been blinded, the insolence of the mob, so marked before, died away, and with it their rage (θράσος) against these men. They left them to rest there...

Psellos's extended treatment of this blinding is occasioned by the fact that he was there throughout—he literally gives us a blow-by-blow account of the "drama" that he was fascinated by, as if compelled to continue watching.[25] Although ostensibly in a position of power as he watches the scene unfold, he is in fact rendered powerless and in tears by the anguish of the two victims. But there are other gazes at work here: the crowd pushing and struggling to be "the first witness of their punishment," Constantine's cool and direct address to the commander of the blinding party, the terrified Michael, watching his companion's mutilation and unable to mirror the older man's bravery, and finally the executioner, seeing the flinching man and forced to bind him securely in order to do his job (blinding, not killing) properly.

Anna Komnena's descriptions of the blindings and mutilations during her father's rise to power and his emperorship are both consistent in conveying the horror of such actions and yet curiously full of detail, providing for her readers a spectacle of punishment. Unswervingly loyal to her father's memory, she presents him as a man who "thought capture was punishment enough for an enemy," willing at times to threaten and even to simulate blindings as part of elaborate ruses to flush out traitors, but distanced (in her text at least) from those occasions when it was actually carried out.[26] For example the rebel Basilacius, captured by Alexius when he was still acting as Domestic of the *scholae*, was taken away *by the emperor's men* (my emphasis) to "some place called Chlempina, and near the spring of water there [they] put out his eyes (τους οφθαλμούς αυτού εξορύττουσιν). Ever since then to this day it has been called 'the spring of Basilacius.'"[27] The topographic detail calls to mind ritual sites of martyrdom, and may even convey ambivalence about the act itself. Anna is less convincing when she tries to remove her father from involvement in the blinding of the rebel Nicephorus Diogenes: Alexius spreads a rumor that Nicephorus had been secretly blinded, in order to dash his supporters' hopes. But then "certain men" blinded him and another conspirator anyway, and Anna remarks coyly that, "I have been unable so far to discover anything for certain" about whether Alexius ordered or consented to this.[28] As we shall see, however, she does give Nicephorus's story a happy ending, retired and apparently reconciled to his lack of sight.[29] A third blinding, of her husband's father Bryennius, is referred to only obliquely; she refers the reader to her husband's own history for the details, but repeatedly absolves Alexius of involvement.[30]

If Anna's Alexius was reluctant to blind, his repeated use of threat, rumor and simulation suggests nevertheless that—to Anna at least—resort to such tactics could be justified in times of war.[31] Anna's lengthy account of the feigned "blinding" of Roussel, early in her book, is graphic in its detail but also remarkably similar to Psellos's earlier set-piece account:

> The man was stretched out on the ground, the executioner brought the branding-iron (σίδηρον) near to his face, and Roussel howled and groaned; he was like a roaring lion. To all appearances he was being blinded. But in fact, the apparent victim had been ordered to shout and bawl; the executioner who seemed to be gouging out his eyes (εξορύττων again) was told to glare horribly at the prostrate Roussel and act like a raving madman – in other words, to simulate the punishment. So he was blinded (απετυφλοῦτο), but not in reality, and the people clapped their hands and noisily spread the news all over the city that Roussel had lost his eyes (την τοῦ Ουρσελίου τύφλωσιν).[32]

Note again the fact that this punishment is being carried out with an audience looking on—there would have been no point in pretending to blind Roussel in secret or private, since the object of the exercise is to convince the crowds of Alexius's authority. So convincing is the pantomime that even Alexius's cousin is fooled:

> [Dokeianos saw Roussel], "wearing the bandages, apparently blinded (τα της τυφλώσεως σύμβολα φέροντα, literally, "bearing the signs of blinding"),

and being led by the hand. He...accused my father of cruelty...[Alexius] took [Dokeianos] to a little room and there uncovered Roussel's head and disclosed his eyes, fiercely blazing. Dokeianos was astonished at the sight; the miracle filled him with wonder and amazement. Again and again he put his hands on Roussel's eyes... When he did learn of his cousin's humane treatment of the man and with his humanity his artifice, he was overcome with joy.[33]

Both accounts are so vivid that it is tempting to suggest they might even have been a favorite story of Anna's father. The description of the fake blinding builds atmosphere with its attention to both visual and auditory cues—the glowing hot iron, the glaring executioner, the roaring, bawling victim and the raving perpetrator, all contributing to imagining the scene. (Sounds had also featured heavily in Psellos's account, too—textual staring is clearly a multisensory experience.)[34] Yet Anna's literary skills derived as much from her reading and education as her imagination: the "big reveal" in front of Dokeianos owes more to hagiography than history—the removal of bandages, the "miracle" filling him with wonder, and the repeated physical touching of Roussel as evidence that yes, his eyes were indeed still intact. In both passages, the reader is immersed in an imbricated series of scenes and actions, all designed to impress with the guile of Alexius in the service of mercy. Witnessing the apparent horror of blinding, we are doubly relieved and impressed—as Dokeianos is—to find it has not taken place at all. But the sheer *fear* of blinding is convincingly displayed in both real and fake situations.

Anna is not done with us yet, however. She inserts her *own* gaze into the text when she recounts the humiliation of the rebel Michael Anemas and his brothers. Having been shaved completely, and their beards cut off, the rebels were mounted sideways on oxen, dressed in sackcloth, and "crowned" with entrails before being driven through the palace courtyard to their blinding. Attention was called to this spectacle by criers walking ahead, singing parodic songs (an inversion of the praises of the emperors), and

> People of all ages hurried to see the show; we too, the princesses, came out for the same purpose secretly...[35].

As Michael gestures toward the palace that he would rather be dismembered and beheaded, however, Anna is overcome with pity and begs her mother, the empress, to intercede, thereby saving Michael's sight.

The elaborate visual and auditory spectacle laid on for the "people" is not meant to be witnessed by the princesses—hence their secrecy in coming out to watch. Whether Anna's memory of the event and her part in it is credible, it is clear that she wants the reader to see the spectacle through her younger eyes, and to be as distressed as she was by Michael's pleading gaze.[36] (Again, there is a strong parallel with Michael Psellos's own feelings of pity for the victims.) The parading of a traitor through the Agora is repeated soon afterwards in another case, but Alexius only "pretended he wished to blind Gregory," settling instead for his hair and beard to be "shaved to the skin" before displaying him.[37] The public parading of enemies and criminals, of course, was nothing new: there are plenty of earlier examples (including the exhibition of the antipope Pope John XVI),[38] and so when the educated Anna was looking for inspiration for her reports, it is not unlikely that she found examples to imitate.

Such set-piece narratives are not just part of Byzantine writing in the twelfth century, however: Orderic Vitalis similarly ramps up the tension in his account of King Henry I of England's condemnation of Luke of La Barre, found guilty of spreading scurrilous songs about the king, to blinding. Here, others spring to Luke's defense, but to no avail. Luke, who "knew that he was condemned to everlasting darkness in this life" and chose instead to die, then

> struggled desperately to injure himself as the officers pinioned him. Finally, beating his head like a madman on the walls and stones as they held him, he perished miserably, greatly mourned by all who knew his valour and merry jests.[39]

The two accounts differ in their outcome: Henry I's failure to be merciful toward Luke of La Barre (and to two knights captured and blinded at the same time) leads to all three being memorialized by Orderic, Luke himself preferring suicide, and the king being presented as unjustly harsh (though Orderic never says so directly). Michael, on the other hand, is spared by Alexius Comnenus on the special pleading of his wife and daughter. For Anna, in fact, her father was almost uniformly merciful when it came to blinding and mutilation: regardless of accuracy (and she admits at one point that she will be accused of favoring her father) her text makes it clear that these are things Others do—the Norman leader Robert Guiscard and his son Bohemond are seen cruelly mutilating to extort money, and blinding or threatening to blind their opponents; she also reports on Alexius and his brother being faced with a plot to "get rid of them by gouging out their eyes on a trumped-up charge;" and, by far the most bizarre, the blinding inflicted on the Sultan of Iconium, Malik-Shah, by the Turks working for his brother, Mas'ud:

> As the instrument normally used for the purpose was lacking, the candela-brum given to Malik-Shah by the emperor took its place—the diffuser of light had become the instrument of darkness and blinding. However, he could still see a small ray of light and when he arrived at Iconium, led by the hand of some guide, he confided this fact to his nurse and she told his wife. In this way the story reached the ears of Mas'ud himself.[40]

Malik-Shah is swiftly eliminated by strangling on his brother's orders.

The Byzantine texts, in fact, mirror a wider development visible in narrative sources in the eleventh, and particularly the twelfth century, that increasingly associates disfigurement and mutilation with injustice or the actions of strangers and enemies. Just as being disfigured risked marginalizing a person, so *inflicting* disfigurement came to be a sign of alterity. It is notable that the examples of deliberate blinding in Abbot Guibert of Nogent's autobiography are carried out by Bishop Gaudry of Laon's "African man" and by Alais, mother of John of Soissons, already discussed.[41] And Guibert notes that the vicious mutilations of eyes and feet that accompanied a dispute between Godfrey of Namur and Enguerrand of Boves left a visible legacy, "as is plainly apparent today to anyone visiting the county of Porcien."[42] Was Guibert staring as intensely as his Byzantine contemporaries? He certainly noticed facial difference: reporting the murder of Gérard of Quierzy, he notes that Gérard had only one eye to turn round on his assailant, and he discusses at length the murder of Bishop Gaudry, the mutilation of his body, and the means used to recognize him (a scar on his neck) when his face was so badly disfigured.[43]

Like Orderic Vitalis, Guibert also recounts stories of disfigurement linked to the supernatural, although the facial injury visible in Guibert's tale of a "benign and simple" monastic novice is somewhat more prosaic than Orderic's story of Walchelin. The novice was pursued by the devil while answering the call of nature and injured his forehead against the privy door: the devil was able to injure his body, Guibert comments, but powerless against the monk's purity of soul.[44]

## DEPICTING DISFIGUREMENT: ICONOGRAPHIC CHALLENGES.

Medieval texts describe, and allow readers to stare figuratively at, the scenes of disfigurement and mutilation they recount. The ubiquity of modern images of people with disfigurements, across the internet and print culture, in collections such as Wellcome Images, as well as in specifically-commissioned projects such as that sponsored by the *Saving Faces* charity, allows for staring and contemplation at one remove from the reality of scarred flesh or missing facial features.[45] Yet in early medieval iconography the actual *appearance* of people is rarely explored in detail. Even depictions of prominent figures, such as those depicted in the bible of the Carolingian Emperor Charles the Bald at S. Paolo fuori le Mure in Rome, or the series of portraits of early Lombard rulers (including the Franks Pippin the Short, Louis the Pious and Lothar I, and Princes Arechis and Adelchis of the Lombards) on the eleventh-century *Codex Legum Langobardorum* at the abbey of Cava near Salerno in Italy, are all facially alike, presented bearded, red-cheeked, furrow-browed in seriousness and, of course, unblemished. Paul Edward Dutton in fact comments specifically on the "fusion" of identities present in the richly decorated bible, with the Charles medallion perhaps representing Charlemagne, or Charles the Bald, or intentionally fusing both men with the biblical King David.[46] The German abbess Herrad of Landsberg's famous series of portraits of her fellow nuns in her twelfth-century text the *Garden of Delights*, similarly, presents a largely undifferentiated series of faces, for all that the sisters are labeled with names to identify them.[47] This reluctance to depict reality is matched by the sheer reticence of medieval iconography before about 1250 to engage with the disfigured face. Mutilated or impaired bodies do occasionally feature in medieval images, especially of the blind and the lame, complete with crutches or other mobility aids. But the maimed face remains elusive. Why? Willibald Sauerländer suggests that:

> ...from the time of Charlemagne (r. as emperor 800–814) to the days of Dante (1265–1321) we encounter not a single portrait in the modern sense... Like nature, the natural face was considered unworthy of transmission to posterity. The soul would be raised to heaven...but flesh and bones... would turn to dust and ashes, and thus the earthly faces of mortals were not remembered in portraiture.[48]

We have met this sentiment before, in Thietmar's remarks about his own face. He tells us what it looks like, but dismisses his appearance as unimportant compared to the purity of his soul. Early medieval iconography, seemingly, has little to contribute to our knowledge of how people really appeared, in their depictions of the uninjured or the afflicted. Andre Grabar and Carl Nordenfalk offer some explanations: after the achievements of late Roman portraiture, Merovingian art, they suggest, reflected the iconoclastic distaste for depictions of the human figure altogether; paintings of the Carolingian period, by contrast, focused on the pedagogical theme of Christ's life on earth. The Charles the Bald bible, with its illustrative material, simply reflects and extends the concern of medieval clerical writers to situate their accounts within a Christian, biblical framework of understanding. Only occasionally do we meet anything approaching a "portrait," such as that of the priestly donor in the ninth-century decoration of the church of S. Benedetto Malles near Bolzano, Italy. Even donor portraits have their problems, not least in examples of twelfth-century "retrospective" paintings and depictions of much earlier donors, a parallel of this period's intense interest in re-asserting claims to property through the editing and outright creation of early donation charters into cartularies.[49] Otherwise, the theme of painting and book illumination was entirely religious and generic. There are depictions of those healed by Christ, so we do have some impairments illustrated in rudimentary ways, but the only really distorted facial features are those of devils in hell.[50]

Images were not totally without meaning of course—even the generic, stern-faced king-portraits in the Cava manuscript were designed to convey authority alongside the legal material copied there, whilst the internal unity of Herrad's community was emphasized by its iconographic uniformity. And the power of images was certainly expressed when people took the trouble to destroy or obliterate them, as occurred during the two waves of iconoclasm—the destruction of holy images—in the Byzantine Empire in the eighth and ninth centuries This, though, was not the same as the defacing of ruler portraits: the iconoclasts expressed opposition to a belief in the power of images as intercessors with God, whilst removing the faces of ruler portraits was a targeted attack on items associated with the deposed or disgraced ruler. Yet it is notable that the faces *were* removed, rather than disfigured: all memory of that person was to be erased. Thus when Empress Zoe was exiled and had her hair cut, the portrait of her in Hagia Sophia, Constantinople, was also removed. When she was restored, so was her portrait.[51]

The stained glass windows at Canterbury cathedral, depicting some of the miracles of Thomas Becket, include the episode of the blinding, castration and subsequent restoration of Ailward of Westoning. Yet, despite one of the panels showing the actual moment of the attack, the artists clearly decided not to portray Ailward after the deed, instead halting at precisely the moment he is looking up at his assailants, bearing down on him with a sharpened implement.[52] Again, just as in textual accounts, the viewer is left to visualize for him- or herself the aftermath of the mutilation.

## SEEING, LOOKING AND SELFHOOD

Clearly, being deprived of sight by violence was a terrifying ordeal, and it excited the curiosity and pity of those who wrote about it. Moreover, as the story of Malik-Shah illustrates, the process of blinding could be botched, leaving partial sight, and there was always the risk that gouging too far could compromise the intended "mercy" of preserving the life of the victim.[53] Yet Garland-Thomson remarks that the "ocularcentric" modern world underestimates "the advantages of blindness, such as being able to navigate without artificial light or engaging fully with other senses such as touch and smell."[54] This sentiment is nicely illustrated by two stories recounted by Gerald of Wales in the twelfth century. One concerns a prisoner at Chateauroux whose eyes had been put out. "From long familiarity with them [he] had committed to memory all the passageways of the castle and even the steps which led up to the towers," and used this knowledge to take hostage the son of the castellan.[55] Here the rehabilitative intention in the blinding clearly had not had any effect. The castellan of Radnor castle, by contrast, having impiously spent the night with his dogs in the church of St Afon and awoken to find himself blind and his dogs mad, initially "passed his days in tedium and distress," before making a pilgrimage to Jerusalem and dying in battle there, so ending his life "with honor."[56] This apparent rehabilitation, of course, is in response to a supernatural event, but as we shall see there are cases of blinding victims who are portrayed as overcoming their pain and sightlessness to pursue other avenues to fulfillment.

The textual staring apparent in some of the extracts presented here highlights the power of sight and the intensity of the stare or gaze. Eyes are, after all, not only able to take in the world, but are also the key to communication with others. As Miller points out, if eyes can give offence by staring for too long, they can also ward off with a glare: "they tell the intruder to back off."[57] This, though, assumes that the person being stared at was capable of returning the look, and this was by no means universally the case in medieval society. In particular, tropes of modesty surrounding women demanded that they kept their eyes cast down before men.[58]

We have already noted that blocking a woman's or girl's way (*wegwo-rin*) attracted a penalty in Frankish and Lombard laws.[59] But what was at stake here? This group of laws has usually been treated as one of a set that envisages, and prohibits, the intrusion of men into the inviolable space occupied by a woman's body.[60] Whilst some laws explore this intrusion literally—violating the spatial boundary by touching the hand, arm or breast, bursting into a house and illegally cutting a woman's hair, abducting her, engaging in sex—way-blocking, it seems to me, operates somewhat differently, and is inextricably bound up with ways of seeing and looking. Several possibilities offer themselves: blocking a woman's way was an inherently threatening act even without touch;[61] blocking a woman's way forced her off a path or road and caused physical discomfort if it involved treading in mud or dirt (assuming that the track itself was recognizably drier or smoother than its edges); or blocking a woman's way involved engineering bumping into her, thereby bringing about a moment of illicit physical contiguity. But this last scenario assumes that *she is not looking where she is going*, that is, that her gaze is a modest one, directed to the ground, not to what lies ahead of her. Did the woman who *was* looking where she was going indirectly challenge men to get in her way? Such is the double standard still employed in asking women to modify their behavior to avoid unwanted male attention.[62]

Much of the early medieval material on representations of disfigurement feature reports of those who were staring at the facially-different person, but what about the man or woman in the mirror? To what extent was staring at oneself even possible in the early Middle Ages? Demaitre's point about townsmen and women becoming more self-conscious of their looks suggests that another phenomenon was taking place. The "discovery of the individual" in the eleventh and twelfth centuries, long-argued by historians from Colin Morris onwards, may not only have included a heightened awareness of social, religious or even racial difference, but also a more constant scrutiny of one's own looks.[63] Certainly we have plenty of later medieval examples not only of iconography featuring mirrors, but also extant examples of mirrors themselves, which had made the transition from polished metal to worked glass in western Europe by the twelfth century.[64] Since the latter would have been a luxury item (the technology of glassmaking being jealously guarded by the artisans of Venice and regulated by the city authorities), part of the veritable boom in consumer goods in medieval towns, there may be a very strong correlation between the chronology of mirror consumption in the thirteenth and fourteenth centuries and the demand for cosmetics and cures identified by Demaitre. Yet this is clearly an elite phenomenon, and whilst evidence survives for the use of mirrors before 1200 (particularly in Muslim Spain), the kind of self-scrutiny portrayed in later medieval texts and iconography does not appear to have been a feature of early medieval culture. It might be objected that anyone could look at himself or herself in a pool of still water, that mirrors were not necessary for an individual to realize he or she looked different. This is certainly true, but if the overwhelming message preached in the churches was of the ephemerality of the flesh and a criticism of vanity, then looking at oneself, facially whole or not, may have been a less obsessive pastime than it is in modern culture. Moreover, the quality of metal and early glass mirrors possibly distorted the reflection so much that there was really little purpose in looking.

We have met textual staring as a phenomenon, encouraging the reader to contemplate and become involved with vivid scenes of other people's suffering. And texts functioned too as a way to encourage readers, particularly those in power, to consider their own behaviors, the so-called "mirrors-for-princes" literature.[65] Mirror metaphors, in fact, were utilized early by church fathers to express the idea of divine wisdom—if Man was made in God's image, then a perfect life would represent a perfect mirror of God.[66]

And if this were true, then fleshly deformity of any kind *did not matter*. After all, the doctrine of heavenly resurrection promised a new start, free of impairments.[67] This, I believe, is why so many of the narrative accounts of disfigurements and mutilations focus on the *process* of disfigurement rather than its result, and do so often at some length, involving the reader in a shared spectacle. Stories of disfigurement and mutilation recounted by medieval authors, bound up as they often are with ideas of morality and justice, are making of disfigured people's faces a mirror of broader *mores* and acceptable or illicit actions. Returning to William Ian Miller's point with which we started, I suggest that any disgust that onlookers felt was centered around the cruelty of disfigurement, not its results. They are commenting on extremes of behavior, working out at what point it is morally wrong to inflict a permanent scar. Legislators are doing the same

thing, and claiming the authority to engage in similar actions, but here
the textual stare is often about how the victim is affected by an illegal
injury, hence the detailed scrutiny and description of pieces of bone, effu-
sions of blood and lasting impairments. A changed face—even a temporarily changed face—signals a breakdown in social relations. A permanently
changed face might require the intervention of the saint if it was unjustifi-
ably changed by the excess force of a powerful perpetrator. If Henry I ever
stopped to stare at those whom he had ordered blinded, did he feel any
remorse for his actions? Perhaps not, but his order to blind is held up to
the reader as one of many examples *not* to follow. One of the main horrors
of disfiguring acts in the early Middle Ages, we might suggest, was the fact
that many *were* so permanent, not amenable to any kind of rehabilitative
treatment. Yet ambivalence remained: a disfigured face could be a lesson
in humility and ultimate salvation. Medical treatment, then, risked going
against God's will (hagiography certainly underlines this). But the early
medieval period was not entirely without recourse to care and rehabilitation, as the next chapter will illustrate.

## NOTES

1. Notker, *Gesta Karoli*, I.18, ed. H. Haefele, *MGH SS rer. Ger. n.s,*
   XII, (Berlin: Weidmann, 1959); Einhard and Notker the
   Stammerer, *Two Lives of Charlemagne*, tr. L. Thorpe (London:
   Penguin, 1969), 111.
2. William Ian Miller, *The Anatomy of Disgust* (Cambridge, MA:
   Harvard University Press, 1997), 19.
3. *Ibid.*, 200.
4. Rosemarie Garland-Thomson, *Staring: How We Look* (Oxford:
   Oxford University Press, 2009), 3. I am grateful to Edward
   Wheatley for pointing me towards Garland-Thomson's work.
5. Garland-Thomson, *Staring*, 33. For her historical perspective,
   Garland-Thomson relies rather uncritically on Lyn H. Lofland, *A
   World of Strangers: Order and Action in Urban Public Space* (New
   York: Basic Books, 1973), which itself seems to make sweeping
   assumptions about the medieval and early modern worlds.
6. *Staring*, 3.
7. The classic case is of course the sixteenth-century story told in
   Natalie Zemon Davies, *The Return of Martin Guerre* (Cambridge,
   MA: Harvard University Press, 1984). See also her "Remaking

impostors: from Martin Guerre to Sommersby," *Hayes Robinson Lecture Series*, 1 (Egham: Royal Holloway University of London, 1997). The transition between community-based recognition and state-controlled documentation is traced by Valentin Groebner, *Who Are You? Identification, Deception and Surveillance in Early Modern Europe* (New York: Zone Books, 2007).

8. William Ian Miller, *Eye for an Eye* (Cambridge: Cambridge University Press, 2006), 101.

9. Garland-Thomson's "baroque staring", described as "shamelessly stimulus-driven, flagrant, open-mouthed, unapologetic... urgent": *Staring*, 50. Miller, *Anatomy of Disgust*, 196, expresses something of the same phenomenon in the "double disgust" felt by observers of cruelty – first, disgust at the perpetrator, then disgust and horror at the sight of the "degraded victim, whether bloody or disfigured."

10. On prurience and saintly torture, see Martha Easton, "Pain, torture and death in the Huntingdon Library *Legenda aurea*," in *Gender and Holiness: Men, Women and Saints in Late Medieval Europe*, ed. Sam Riches and Sarah Salih (London: Routledge, 2005), 49–64. Extended contemplation of images of such martyrdom was, of course, increasingly central to affective, devotional activity in the later medieval period.

11. *GT*, IX.9. The motif of stretching over a doorsill recurs in *Theophanis Chronographia*, AM6203/710–11 CE, ed. C. de Boor, 2 vols (Hildesheim: Georg Olms, 1963), when Justinian II's son Tiberius is killed in the same way.

12. Miller, *Eye for an Eye*, 58.

13. Garland-Thomson, *Staring*, 9 (quote), 28 (Foucault) and 41 (gender, citing Laura Mulvey, *Visual and Other Pleasures: Theories of Representation and Difference* (Bloomington: Indiana University Press, 1989)).

14. Miller, *Anatomy of Disgust*, 82.

15. James Partridge, *Changing Faces: the Challenge of Facial Disfigurement* (London: Penguin, 1990), 89–90.

16. Gerald of Wales, *The Journey through Wales*, II.7, tr. L. Thorpe (London: Penguin, 1978), 190–1.

17. Garland-Thomson, *Staring*, 51.

18. Luke Demaitre, "Skin and the city: cosmetic medicine as an urban concern," in *Between Text and Patient: The Medical Enterprise in Medieval and Early Modern Europe*, ed. Florence Eliza Glaze and Brian K. Nance (Florence: SISMEL-Edizioni del Galluzzo, 2011), 97–120, at 110.

19. "Worried well" has taken root in both media and clinical reports, as the numerous online articles and 33 specific title entries on the PubMed database attest.

20. *Leechdoms, Wortcunning and Starcraft of Early England*, 3 vols, ed. O. Cockayne (London: Longmans Green, 1864, 1865 and 1866), I, 87. Cockayne translated *neb* as "face." "Complexion" is an alternative here.

21. For his account, see above, Chap. 3.

22. The following translated excerpts are drawn from *Fourteen Byzantine Rulers: the* Chronographia *of Michael Psellos*, tr. E. R. A. Sewter (London: Penguin, 1979), V.40–50, 145–151.

23. Greek: καὶ την γε σκηνήν απέθαύμαζου: Michele Psello, *Imperatori di Bisanzio (Cronografia)*, ed. and tr. Salvatore Impellizari, Ugo Criscuolo and Siliva Ronchey, 2 vols (Milan: Fondazione Lorenzo Valla/Mondadori, 1984), I, 234.

24. Τω μεν ουν κατά μέρος οι οφθαλμοι διεκόπτοντο: Michele Psello, *Imperatori*, 240.

25. Garland-Thomson, *Staring*, 27, points out that "fascination" is etymologically linked to the Latin for being "bewitched" or caught in the evil eye.

26. Anna Comnène, *Alexiade*, I.6, ed. and tr. Bernard Leib, 3 vols (Paris: Les Belles Lettres, 1967) [hereafter *Alexiad*]. English translations throughout from Anna Komnena, *Alexiad*, tr. E. R. A. Sewter (London: Penguin, 1969) [hereafter Sewter], here at 45.

27. *Alexiad*, I.9 (Sewter, 52). Greek: *Alexiade*, ed. Leib, I, 36.

28. *Alexiad*, IX.9 (Sewter, 289).

29. Below, Chap. 7.

30. *Alexiad*, I.7: Alexius hands Bryennius over to Borilos, envoy of the emperor, who "did what he did": Sewter, 46; VII.2 Alexius "handed [him] over to Borilos with his sight undamaged": Sewter, 219.

31. Threat: *Alexiad* XII.8: Isaac Contostephanos sent to intercept the Norman leader Bohemond at Dyrrhachium with the threat that his eyes would be gouged if he failed to arrive there before Bohemond crossed the Adriatic. Rumor: the case of Nicephorus Diogenes, already discussed. Simulation: the case of Roussel, discussed here, and of Alakaseos, who pretended to have been mistreated by the emperor to flush out another traitor: *Alexiad*, X.4.

32. *Alexiad* I.3 (Sewter, 36). Greek: *Alexiade*, I, 15.

33. *Alexiad* I.4 (Sewter, 37). Greek: *Alexiade*, I, 16.

34. William Ian Miller, *Humiliation and Other Essays on Honor, Social Discomfort and Violence* (Ithaca/London: Cornell University Press, 1998), 66, comments that noise functions as part of the sign system of pain, where groans and screams replace words.

35. *Alexiad*, XII.6, (Sewter, 384–5); τὸν δε Ανεμαν καὶ τοὺς σὺν αυτῶ ὡς προταιτὶους καὶ την εν χρω κουραν της κεφαλῆς καὶ τοῦ πώγωνος ψιλώσας δια μεσης πομπεύσαι της αγοράς παρεκελεύσατο, είτα εξορυχθῆναι τοὺς οφθαλμούς: *Alexiade*, III, 72–3.

36. The power of face-to-face looking between victim and spectator, Garland-Thomson comments, led to the hooding of those going to execution from the seventeenth century onwards: *Staring*, 54.

37. *Alexiad*, XII.8 (Sewter, 388); ...την εν χρω κουρειαν κειραμένου την κεφαλήν τε καὶ του πώγωνα: *Alexiade*, III, 77.

38. Above, Chap. 3.

39. *Orderic*, XII.39 (VI, 352–6).

40. *Alexiad* I.11 and V.5 (Robert); XI.10 (Bohemond); II.4 (threat to Alexius); XV.6 (Malik-Shah, Sewter, 490–1).

41. *Self and Society in Medieval France: the Memoirs of Abbot Guibert of Nogent*, II.7, ed. and tr. John Benton (New York: Harper, 1970), 170 (African). For Alais see above, Chap. 5.

42. *Self and Society*, II.3, 150.

43. *Self and Society*, III.5, 159 (Gérard), 8 and 9, 176 and 181 (Gaudry).

44. *Self and Society*, II.5, 137–8.

45. http://savingfaces.co.uk/news-media/art-project/35-news-media/art/15-art-exhibition [Accessed 12 July 2015].

46. Bible: Andre Grabar and Carl Nordenfalk, *Early Medieval Painting* (Paris: Skira, 1957), 153. Most of the Lombard portraits are available to view on the Getty Images website: www.getty.co.uk [accessed 11 April 2015]. Paul Edward Dutton and Herbert Kessler, *The Poetry and Paintings of the First Bible of Charles the Bald* (Ann Arbor: University of Michigan Press, 1997), 43.

47. Moreover, the names allow for identification of some of the women: Fiona Griffiths, *The Garden of Delights: Reform and Renaissance for Women in the Twelfth Century* (Philadelphia: University of Pennsylvania Press, 2006), 28.

48. Willibald Sauerländer, "The fate of the face in medieval art," in *Set in Stone: the Face in Medieval Sculpture*, ed. C. T. Little (New York: Metropolitan Museum, 2006), 3–17, at 3–4.

49. Retrospective portraits of Charlemagne as donor are visible, for example, twelfth-century decorative schemes: Thomas E. A. Dale, *Relics, Prayer and Politics in Medieval Venetia: Romanesque Painting in the Crypt of Aquileia Cathedral* (Princeton: Princeton University Press, 1997), 40–41.

50. Grabar and Nordenfalk, *Early Medieval Painting*, 58 (portrait), 126 (Merovingians), 17 (Carolingians) and 56 and 79 (Christ healing).

51. Carolyn L. Connor, *Women of Byzantium* (New Haven: Yale University Press, 2004), 236.

52. Canterbury Cathedral, Trinity Chapel, North Aisle, North Window, panels 16–19.

53. *Gesta Guillelmi of William of Poitiers*, I.3, ed. and trans. R. H. C. Davis and M. Chibnall (Oxford: Clarendon Press, 1998), reports that the attempted blinding of Alfred, son of Aethelred, in 1036 with a knife went wrong, damaging his brain and thus killing him.

54. Garland-Thomson, *Staring*, 25–6.

55. *The Journey through Wales*, I.11, tr. Thorpe, 142–3.

56. *ibid.*, I.1, tr. Thorpe, 77–8.

57. *Eye for an Eye*, 136.

58. Sarah Alison Miller, *Medieval Monstrosity and the Female Body* (London: Routledge, 2010), explores the longevity of this theme from the Church Fathers to the *De Secretis Mulierum* of the late-thirteenth/early-fourteenth century.

59. *Pactus Legis Salicae*, XXXI.2, ed. K. Eckhardt, *MGH LL nat. Germ.*, IV.1 (Hannover: Hahn, 1962), 121; *Lex Salica*, XXXVIII.2, ed. K. Eckhardt, *MGH LL nat. Germ.*, IV.2 (Hannover: Hahn, 1959), 215; *Leges Langobardorum*, Rothari 26 and 171, ed. F. Bluhme in *MGH LL*, IV, ed. G. H. Pertz (Hannover: Hahn, 1868),17 and 86.
60. See above, Chap. 5, for more on this "jurisdictional space."
61. For a modern presentation of way-blocking a young woman, compare the dark [and threatening] spatial dynamics in the pop video for Michael Jackson's "The Way You Make Me Feel," (dir. J. Pytka, 1987), contrasting markedly with the breezy tone and lyrics of the song itself.
62. See the brief controversy over the now-withdrawn rape awareness campaign by Sussex Police in the UK to encourage groups of women on a night out not to "leave their mate behind": http://www.bbc.co.uk/news/uk-england-sussex-32255606, accessed 11 April 2015.
63. Colin Morris, *The Discovery of the Individual, 1050–1200* (New York and London: Harper and Row, 1972).
64. Mark Pendergast, *Mirror, Mirror: A History of the Human Love Affair with Reflection* (New York: Basic Books, 2003), 117–118.
65. The literature on these texts is extensive: Herbert Grabes, *The Mutable Glass: Mirror-Imagery in Titles and Texts of the Middle Ages and English Renaissance* (Cambridge: Cambridge University Press, 1982); *Le prince au miroir de la littérature politique de l'Antiquité aux Lumières*, ed. F. Lachaud and L. Scordia (Rouen: Publications des universités de Rouen et du Havre, 2007), especially Rachel Stone, "Kings are different: Carolingian mirrors for princes and lay morality," 69–86; Linda Darling, "Mirrors for princes in Europe and the Middle East: a case of historiographical incommensurability," in *East Meets West in the Middle Ages and Early Modern Times: Transcultural Experiences in the Premodern World*, ed. A. Classen (Berlin: DeGruyter, 2013), 223–242.
66. Pendergast, *Mirror Mirror*, 120–121, discusses some early examples of ecclesiastical texts using this image.
67. I am grateful to Kristi Upson-Saia for advice on this point. See her "Resurrecting deformity: Augustine on wounded and scarred bodies in the heavenly realm", in *Disability in Judaism, Christianity,*

*and Islam: Sacred Texts, Historical Traditions, and Social Analysis,* ed. Darla Schumm and Michael Stoltzfus (New York: Palgrave Macmillan, 2011), 93–122; Candida Moss, "Heavenly healing: eschatological cleansing and the resurrection of the dead in the holy church," *Journal of the American Academy of Religion,* 79 (2011): 991–1017. Caroline Walker Bynum, *The Resurrection of the Body* (New York: Columbia University Press, 1995), 116, highlights that the mosaic of the Last Judgment at Torcello Cathedral near Venice depicts only the blessed rising whole, whilst the damned "are shown in a state of fragmentation that is a symbolic expression of their sins."

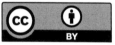

CHAPTER 7

# Paths to Rehabilitation? The Possibilities of Treatment

As previous chapters have established, heads and faces might be deliberately targeted in cases of injury; marking of the head and face formed
part and parcel of many legal sanctions against thieves, traitors and sexu-
ally transgressive men and women, but almost all early medieval lawcodes
penalized similar interpersonal violence. Facial and head wounds opened
a person to stigma and ridicule, and honor was bound up in facial appearance, women's faces were a site of particular meaning, and episodes of
mutilation and disfigurement were sometimes written up as if staring at
the process and its aftermath, even if the author were not there to witness the actual deed. Whilst clerics argued that the flesh was less important than the spirit in the life to come, fleshly considerations were still
important to social status among the secular elite in this life. It is relatively
safe to assume, therefore, that if anything *could* be done to improve the
appearance of an injured or disfigured face, recourse might be had to the
appropriate persons. Otherwise, as we have seen, the main option was to
conceal the injury as far as possible. This chapter, therefore, will explore
the possibilities, in some specific cases of head and facial injury, for treatment and/or rehabilitation. Before doing so, however, it is important to
try and establish the nature of medical and surgical knowledge in early
medieval Europe, in order to provide a broader context for the few cases
that have survived in the evidence.

---

This chapter began life at the Leeds International Medieval Congresses in 2013
and 2014, where it benefited from the insights of varied audiences.

© The Author(s) 2017
P. Skinner, *Living with Disfigurement in Early Medieval Europe*,
DOI 10.1057/978-1-137-54439-1_7

## LOOKING FOR EARLY MEDIEVAL SURGERY: A NEEDLE IN A HAYSTACK?

The early Middle Ages have not been considered a high point of medical knowledge or practice, nor does this chapter claim to offer a wholesale or comprehensive revision of existing scholarship. What is at issue here is the limiting force of older views such as Stanley Rubin's comment at a colloquium in 1986 that practitioners in Anglo-Saxon England "learnt their skills on a trial and error basis," and that "Their practice was an amalgam of empirical herbal techniques, Classical precedent and philosophy, ritual incantations with a very strong superstitious overlay, plus a very basic form of faith healing. *Yet even among all this worthless matter a whisper of rational expertise can be determined*" [my emphasis].[1] Sean McGlynn, too, seems to accept older views of medical expertise in the early Middle Ages when he comments that "the lack of medicinal knowledge and good practice could make even a minor wound potentially dangerous."[2] Peregrine Horden is less judgmental at least, but comments that our knowledge of medical practice pre-1200 is "all mutability," that is, there is no over-arching scheme to mirror later scholastic medicine, but early medieval medicine "is, to some extent, ancient medicine (e.g. Dioscurides) continued by other means."[3] The major problem dogging the study of early medieval medicine, however, is hindsight—all of these authors know what happened in the twelfth and thirteenth centuries, when ancient texts and "rationality" were restored to Western medical practice after a long hiatus. But whilst the period c.400–c.1100 in Western Europe clearly did see a comparative dip in scholarly activity around medical knowledge, this does not mean that medical practice was therefore in some way "inferior."[4]

An example of such ancient knowledge was excerpted and collected, and is visible in three *receptaria* preserved in the monastic archives of St Gall and Bamberg. Published by Julius Jörimann in 1925, two (which I shall term *St Gall A* and *B*) are preserved (one incompletely) in *Codex Sangallensis* 44, a ninth-century collection written in Carolingian miniscule, and the third in Bamberg, dating to the tenth century and written in fine book hand. The Bamberg codex shares some common material with the earlier part (i.e. before the section with the recipe books) of the *Codex Sangallensis*.[5] Jörimann suggests that these collections contain remedies for the use not of a "professional" doctor, but a monk with medical skills who could apply the recipes to his brethren in the cloister.[6] His comment again reveals the explicit devaluing of practitioners vs. professionals in early medical history, but if these collections were indeed for actual use, the inclusion, in two out of the three, of gynecological recipes suggests that the copying and excerpting were not entirely shaped by likely patients.

What is interesting about the texts, however, is the apparent concern for personal appearance that emerges from them. Arranged in a head-to-toe order, *St Gall A* contains remedies for stains (*maculas*) in the eyes, head injuries and injured noses (*nares vulnerosas*), lesions near the eyes and nose and pustules. *St Gall B*, whilst incomplete, adds remedies for scurf, lice and fleas in the hair, eyes that have been hit/injured (*ad percussum oculum*) and chapped lips and face in the winter. Bamberg addresses baldness, alopecia and scurf, and has a recipe to remove stains on the face. There are parallels here with the Anglo-Saxon leech books, which Rubin long ago suggested demonstrated a high concern for personal appearance.[7] These medical texts, at the very least, *theorized* what to do to improve facial appearance: there are numerous remedies found in the Anglo-Saxon *Leechbook* for pustules, ulcers and blotches on the face, as well as for loss of hair. Perhaps most surprising of all is a surgical procedure for the correction of disfigurement caused by a hare lip:

> For hare lip: pound mastic very small, add the white of an egg and mingle as thou dust vermilion, cut with a knife the false edges of the lip, sew fast with silk, then smear without and within the salve, ere the silk rot. If it draw together, arrange it with the hand; anoint again soon.[8]

That the copyist of the *Leechbook* included surgery such as this may be linked to the likelihood that any such operation would have been carried out on an infant or young child. A risky action, perhaps, but if it succeeded, it might assist the child to attain full social adulthood, particularly if it also ameliorated any speech impairment caused by the condition.[9] Throughout the book our attention has been drawn to the fact that the writers of early medieval narratives and law codes cared about, observed and imputed meaning to facial appearance. Whether or not the *Leechbooks* and continental medical texts represent evidence of medical practice is rather less important than the fact that they correspond, in their ideas about the face, with other sources. Gariopontus' revolutionary head-to-toe *Passionarius* was known in England by the end of the eleventh century, and extracts were also copied into the Old English translation of the *Peri Didaxeon*.[10] Despite the obvious scholarly interest in such texts, we should not discount the possibility that some remedies and procedures were actually tried out.[11] Early medieval *non-medical* sources, such narrative texts, laws and archaeology, after all, point to a rather more sophisticated medical—and surgical—environment than has previously been credited in the early medieval period.

Medicine and surgery have been understood and studied as almost separate areas of care. Surgery had a long history, from antiquity,[12] of being viewed as a separate, practical—and subject—branch of medicine. The distinction seems to have disappeared in early medieval Western Europe, judging by examples to be discussed below, but persisted in areas of Muslim rule, where the inheritance of antiquity was far more direct. The difference between the two fields is expressed most clearly in texts such as that of the Egyptian physician Ibn Ridwan (d.1068), who commented:

> I divide the teaching of medicine into two parts: one is theory, which is to be studied either from the books of Hippocrates or those of Galen... The other is practice, by which I mean the study of bone-setting, the restoration of dislocations, incision, suturing, cautery, lancing, eye remedies and all other manual procedures.[13]

Put simply then, surgery was conceived as the care of the external body, a response to trauma, wounding, or the visible lesions caused by disease. The knowledge required to do this effectively might vary between practitioners, and there were certainly, in the Muslim world, texts instructing the surgeon, but the overarching framework for understanding early medieval surgery in Western Europe before c.1200 is as a practical skill, rather than a theorized vocation. The description of surgical procedure on view in *Bald's Leechbook*, for example, does not link it in any way to the general health of the person being operated on. But this text is exceptional in many ways, both in terms of its content and the level of scrutiny it has received from historians.[14] In fact, early medieval European medical texts more usually feature lists of remedies, rather than the surgical procedures that are included in Bald. Rubin concedes that "even in Anglo-Saxon times there was some form of medical education."[15] And as we shall see, the early medieval doctor was expected to be a general practitioner of sorts, skilled in all aspects rather than specializing in one.

The distinction between medicine and surgery resurfaced in Europe and was reinforced during the course of the twelfth and thirteenth centuries. The advent of "rational" surgery, evident in western writers such as Theoderic of Bologna, confined surgical intervention to a last resort after diet, regime and medicines had been tried.[16] The invisibility of early medieval surgeons in Western Europe, then, stems from the fact that documented specialism in a field only became common after 1100. Again, this has led to relative neglect, until relatively recently, on the part of historians, in tracing earlier evidence of surgical practice.[17] Yet the early Middle Ages in Western Europe are not devoid of surgical texts, and Horden's own work has demonstrated that looking for information in other types of early medieval sources can produce quite startling insights into the sophistication of care and cure at this time, extending even to "alternative" therapies such as the use of music.[18]

Even if we do not have early medieval references to "professional" surgeons, therefore, the existence of such a group of skilled practitioners should not be dismissed as fanciful. Clare Pilsworth's work on the apparent prestige of medical experts in Lombard Italy suggests that competent practitioners existed long before the advent of the "rational" surgical profession in the late twelfth and early thirteenth centuries, and at the very least were viewed as respected members of their local communities.[19] Moreover, the definition of a medical profession, commonly thought to be a phenomenon of the twelfth and thirteenth centuries, needs to be reconsidered in the light of numerous examples of paid doctors earlier on, and the evidence, albeit slim, of regulation and of doctors being encouraged to indemnify themselves against accusations of malpractice. The early Welsh poem, the *Prophecy of Britain*, famously declares of the battle between Britons and Saxons, "no fee for the doctor will come of their deeds." Rhetorical flourish or evidence of potentially redundant battlefield surgeons?[20] We shall return to this issue.

As Horden, Banham and others have demonstrated, the copying and excerpting of medical texts continued throughout the early middle ages,[21] but the relative paucity of material, in comparison with the intensity of activity in the twelfth century,[22] is revealing: it is unlikely that text survival is a reliable indicator of the levels of competency or the distribution of practical competence. Ideas about wound care, on the other hand, occur frequently in non-medical texts: a rich source to mine is the abundance of legal codes from early medieval Europe, which list in some detail the penalties to be imposed for various injuries to the body.[23] Whilst the severity of the wound, and its care, might be determined by bleeding—several early medieval laws draw a distinction between a wound that could or could not be staunched,[24]—the laws are primarily concerned with the compensation payable for injury, and this financial penalty might also include calling for a doctor,[25] or offering the victim some kind of sick maintenance.[26] The clear overlap between versions of the same code, and between codes intended for different ethnic groups, prevent any sense of where such assistance might be more common, but all assume the existence of paid doctors (*medici*) to attend to injuries and/or to testify to their severity. This legal function mirrors Pilsworth's findings about the status of Lombard doctors. The esteem in which medics were held in this period is also possibly illustrated by the elevation of one, Deroldus, to the bishopric of Amiens in 929.[27]

## Healing in Action?

At the same time as providing evidence of the existence of such trusted figures, the source material is frustratingly reticent about describing treatment practices. We are certainly not lacking in references to serious and superficial head and facial wounds (one has only to read Gregory of Tours' accounts of the endemic violence in Merovingian Francia)[28] but their concern, as we have seen, is less with the medical after-effects than with the responses that such wounds might elicit. A rare reference to medical treatment in Gregory in fact indicates that not all care was designed with beneficial effects in mind. Describing the arrest and downfall of Count Leudast of Tours, whose earlier mutilation was discussed above, Gregory reports that Queen Fredegund's men struck him on the head, cutting away most of his hair and scalp, and that he broke his leg in the process of fleeing his assailants. King Chilperic ordered that he receive medical attention (*ut studeretur a medicis*) until his wounds were cured, and then be put to lingering torture. When his wounds began to fester, Leudast was put to death on the orders of the queen. Gregory, whose own hostile relationship with Leudast was longstanding, expresses satisfaction at the death.[29] Exploring the medical aspect of this account, however, the idea that a victim should be rendered fit enough to undergo further bodily punishment (Miller's "keep him alive for scoffing"?) does not appear to have caused any moral qualms on Gregory's part, and we do not know what the doctors implicated in this process thought of their orders.[30] Presumably fear of the king and queen prevented protest, but the fact that only the wounds inflicted by the torturers are described as festering signals some competence of care at least, even if the ethics of the doctors' actions were questionable.

We see doctors in action in early ninth-century narrative accounts from Francia as well. When a fragile wooden arcade collapsed on Emperor Louis the Pious and his attendants in 817, the king's bruised chest, injury to the back of his right ear and injury to his groin from a piece of flying wood were quickly dealt with "through the diligence of his physicians (*medicorum*)" and he was able to go hunting less than three weeks later.[31] Louis's eponymous son, Louis the German, also met with misfortune, falling from a second storey; not giving his physicians (*medici*) enough time to heal him, however, he then had to have rotting flesh cut out from his (unspecified) wounds and remain laid up at Aachen.[32] "Rotting flesh" may serve as a catch-all term for any type of infection, but this passage is valuable for confirming that "the same *medici*" had to deal with the surgical intervention—it is tempting to surmise that if the distinction between medical and surgical practice was not manifest at the level of court physicians, the same was also true lower down the social scale.[33] The sources are silent, however, on the care received by King Louis IV of Francia on his deathbed in 954 after a fall from a horse. Flodoard reports that he was gravely injured, and lay sick at Rheims for a long time, afflicted by "elephantiasis," before dying. Given that this term was used by ancient physicians and their medieval heirs as a term for leprosy or skin lesions in the early Middle Ages, however, one wonders whether Louis' fall was a result of an existing illness, rather than its cause.[34]

Leaving the court environment, physicians become rather more elusive (except in stock tales about their inability to provide a cure in hagiographic texts, which were all-too-often utilized by earlier historians of medicine as evidence of the "ignorance" of medieval medicine).[35] We have already seen that early medieval lawcodes contained detailed clauses about injuries to the head and face.[36] When looking specifically for medical practice in the laws, it is striking just how many references to medical practice and medics there are. These can be broken down into earlier regulation of medical practice, and the evidence for doctors being called in to treat illegally-inflicted wounds and/or attest to their severity.

Book XI of the seventh-century Visigothic lawcode, for example, has no less than eight clauses relating to physicians and their practice, including bleeding and the removal of cataracts from eyes (for which the reward is high: 5 *solidi*.) The laws assume that a medic will be called to treat the sick and wounded, recognize those who pass on their knowledge to others, and offers protection to the doctor whose patient dies.[37] Elsewhere in the code, wounds requiring compensation are categorized as slight, drawing blood or down to the bone.[38] This code has of course been recognized as one of the most "Roman" of lawcodes, and the regulation of physicians echoes—but does not reproduce, textually, Book 13 of the Theodosian lawcode. (The latter regulates the appointment of doctors and their exemption from municipal and public office, rather than their practice as such.)[39] At a most basic level, even if the Visigothic kingdom was not teeming with doctors, it is clear that the rhetoric of royal authority in the lawcodes was thought to be enhanced by encouraging their practice and, crucially, the training of future generations. The flourishing intellectual and medical culture of Al-Andalus, then, may have benefited from and built on pre-existing foundations of practice.

Almost contemporary Lombard law, whilst it does not regulate medics in quite the same way, nevertheless reiterates, from Rothari's edict in 643 to Liutprand's recension in the early eighth century, that "He who causes injuries should seek the doctor (*Qui plagas fecerit, ipse querat medicus* [*sic*])." Moreover, the assailant is charged to pay the doctor's fees and tip "as will be decided by learned men (*per doctos homines arbitratum fuerit*)."[40] "Learned men" might suggest either those versed in the law or previous cases, or may hint at other doctors being called in to give their opinion on the injury itself before costs of care were calculated. A striking element in these laws is the fact that the doctor is assumed to be called for injuries to slaves or semi-free (and the fee and tip excluded from the compensation amounts quoted), but is not mentioned in the list of compensations for injuries to freemen. Why should this be? One possibility is that medical care here is being expressed as an additional cost in the restoration of an asset, that is, the slave or semi-free peasant, to working order.

Both codes indicate, therefore, that doctors were thought to be available, and assume that *medici* would be able to treat wounds, that is, undertake the work that would later be left to surgeons.[41] The clauses considered so far are less explicit (with the exception of the clause on cataract removal) about the treatments they offered. For more detail we have to turn to the laws of the Alemans. Although the attribution of this code in different manuscripts to an unidentified King Clothar (II – 613–628, III – 657–673 or IV – 717–719) or to Duke Lantfrid (709–730) makes precise dating of the laws difficult (their modern editor plumps for early eighth century),[42] their medical content is quite striking. Law 57 [59] is worth drawing attention to for its detailed, gradated description of head injury and to the role of the doctor in providing care and subsequent testimony:

1. If anyone out of anger hits another, called "pulislac" by the Alemans, let him compensate with one solidus. (*Si quis alium per iram percusserit, quod Alemanni "pulislac" dicunt, cum uno solido componat*).[43]

2. If blood is shed, that touches the ground, let him compensate with 1½ solidi. (*Si autem sanguinem fuderit, ut terra tangat, conponat solido uno et semis.*)

3. If he should hit him so that the head appears and is scratched, he compensates with 3 solidi. (*Si autem percusserit eum ut testa apparet et radatur, cum 3 solidis componat.*)

4. If a broken bone should be taken from the head, and that bone makes a sound in a shield across a road 24 feet wide, let him compensate with 6 solidi. (*Si autem de capite ossum fractum de plaga tullerit, ita ut super publica via lata 24 pedis in scuto sonaverit ille ossus, cum 6 solidis componat.*)

5. If however the doctor loses [the bone] and cannot present it, then he should bring two witnesses who saw that bone was taken from the wound, or the doctor himself should prove that it is true that bone was taken from the wound. (*Si autem ipsum perdit medicus et non potest eum praesentare, tunc duos testes adhibeat, qui hoc vidissent, quod de illa plaga ossus tullisset, aut ille medicus hoc conprobet, quod verum fuisset, quod de ipsa plaga ossus tullisset.*)

6. If the head is scalped/cut into, so that the brains appear and the doctor has to touch them with a quill or a cloth, 12 solidi should be paid. (*Si autem testa trescapulata fuerit, ita ut cervella appareant, ut medicus cum pinna aut cum fanone cervella tetigit, cum 12 solidis conponat.*)[44]

7. And if the brain should come out of the wound, as often happens, so that the doctor staunches it with medicine and silk, and afterwards [the victim] recovers, and this is proven to be true, 40 *solidi* are to be paid. (*Si autem ex ipsa plaga cervella exierunt, sicut solet contingere, ut medicus cum medicamento aut cum sirico stuppavit, et postea sanavit, et hoc probatum est., quod verum sit, cum 40 solidis componat.*)[45]

A very similarly-structured list is included in the *Lex Frisionum*, Title XXII, compiled nearly a century later. This, though, has some important differences. It envisages that head injuries could cause impairment:

1. If anyone hits someone else on the head out of anger, and makes him deaf, he should give 24 *solidi*. (*Si quis alium per iram in capite percusserit, ut eum surdum efficiat, 24 solidos componat.*)

2. If he is made mute but can nevertheless still hear, 18 solidi should be paid. (*si mutus efficiatur, sed tamen audire possit, 18 solidos componat.*)

3. If anyone hits someone, which they call "durslegi", he should pay ½ *solidus* compensation. (*Si quis alium ita percusserit, quod "durslegi" vocant', dimidium solidum componat.*)

4. If he should shed blood, he should pay 1 *solidus*. (*Si autem sanguinem fuderit, componat solidum 1.*)

5. If he should hit him so that the head appears, he should pay 2 *solidi*. (*Si eum percusserit ut testa appareat cum 2 solidis componat.*)

6. If the skull is perforated, he should pay 12 *solidi*. (*Si os perforatum fuerit, 12 solidos componat.*)

7. If his sword should touch the membrane around the brain, he should pay 18 solidi. (*Si membranam, qua cerebrum continetur, gladius tetigerit, 18 solidos componat.*)

8. If the membrane is ruptured, so that the brain can come out, he should pay 24 *solidi*. (*Si ipsa membrana rupta fuerit, ita ut cerebrum exire possit, 24 solidos componat.*)

71. If from the wound there comes out a bone of such size, that thrown into a shield across a public road its sound can be heard, 4 *solidi* should be paid. (*Si de vulnere os exierit tantae magnitudinis, ut iactum in scutam trans publicam viam sonitus eius audiri possit, 4 solidis componatur.*)

72. If 2 bones: 3 *solidi*;

73. If 3 bones: add one *solidus*;

74. If smaller bones but they sound in the shield, half the above payments.[46]

Clearly, the detailed clauses on head injury share much with the Alemannic model, but the Frisian laws are silent on the care of doctors until some later additions relating to injuries to the stomach (the "judgment of Wulemar," 1 and 2). As we have seen from the Lombard material, however, the presence or absence of references to medics may not be determined by their relative accessibility in a particular region. The *Lex Baiwariorum*, for instance, repeats clauses about wounding, but the need to call a doctor—"ut propter hoc medicum inquirat"—is only mentioned as a measure of the compensation to be paid.[47]

Slightly later in date, the regulation of medical practice also appears in the Welsh laws, with the role of the court doctor outlined in some detail.[48] Dating anywhere between the tenth and twelfth centuries, the laws outlining the duties of the king's physician (*meddyg*) provide some striking points of comparison with earlier laws. The court physician is supported by the king and queen in return for treating members of the court free of charge, except for the three "dangerous wounds"—a blow to the head reaching the brain, a blow to the body reaching the bowels and a broken arm or leg. For treating these, the medic can charge set fees, which are outlined in the laws. Further treatments, such as bleeding, applying herbs to swellings and applying "medication with red ointment" are also given set charges.[49] What was this precious "red ointment"? Cule says it is a mistranslation of a treatment for a major blood vessel: if so, it would represent a substantial fee.[50] We shall return to this issue.

Rather like the Visigothic laws, Welsh law advises the physician to take assurances from his patients' families before undertaking treatment, in order to avoid repercussions if the patient dies. And like the Alemannic codes, the doctor—and here we may be moving beyond simply the court physician—is also involved in disputes following serious injury. Again, the assumption is that the doctor should keep any extracted bone from a skull injury, so that if there is a dispute about its size (indicating seriousness of injury), he can "take a brass bowl, and let him set his elbow on the ground with his hand above the bowl, and if its sound is heard, 4d, and if it is not heard there is no right to anything."[51] The physician's fees are also repeated, although there is a difference of two and a half pence per day between the food for the court physician and any other person!

The similarities between Welsh and earlier continental laws on these issues have not gone unnoticed. Although Thomas Glyn Watkin's extensive survey of Welsh legal history identified some possible lines of transmission (he notes, for example, that the Theodosian code was known in Britain, despite postdating the Roman withdrawal), they have remained brief comments in footnotes. Yet, medieval Wales was a cosmopolitan place, and had links not only with other Celtic regions such as Ireland and Brittany (all three sharing specific legal terminology relating to honor-price, as we have seen), but also with England and Francia, particularly the court of Gwynedd's links with that of Charles the Bald.[52] The medical motifs visible in Welsh law might simply derive from a shared, Indo-European past that valued ritual (the clang of a bone in a metal receptacle) and had taboos (blood reaching the ground, polluting the kingdom). But I wonder whether they are in fact more valuable in demonstrating the earlier, oral stratum of the law as well, one receptive to the idea of specially-appointed medical men, and aware that some wounds, and illnesses, just could not be cured? How far did shared medical ideas travel, particularly but not exclusively relating to head injuries? This is where the question of "red ointment"/"major blood vessel" comes in again, for the serious wound to a vein is included in Bavarian laws requiring the presence of the doctor. Does legal medicine represent medicine on the ground? I suggest that the ubiquity of references to doctors in some texts, their absence in others, and the occasional glimpse into practice argues against seeing these simply as textual reproductions.

## Medical Language

Letters, too, offer a rich seam of what might be best-termed quasi-medical information and the use of medical metaphors. Like their Biblical models, these tend to contrast earthly healing with spiritual rewards, but are nevertheless useful for exploring recurring themes. Charlemagne's biographer Einhard reflects on whether the "wound" of his wife's death will ever heal over to a scar with the medicine of consolation.[53] In Gerbert of Aurillac's letters, among others, there is ample evidence of medical terminology being utilized in a metaphorical sense to persuade erring members of the church to have a care for their spiritual health. For example, in a letter to Thibaud, Bishop of Amiens in 976, he rebukes the bishop for refusing to attend synods, and says that "The reverend 'physicians,' well acquainted with your ailments... and that pseudo-archbishop who... infected you as if by certain contagion, agreed upon the dishonor as far as you are concerned... the judgment of Pope Benedict VII found you incurable."[54] A letter written for Bishop Dietrich of Metz in 984 condemning Duke Charles for his betrayal includes: "you pour forth the disease of your utterly wicked heart... Eager to care for your wounds, hitherto I poured oil and wine upon them by mixing soft words... unless you repent, by the sword of the Holy Spirit, entrusted to me, I will cut you off along with your putrescent members." A wandering monk, too, was to be given "honeyed doses, according to the manner of a good physician lest, when the bitter antidotes are administered, the patient... should begin to tremble for his safety."[55] In terms of his own medical practice, as we have seen, Gerbert drew a line between knowledge, of which he had plenty,[56] and practical remedies, which he was reluctant to put into effect.[57]

Slightly later, Fulbert of Chartres (c. 970–c.1030) envisages a more robust, "surgical" intervention to bring Bishop Hubert of Angers, whom he had excommunicated, to penitence. In his letter to the bishop, Fulbert refers to "the scalpel of prudence (*falce discretionis*)" cutting away Hubert's sins, before launching into a lengthy series of medical metaphors for treating the now open "wounds."[58] Metaphorical, certainly, but hinting at some very simple wound management open to those less well-educated than Fulbert and his circle: cutting away bad flesh, cauterizing but then applying emollients to the wound before adding honey, whose antiseptic qualities both protected and healed.[59] A letter of 1031 of Ebbo, schoolmaster at Worms cathedral, also exemplifies the common use of medical terminology, but illustrates the division, already met in Thietmar, between the relative unimportance of the body when compared with the soul: "For as it says in proverbs, a friend out of duty disagrees with the doctor, for whilst [the doctor] can heal the scars of the body, so [the friend] if he wishes well can cure the sicknesses of the soul."[60]

Although medieval letters were written with an eye to demonstrating the writer's erudition and learning as well as conveying information and maintaining social relations, it is clear that their mainly clerical authors combined Classical allusions, biblical *topoi* and familiar home remedies to articulate their spiritual lessons. They are very comfortable with medical language; Orderic Vitalis, for example, terms the evangelist Luke the *spiritualis archiatros* or chief doctor of souls, and opined that, "A wise physician treats a sick man with a mild medicine, for fear that if he goads the sick man with the pain of too drastic a remedy he may kill instead of curing him."[61] Here he is again referring to the care of souls, but he is also informative on some of the medical care for the body available in his own day, good and bad. His famous portrait of Ralph, the "Ill-Tonsured," is of a skilled medic who had "spent much of his time out of the study in the battle-field," (and so by implication was ill-suited to be a monk, hence his nickname?) and could treat victims of disease and accident. Operating as Ralph was during the latter part of the eleventh century and early twelfth, Orderic's text is valuable evidence that the split between medic and surgeon had not yet occurred. By contrast, the personal physician of King Henry I of France, he reports, was called "Blockhead" (*Surdus*—literally "Deaf"). Although he prescribed the ailing king a medicine, Henry died after drinking water: presumably the attack on the doctor was for lack of care or close observation, rather than the prescription itself.[62]

Self-care of sorts features in the twelfth-century *Life* of St Ulrich of Zell (d. 1093). It recounts how the prior gave himself a severe headache though his long, nocturnal vigils and his continuous work writing (*per longas vigilias noctium, per scribendi laborem continuum, gravissimum capitis dolorem incurrebat*). Not realizing this was a divine test, he decides to self-treat, washing his head "several times" with wormwood (*aliquoties caput lavit absinthio*). But he accidently pierced his eye with the stick (*festuca*) with which he was applying the remedy, and could not get it out. For six months he wept copious tears (*guttatim effluxit*) from the eye, but recognized that this temporary lack of external light and vision was a test to make him see the inner light more clearly (*non est. contristatus pro exterioris luminis detrimento: quia quanto carnalis visus obscurior, tanto mentis acies ad contemplandum superni luminis claritatem fuerat perspicacior*).[63]

## Case Study: Serious Head Injury in Battle

All of this tangential evidence suggests that basic remedies were known and doctors were available (for a fee), and that many of their procedures, whilst clearly empirical, were not entirely without skill and knowledge.

Removing bone from skull injuries, for example, was clearly understood to relieve pressure on the brain and may have been a widespread practice, whether or not the *dura mater* had been punctured. Whilst thirteenth-century surgical manuals such as that of Theoderic of Bologna (c. 1267) urged haste in dealing with bone fragments, they were clearly not introducing a new method of treatment.[64] Indeed, a clause in the mid-thirteenth-century Assizes of the Kingdom of Cyprus explicitly criticizes any doctor who did *not* know how to undertake this procedure competently: "should the doctor not have known how to open the wound, but treated it in such a way that the fractured bones came into contact with the brain," resulting in the patient's death, the doctor was liable to pay compensation.[65]

Whilst surgical texts might be lacking from the early medieval period, surgical knowledge clearly was not. Archaeological evidence from early medieval sites reinforces the evidence of competent surgery, and demonstrates that even serious head wounds were survivable, and that some must have been treated. Two warrior burials recently found in central Italy showed severe, but partly healed, head traumas.[66] Had these men received care from a surgeon? Certainly there would have been a need to remove splinters of skull, and in a case from the cemetery of the deserted medieval village at Wharram Percy, Yorkshire, there was some evidence of additional trepanation.[67] This individual, dating from the tenth/eleventh century, is particularly exciting, as the location of the cemetery suggests that there was access to medical care in a relatively rural setting. Caution is required here, however, for the trepanation process can be interpreted as a religious ritual as well as one with a curative aim. Yet a sample of Anglo-Saxon cases studied by Parker suggests that, pagan or Christian, the procedure had been carried out with a medical aim as well as or rather than a ritualistic one, and there was a high success rate, evidenced by the partial healing evident in many of the skulls. Parker does not, however, speculate as to the reasons for the trepanning: blunt force injury and the need to access impacted bones is not mentioned at all.[68] Exploring the later world of the crusade surgeon, Piers Mitchell cites a survey of cemetery evidence dating from the sixth to eighth centuries in Germany, in which approximately thirty of the deceased had cranial fractures and three-quarters of these had healed, again indicating survival.[69] As Mitchell comments, further work on archaeological sites can only expand the sample of remains to inform our knowledge of the survivability of head injuries, whether sustained in warfare or through rather more mundane accidents. Blunt force cranial injury, of course, is not quite facial disfigurement. Nor does it all have to be the result of interpersonal violence (although it is often reported as such). Falls, and items falling on the head, could produce equally serious breakage of the skull.

More likely causes of disfigurement were assaults with bladed weapons: we have already met one or two of these. Literary sources portray survivors, such as Wulf Wonreding in Beowulf, who, though injured by a "keen wound" from a sword to his head through his helmet, was nevertheless "bound up" and recovered from it.[70] Bernard Bachrach, basing his discussion on Rabanus Maurus's ninth-century text *De Procinctu Miliciae*, suggests that infantry soldiers were trained to jab short swords and cause puncture injuries, first at the head and face of the enemy, then at other parts of his body. This, he argues, was a more effective means of disabling and killing than using a slashing motion with the sword, which risked hitting only bone and shield and possibly one's own comrades.[71] Yet Rabanus drew heavily on the fifth-century Roman author Vegetius's *De Re Militari*, which may explain his emphasis on Roman-style short swords. Slashing injuries in early medieval skeletal remains attest to longer weapons in individual combat. Archaeological studies seem to concur that the "primary target on the body" in close combat was the head which, if the individual was lacking or had lost his helmet, was the least protected part of his body,[72] and remains quite commonly display blunt-weapon injury to the skull (such as might have been made by staves or spear shafts) alongside blade injuries. The potential for bruising and superficial cuts and lacerations, however, was greater than is revealed by the archaeological evidence, which mainly picks up the blows that hit home to the bone in a fatal, or near-fatal manner.[73] Earlier sources rarely describe these in much detail,[74] but the literary and rhetorical skills of later poetry make much of such glancing blows, emphasizing the dangers of hand-to-hand combat. Robert of Courcy was wounded and lost his right eye in battle.[75] Another type of head wound that shows up in the evidence is a direct hit by a projectile, whether an arrow in the face, often the eye area, or missiles such as stones either thrown from above or shot by machine.[76] Arrow wounds were particularly difficult to treat, and those recorded in the written evidence were usually fatal, compounded, in many cases, by the difficulty of removing an arrowhead that might be barbed or poisoned.[77] Richard of Acerra's arrow wound through both cheeks, discussed above and apparently successfully treated by a "medicus" and two female assistants, seems an entirely exceptional case when compared with the many full-frontal arrow strikes documented in the evidence. Richer son of Engenulf of Laigle was fatally wounded just beneath the eye by an arrow shot by "a certain beardless boy."[78] Hugh, earl of Shrewsbury, despite being "clad in iron from the top of his head to the souls of his feet," was hit in the right eye by an arrow that penetrated his brain and killed him when fighting pirates from the Orkneys, "so that he fell mortally wounded into the sea."[79]

## Blinding, Disfigurement and Aftercare: Living with a Changed Face

If the theatre of warfare seems an obvious place to look for medics at work, the many examples of judicial mutilations and other blindings scattered throughout this book also demand attention as potential theatres of surgery. If the idea was to inflict a lasting punishment, the person needed to heal sufficiently to act as a living example to others. Branding was its own form of cautery, but were cut wounds—ears, noses and lips—also cauterized, as some of the metaphorical material explored above envisages? Limited evidence of the use of cautery has emerged from an eighth-tenth-century grave in Pisa, but the report authors' speculation as to why it was used relies upon evidence from medical texts that were unknown in the West at this date.[80]

Blinding could be carried out without recourse to extraction of the eyes, but most of the examples do seem to involve heated brands or spiked implements, and as we have seen, care was needed to ensure these did not penetrate beyond the eye sockets and kill the unfortunate victim, even if the eyes were "discrete and as such neatly and discretely extractable" in Miller's words.[81] But what happened next? In the extended scene recounted by Psellos, the two victims are "left to rest" after their ordeal, but presumably they might seek assistance to deal with the pain and bleeding. Anna Komnena relates that the blinded rebel Nicephorus Diogenes was "frantic with pain" after his ordeal.[82] The most detailed account of possibly medical intervention, however, occurs in a hagiographical context. I alluded above to the case of Ailward of Westoning, pictured in the Canterbury cathedral Becket windows as the victim of an unjust blinding and castration, and cured by the saint. In two narrative text versions of the miracle, some form of aftercare treatment with an emollient, wax and bandages wrapped around the victim's eye sockets is mentioned. William of Canterbury reports that Ailward had a vision of St

Thomas ten days after the blinding, and feeling his left eye itching (*pruriente sinistro oculo*) he scratched at the wax and emollient that had been applied to eliminate the pus (*scalpens ungue ceram summovit et malagma quod appositum fuerat ad purulentias extrahendas*).[83] Does this add veracity to the miracle story by introducing a "realistic" medical detail, or was this apparent "sealing" of the sockets a standard practice once eyeballs were removed? Benedict of Peterborough's slightly later account adds the detail that Ailward's eyes were bandaged (as he wonders whether his vision will come true once the bandage is removed), but confuses the issue too. Whilst William separates out the wax and the emollient, Benedict combines them into "waxy emollient (*malagma cereum*)" and adds that it had been applied "either to extract the pus from the empty sockets or to close the lids themselves (*quod sive ad extrahendas orbium vacuorum purulentias seu ad ipsa cilia claudenda fuerat appositum*)."[84] Certainly there is other limited evidence of bandaging being applied after blinding (in Anna Komnena's accounts), but whether this was to assist in healing, or simply an aesthetic choice to cover the wounds is never stated.

Focusing on the aesthetic demands a brief consideration of cosmetic aids. Demaitre has noted that the later Middle Ages saw an upsurge in medical texts dealing with apparently minor skin conditions and lesions. Remedies for ulcers and pimples on the face feature in the fourth-century *Herbarium* of Pseudo-Apuleius, translated into Anglo-Saxon in England in the tenth, and in Bald's *Leechbook*, but they were intended to heal such conditions, not conceal them.[85] There is no consideration in this text of concealing or reducing scarring, for example. The rising concern with appearance may, however, be indicated by the numerical increase in such recipes, from three in the Apuleius to nineteen in the *Leechbook*. Specific concern with cosmetic appearance seems to have been focused on women: the twelfth-century *De Ornatu Mulierum* (On Women's Cosmetics), produced in Salerno in the twelfth century, starts with a series of recipes about hair (both conditioning and colouring, and depilation) before moving on to the face. Adorning the face, the text points out, "embellishes even ugly women (*deformes mulieres palliat*)."[86] There follow recipes for diminishing blotches and freckles, whitening the complexion, curing scabies and attending to sunburn, but again, dealing with the after-effects of disfiguring conditions or scars is not considered explicitly.[87] It seems that concealing facial scars with preparations was not, yet, a technique to "pass."

Modern surgical care packages for disfigured people address not only the physical challenges their acquired disfigurement presents, but also the psychological trauma of waking with a new face (a trauma that, arguably, is repeated several times if surgery takes place in stages). To what extent is there any evidence of emotional or psychological support in the early Middle Ages? From the preceding discussion, it seems that in the early Middle Ages the circumstances of the disfiguring injury strongly shaped responses toward it, a phenomenon that arguably persists today. Military heroes (even unlikely ones like Bishop Michael of Regensburg, discussed above) or unjustly or illegally injured people (mutilated hostages) evoked some pity or sympathy and even—in the case of Genoese archers—financial support. Those who brought their disfigurement upon themselves, however, including not only criminals (like Septimina and Droctulf) but also irresponsible youths (Young Charles), seem to have been given rather shorter shrift. Ailward, according to Benedict's account, spent a day in Bedford sitting against the wall of a house "without any favor of humanity being shown towards him (*nullo sibi collato humanitiatis beneficio*)." Here the pathos of the broken man and his accompanying young daughter is designed of course to evoke even more pity before the miraculous intervention of Thomas.

Many cases feature those who were already socially visible elites, whose fate might usefully serve as an object lesson in humility. But their changed circumstances could also bring new opportunities. This is at least the tenor of Anna Komnena's report of the blinded Nicephorus, mentioned earlier. After withdrawing to his estates (wealth clearly cushioned the blow of his fall from favor), Anna recounts that he "found satisfaction... devoting all his energies to the study of ancient literature, read to him by others. Deprived of his own sight, he used the eyes of strangers for reading... Later he...even studied the celebrated geometry (an unprecedented feat) by getting a philosopher he had met to prepare the figures in relief. By touching these with his hands he acquired knowledge of all the geometrical theorems and figures. Thus he rivaled Didymus... I myself have seen the man and marveled at him..."[88] Anna's text is a classic example of the "triumphing over adversity" model, yet her account also objectifies Nicephorus, particularly that last sentence that sets him up almost as an exhibit to be visited and "seen."[89]

No doubt Nicephorus's already high status and obvious wealth (he retired to his estates) cushioned the blow of his sightlessness, as well as persuading Anna to visit him. Lower-status victims of disfigurement were in a much more vulnerable position, and living with their condition required that they promote a fascinating back-story to make it into the written records at all. Walchelin the badly-burnt priest is a case in point, emphasizing the supernatural origin of his wounds (and thus again inviting wonder, not rejection). Ailward's initial day of dejection in Bedford, albeit a hagiographical tool to evoke pity in the reader, probably reflects far more accurately the social norm of living with an acquired disfigurement if one were only a peasant farmer. Yet another hagiographic text featured an alternative outcome. The eleventh-century *Life* of the sixth-century St Cadog of Wales features a "rustic" who dared to look through a spyhole to the tombs of Cadog's disciples in a Scottish monastery, despite the warnings of the custodian priests that Cadog would punish him for his presumption: "Go," they say, "and may St Cadog make a sign of his revenge appear on you [ *Vade, et faciat sanctus Cadocus quatinus signum ultionis appareat in te*]." Peering through the opening, the peasant's eye immediately "burst, and hung down his face suspended on the optic nerve [*crepuit, et per neruum octicum facie tenus depependit*]." Far from being defeated by this punishment, he subsequently "traveled from place to place throughout the province of *Lintheamina*, covering his broken eye. And many people gave him alms, in order that he should show them the torn apart eyeball. And from this more and more of his countrymen learnt to fear God, and reverently worship him through his saint [ *Giravit equidem itidem rusticus de loco ad locum per totam provinciam Lintheamine, erutum oculum tegens. Plures mercedem ei largiebantur, ut eis diuulsum ocelli orbiculum ostenderet. Exin magis ac magis compatriote discebant Deum metuere, et cum sancto suo reverenter glorificare*]."[90]

For the rustic, his impairment represented an opportunity, and whilst at first sight his wandering and seeking alms mirrors that of the blinded priest Wipert, discussed earlier, his showman-like action in concealing and then revealing his eyeball seems to represent social elevation of a kind rather than humiliating punishment. For those already in socially-elevated positions, however, death was indeed written up as preferable to disfigurement or impairment (Emperor Michael, Luke of La Barre), but we cannot discount the idea that faith supported the survivors in ways that the texts just do not make explicit. (This, after all, was the purpose of hagiographic tales of exceptional cures.) Were people with disfigurements reminded that their humility or humiliation on earth would be rewarded in heaven, and did this help at all with the day-to-day battle of living with disfigurement? In the concluding chapter, the continuities and changes across time will be briefly considered as a starting point for more work on the history of disfigurement.

## NOTES

1. Stanley Rubin, "The Anglo-Saxon physician," in *Medicine in Early Medieval England: Four Papers*, ed. Marilyn Deegan and D. G. Scragg (Manchester: Centre for Anglo-Saxon Studies, 1987), 7–15, quote at 9.
2. Sean McGlynn, *By Sword and Fire: Cruelty and Atrocity in Medieval Warfare* (London: Weidenfeld and Nicolson, 2008), 11.
3. Peregrine Horden, "Medieval medicine," in *The Oxford Handbook of the History of Medicine*, ed. Mark Jackson (Oxford: Oxford University Press, 2011), 51–2.
4. A recent and sustained polemic against such assumptions about the early middle ages is Clare Pilsworth, *Healthcare in Early Medieval Northern Italy: More to Life than Leeches* (Turnhout: Brepols, 2014).
5. J. Jörimann, *Frühmittelalterliche Rezeptarien* (= *Beiträge zur Geschichte der Medizin, Heft 1*) (Leipzig and Zurich: Orell Füssli, 1925).
6. Jörimann, *Frühmittelalterliche Rezeptarien*, 81.
7. Stanley Rubin, *Medieval English Medicine* (London: David and Charles, 1974), 147.
8. Leechbook I, in *Leechdoms, Wortcunning and Starcraft of Early England*, ed. O. Cockayne, 3 vols (London: Longmans and Green, 1864–6), II.19–26 (head, 17 recipes), 27–38 (eyes), 53–4 (facial blotches), 59 (hare lip), 77–81 (pustules and blotches), 155 (hair loss or excess hair).
9. I have alluded to the issue of congenital impairment in children above.
10. F. Eliza Glaze, "Gariopontus and the Salernitans: textual traditions in the eleventh and twelfth centuries," in *"La Collectio Salernitana" di Salvatore de Renzi*, ed. D. Jacquart and A. Paravicini Bagliani (Florence: SISMEL Galluzzo, 2009), 149–90, at 165. Online at http://coastal.academia.edu/FlorenceElizaGlaze/ Papers/558742/_Gariopontus_and_the_Salernitans_Textual_

Traditions_in_the_Eleventh_and_Twelfth_Centuries_   [Accessed 21 August 2012]. On the OE Peri Didaxeon (British Library, Harley MS 6258 B, ff 55v-66v), see L. Sanborn, "Anglo-Saxon medical practices and the *Peri Didaxeon*," *Revue de l'Université d'Ottawa*, 55 (1985): 7–13.

11. Not only tried out, but in some manuscripts clearly collected for use "by any able and experienced individual, whether in the home, monastery or clerical community": Pilsworth, *Healthcare*, 93.

12. The preface to Celsus, *De Medicina* states that medicine is made up of diet/regimen (*rictu*), remedies (*medicamenta*) and operations (*manu*): cited in Michel Foucault, *Care of the Self: the History of Sexuality vol. 3*, tr. R. Hurley (London: Penguin, 1990), 100.

13. Ibn Ridwan, *Useful Book*, 103, 5–9, tr. A. Z. Iskandar, "An attempted reconstruction of the late Alexandrian medical curriculum," *Medical History*, 20 (1976): 243, quoted in Peter E. Pormann and Emilie Savage-Smith, *Medieval Islamic Medicine* (Edinburgh: Edinburgh University Press, 2010), 84.

14. M. L. Cameron, "Bald's Leechbook: its sources and their use in compilation," *Anglo-Saxon England*, 12 (1983): 153–182; *id.*, "Bald's Leechbook and cultural interactions in Anglo-Saxon England," *Anglo-Saxon England*, 19 (1990): 5–12; Audrey Meaney, "Variant versions of Old English medical remedies and the compilation of Bald's Leechbook," *Anglo-Saxon England*, 13 (1984): 235–268; Richard Scott Nokes, "The several compilers of Bald's Leechbook," *Anglo-Saxon England*, 33 (2004): 51–76; Stephanie Hollis, "The social milieu of Bald's Leechbook," *AVISTA Forum Journal*, 14 (2004): 11–16; Maria A. D'Aronco, "The transmission of medical knowledge in Anglo-Saxon England: the voices of manuscripts," in *Form and Content of Instruction in Anglo-Saxon England in the Light of Contemporary Manuscript Evidence, Papers presented at the International Conference, Udine, 6–8 April 2006*, ed. by Patrizia Lendinara, Loredana Lazzari, and Maria A. D'Aronco, (Fédération Internationale des Instituts d'Études Médiévales, Textes et Études du Moyen Âge, 39, Turnhout: Brepols, 2007), 35–58

15. Rubin, "Anglo-Saxon physician," 8. Despite its air of disparagement, Rubin's is a useful overview.

16. E. Campbell and J. Cotton, tr., *The Surgery of Theoderic, c. AD 1267* (New York: Appleton-Century-Crofts, 1955), Introduction,

4 and 5. See more generally Michael McVaugh's influential study, *The Rational Surgery of the Middle Ages* (Firenze: SISMEL-Edizioni del Galluzzo, 2006).

17. Texts still dominate the field, however, as essays in the recent volume *Between Text and Patient: the medical enterprise in medieval and early modern Europe*, ed. Florence Eliza Glaze and Brian Nance (Florence: SISMEL-Edizione del Galluzzo, 2011), illustrate.

18. Peregrine Horden, "Religion as medicine: music in hospitals," in *Religion and Medicine in the Middle Ages*, ed. Peter Biller and Joseph Ziegler (York: University of York, 2001), 135–153, reprinted in *id.*, *Hospitals and Healing from Antiquity to the Later Middle Ages* (Aldershot: Variorum, 2008); *Music as Medicine: the history of music therapy since antiquity*, ed. Peregrine Horden (Aldershot: Ashgate, 2000), including his "Commentary on Part II, with a note on the early middle ages," 103–108.

19. Clare Pilsworth, "'Could you just sign this for me John?' Doctors, charters and occupational identity in early medieval northern and central Italy," *Early Medieval Europe*, 17 (2009): 363–388.

20. *The Earliest Welsh Poetry*, tr. Joseph P. Clancy (London: Macmillan, 1970), 109. The poem is thought to date to c. 930.

21. Debby Banham, "A millennium in medicine? New medical texts and ideas in England in the eleventh century," in *Anglo-Saxons: Studies presented to Cyril Roy Hart*, ed. Simon Keynes and Alfred P. Smyth (Dublin: Four Courts Press, 2006), 230–242; Peregrine Horden, "The year 1000: medical practice at the end of the first millennium," *Social History of Medicine*, 13 (2000): 201–219. See also Anne van Arsdall, "The transmission of knowledge in early medieval medical texts: an exploration," in *Between Text and Patient*, ed. Glaze and Nance, 201–216 and Maria Amalia D'Aronco, "How 'English' is Anglo-Saxon medicine: the Latin sources for Anglo-Saxon medical texts," in *Britannia Latina: Latin in the Culture of Great Britain from the Middle Ages to the Twentieth Century*, ed. Charles Burnett and Nicholas Mann (London: Warburg Institute, 2005), 27–41.

22. See Monica Green's report on her project to collate twelfth-century materials at http://www.academia.edu/4613362/_Medical_Manuscripts_from_the_Long_Twelfth_Century_Manuscripts_on_My_Mind_News_from_the_Vatican_Film_Library_No._8_January_2013_p._11 [Accessed 2 October 2013].

23. See above, Chap. 3 and below, Appendix 2; wound care is extensively discussed in *Wounds and Wound Repair in Medieval Culture*, ed. Kelly de Vries and Larissa Tracy (Leiden: Brill, 2015), and has already formed the focus of *Wounds in the Middle Ages*, ed. Anne Kirkham and Cordelia Warr (Aldershot: Ashgate, 2014). The latter, however, virtually ignores the period before 1200.

24. *Pactus Legis Salicae*, XVII.7, ed. K. Eckhardt, in *MGH Leges Nat. Germ.*, IV.1 (Hannover: Hahn, 1962), 78. It derives indirectly from a biblical model: a wound that could not be staunched, after all, would drip blood on the ground, polluting it and demanding expiation: Numbers 35:33.

25. *Pactus Legis Salicae*, XVII.7; *Lex Salica Carolina*, XXII.4, ed. K. A. Eckhardt, *MGH LL nat. Germ.* IV.2 (Hannover: Hahn, 1969). Doctors' fees are mentioned in *Leges Langobardorum*, ed. F. Bluhme in *MGH LL*, IV, ed. G. H. Pertz (Hannover: Hahn, 1868), Rothari cc. 79, 81, 82, 83, 84, 103, 106, 107. *Ibid.*, Rothari c. 128 states that "he who struck the blow should seek the doctor; if he has neglected to do this, the man struck or his lord should find the doctor [and the perpetrator pays the bill]."

26. The victim in Irish law was eligible for sick maintenance by his/her assailant if s/he did not recover quickly: Fergus Kelly, *A Guide to Early Irish Law* (Dublin: Institute for Advanced Studies, 1988), 130. On early Anglo-Saxon provision, see Lisi Oliver, 'Sick maintenance in Anglo-Saxon law', *Journal of English and German Philology*, 107.3 (2008): 303–326.

27. *The Annals of Flodoard of Reims, 919–966*, tr. Steven Fanning and Bernard Bachrach (Toronto: Toronto University Press, 2011), 18.

28. *GT*, I.1; e.g. the regular removal of noses and ears (V.18, VIII.29, IX.38, X.15); the punishment of branding to the face (IX.38).

29. Above, Chap. 4, note 32; *GT* VI.32.

30. William Ian Miller, *Eye for an Eye* (Cambridge: Cambridge University Press, 2006), 151.

31. *Annales Regni Francorum*, s.a. 817: *MGH SS rer. Ger.*, VI, ed. G. H. Pertz (Hannover: Hahn, 1895).

32. Annales Bertiniani, s.a. 870, *MGH SS*, I: *Annales et Chronica Aevi Carolini*, ed. G. H. Pertz (Hannover: Hahn, 1826): *minus necessario curari a medicis sustinens, computrescentem carnem ab eisdem medicis secari fecit.*

33. Rubin, "Anglo-Saxon physician," 9, concurs that in England, too, the terms physician and surgeon would have been interchangeable in the early middle ages.

34. *Annals of Flodoard*, s.a. 954, tr. Fanning and Bachrach, 60. "Elephantiasis": Timothy Miller and John Nesbitt, *Walking Corpses: Leprosy in Byzantium and the Medieval West* (Ithaca and London: Cornell University Press, 2014), 8–9.

35. See Patricia Skinner, "A cure for a sinner: sickness and healthcare in medieval southern Italy," in *The Community, the Family and the Saint: Patterns of Power in Early Medieval Europe*, ed. J. Hill and M. Swann (Leeds/Turnhout: Brepols, 1998), 297–309, for a specific representation of competition between doctors and the local saints in southern Italy.

36. See above, Chap. 3 and below, Appendix 2.

37. *Leges Visigothorum*, Book XI, Title 1, ed. K. Zeumer *MGH LL nat. Germ.*, I: (Hannover and Leipzig: Hahn, 1902), 400–403.

38. *Ibid.*, Book VI, Title IV.1, 262–3.

39. *The Theodosian Code and Novels, and the Sirmondian Constitutions*, ed. and tr. C. Pharr (New Jersey: The Lawbook Exchange, 2001), Book XIII.

40. *MGH LL IV: Leges Langobardorum*, Rothari 128 and Liutprand 68, ed. F. Bluhme (Hannover: Hahn, 1868), 30 and 249.

41. Pilsworth, *Healthcare*, 177–215, collects the evidence for northern Italian medical practitioners termed *medici* in the early middle ages.

42. *MGH LL. nat. Germ. V.1*, ed. K. Lehman (Hannover: Hahn, 1966), 8.

43. I have used 'he' and 'him' here and throughout the translations: see above, Chap. 5, for a discussion of the gendering of language in the lawcodes.

44. The translation of *pinna* as 'quill' conveys the sense of a fine surgical tool, and is mirrored in the brand-name of modern 'Feather' micro-scalpels: http://www.pfmmedical.com/en/productcatalogue/featherR_micro_scalpels/index.html, [Accessed 11 April 2015]. Pilsworth, *Healthcare*, 109–110, discusses this passage and its translation.

45. *MGH LL. nat. Germ. V.1*, ed. K. Lehman (Hannover: Hahn, 1966), 116–117. I have benefited from the comments of Wendy Turner on my understanding of brains 'coming out of the wound':

this is more likely to mean a swelling, due to injury or rupture of the *dura mater*, rather than literally a spilling of cerebral matter.

46. *Lex Frisionum*, ed. K. de Richthofen, in *MGH LL*, III, ed. G. Pertz (Hannover: Hahn, 1863), 631–700.

47. *Lex Baiwariorum*, ed. E. Liber, V.3, *MGH Leg. nat. Germ. V.2:* (Hannover: Hahn, 1926), 339.

48. Welsh law also notes blood dripping to the ground, especially the 'complete blood' from a head wound: *The Laws of Hywel Dda (The Book of Blegywryd)*, tr. M. Richards (Liverpool: Liverpool University Press, 1954), 109.

49. *The Laws of Hywel Dda: Law Texts from Medieval Wales*, I.3, ed. and tr. Dafydd Jenkins (Llandysul: Gomer Press, 1986), 24–26. And see John Cule, "The court mediciner and medicine in the laws of Wales," *Journal of the History of Medicine and Allied Sciences*, 21 (1966): 213–266.

50. See also Geoffrey Hodgson, "Dermatology and history in Wales (Cymru)," *British Journal of Dermatology*, 90 (1974): 699–712.

51. *Laws of Hywel Dda*, III.8, tr. Jenkins, 196–198.

52. T. G. Watkin, *The Legal History of Wales* (Cardiff: University of Wales Press, 2007), 46–7.

53. Einhard, letter to Lupus, 836, ed. E. Dümmler, *MGH* Epistolae Merovingici et Karolingici Aevi, IV (Berlin: Weidmann, 1925), 10.

54. *The Letters of Gerbert with his Papal Privileges as Sylvester II*, Letter 1, tr. Harriet Pratt Lattin (New York: Columbia University Press, 1961), 35.

55. *Letters of Gerbert*, letters 39 (76–78) and 74 (113).

56. E.g. we know he was interested in the *Ophthalmicus* of Demosthenes: *Letters of Gerbert*, letter 16 (55).

57. E.g. he offers prayers and medical information to Archbishop Egbert in 988: *Letters of Gerbert*, letter 122 (154); and in letter 178 he specifically states that since his correspondent lacks a physician "and we the materials for healing, we have refrained from describing the remedies which the most skilled physicians judge to be useful for an infected liver."

58. *The Letters and Poems of Fulbert of Chartres*, ed. and tr. F. Behrends (Oxford: Clarendon Press, 1976), letter 71: *Deinde amputationis illius vulnera recentia, ne aliquam aliam passionem generent, penalis cauterio timoris ustulabis...* Such metaphors predate the

medieval period of course: Michel Foucault, *The History of Sexuality, III: the Care of the Self* (New York: Pantheon, 1986), 55, quotes Seneca's Letters to Lucilius, 64.8, outlining much the same scalpel and soothing procedure.

59. Ilana Krug, "The wounded soldier: honey and late medieval military medicine," in *Wounds and Wound Repair*, ed. DeVries and Tracy, 194–214, discusses its healing qualities.

60. *Nam ut solet in proverbiis dici, parum amicus ab officio discordat medici, sicut enim iste corporis sanat cicatrices, ita ille si bene vult animi curat dolores*: *MGH Die Briefe in der deutschen Kaiserzeit III: die ältere Wormser Briefsammlung*, letter 15, ed. W. Bulst (Weimar: Böhlau, 1949), 31–32.

61. *Orderic*, II.16, (I, 189) and VIII.26 (IV, 316–7).

62. *Orderic*, III.ii.69–70 (Ralph) and III.ii.79 (Surdus), (II, 74–77 and 88–9 respectively).

63. *Vita S. Udalrici Prioris Cellensis*, in *MGH SS*, XII, ed. G. H. Pertz (Hannover: Hahn, 1856), 258.

64. *The Surgery of Theoderic, c. AD 1267*, II.6, tr. E. Campbell and J. Cotton (New York: Appleton-Century-Crofts, 1955), 122. He was pessimistic, however, about the patient's chances of survival if the brain had also suffered injury: *ibid.*, II.3, 110.

65. *The Assizes of the Lusignan Kingdom of Cyprus*, Codex I, clause 225, tr. Nicholas Coureas (Nicosia: Cyprus Research Centre, 2002), 181.

66. M. Rubini and P. Zaio, "Warriors from the East: skeletal evidence of warfare from a Lombard-Avar cemetery in Central Italy (Campochiaro, Molise, 6th-8th century AD)," *Journal of Archaeological Science*, 38 (2011): 1551–1559.

67. Stuart Mays, "A possible case of surgical treatment of cranial blunt force injury from medieval England," *International Journal of Osteoarchaeology*, 16 (2006): 95–103: the skull surrounding the injury hole had clearly been scraped to permit lifting of the damaged bone.

68. S. J. Parker, "Skulls, symbols and surgery: a review of the evidence for trepanation in Anglo-Saxon England and a consideration of the motives behind the practice," in *Superstition and Popular Magic in Anglo-Saxon England*, ed. D. Scragg (Manchester: Manchester Centre for Anglo-Saxon Studies, 1989), 73–84.

69. Piers Mitchell, *Medicine in the Crusades: Warfare, Wounds and the Medieval Surgeon* (Cambridge: Cambridge University Press, 2004), 112.
70. *Klaeber's Beowulf, 4th Edition*, ed. R. D. Fulk, Robert E. Bjork and John D. Niles (Toronto: Toronto University Press, 2008), lines 2973–6. The date of the poem is still, clearly, a controversial issue: *The Dating of Beowulf: a Reassessment*, ed. Leonard Neidorf (Woodbridge: Boydell, 2014).
71. Bernard S. Bachrach, *Early Carolingian Warfare: Prelude to Empire* (Philadephia: University of Pennsylvania Press, 2001), 89.
72. Quote from E. T. Brødholt and P. Holck, "Skeletal trauma in the burials from the royal church of St Mary in medieval Oslo," *International Journal of Osteoarchaeology*, 22.2 (2012): 213; vulnerability: Piers Mitchell *et al.*, "Weapon injuries in the twelfth century crusader garrison of Vadum Iacob castle, Galilee," *International Journal of Osteoarchaeology*, 16.2 (2006): 153.
73. Influential in setting the agenda for recognizing peri-mortal injury (i.e. injuries likely to have caused death within a few days) was S. J. Wenham, "Anatomical interpretations of Anglo-Saxon weapon injuries," in *Weapons and Warfare in Anglo-Saxon England*, ed. S. Chadwick Hawkes (Oxford: Oxford University Committee for Archaeology, 1989), 123–139. See e.g. P. Patrick, "Approaches to violent death: a case study from early medieval Cambridge," *International Journal of Osteoarchaeology*, 16.4 (2006): 347–354, who comments that the individual under scrutiny, who had suffered three weapons injuries from sword blows to the cranium, did not long survive the attack. Contrast, however, the cases from early medieval Maastricht in the Netherlands, discussed by Raphael Panhuysen, "Het scherp van de snede: sporen van geweld in vroegsmiddeleuws Maastricht," *Archeologie in Limburg*, 92 (2002): 2–7, where two cases of blade injuries to the skull showed signs of healing.
74. The ninth-century Byzantine chronicler Theophanes, however, highlights the spear injury picked up by Emperor Heraclius in a battle against the Persians in AM6118 (625/6 CE): *The Chronicle of Theophanes Confessor: Byzantine and Near Eastern History, AD284–813*, ed. and tr. C. Mango and R. Scott with the assistance of R. Greatrex (Oxford: Clarendon Press, 1997), 449.
75. *Orderic*, X.7.

76. In a moralizing tale of an impious man named Constantine who threw a stone at an icon of the Virgin, Theophanes reports that he was killed at the siege of Nicaea in 725/6 by a stone which broke his head and face: *The Chronicle of Theophanes*, AM6218, 559–60.

77. Poison: *Lex Baiwariorum*, IV.21. But the later development of streamlined mail-piercing arrowheads, ironically, may have made them easier to remove, even by the victim himself: Mitchell *et al.*, "Weapon injuries," 152.

78. Richard: above, Chap. 4; *Orderic*, VII.10 (48–9).

79. Gerald of Wales, *The Journey through Wales*, II.7, tr. L. Thorpe (London: Penguin, 1978), 188.

80. A. Fornaciari and Valentina Giuffra, "Surgery in the early middle ages: evidence of cauterisation from Pisa," *Surgery*, 151 (2012), 351–2. I thank Monica Green for pointing out the article's deficiency in terms of textual expertise.

81. Miller, *Eye for an Eye*, 29.

82. *Alexiad*, IX.10; English translation Anna Komnena, *Alexiad*, tr. E. R. A. Sewter (London: Penguin, 1969), 290.

83. The Latin term "malagma" clearly deriving from the Greek μαλακός for "soft."

84. Both William of Canterbury's account (c. 1172) and that of Benedict of Peterborough (c. 1181) are reproduced in *English Lawsuits from William I to Richard I volume II: Henry II and Richard I*, case 471B, ed. R. C. Van Caenegem (London: Selden Society vol 107, 1991), 507–514.

85. *Herbarium Apulei Platonici*, c.2.18–19 (ulcers and blisters), XX.8 (ulcer on nose), XXII.3 (women's pimples), in *Leechdoms*, ed. Cockayne, I, 87, 117, 119. *Leechbook* I, cc. 8 (facial blotches), 32–33 (pustules, including leprosy) in *Leechdoms*, ed. Cockayne, II, 53–4, 77–82.

86. *De Ornatu Mulierum*, c.272, in *The Trotula: a Medieval Compendium of Women's Medicine*, ed. Monica H. Green (Philadelphia: University of Pennsylvania Press, 2001), 176–177.

87. *Ibid.*, cc. 273 (freckles), 276 and 286 (refining skin), 278, 280, 282–4 (whitening skin), 288 (scabies) and 290 (sunburn), in *The Trotula*, 176–183.

88. *Alexiad*, IX.10 (tr. Sewter, 290).

89. On the broader history of such voyeurism, though regrettably neglecting the medieval period, see Rosemarie Garland-Thomson, "From wonder to error: a genealogy of freak discourse in modernity," in *Freakery: Cultural Spectacles of the Extraordinary Body*, ed. R. Garland-Thomson (New York: New York University Press, 1996), 1–19. And see note 87.

90. *The Life of St Cadog / Vita Sancti Cadoci*, c.36, in *Vitae Sanctorum Britanniae et Geneaologiae*, ed. A. W. Wade-Evans (Cardiff: University of Wales Press, 1944), 24–141. Caroline Walker Bynum, "Wonder," *American Historical Review*, 102 (1997): 1–17, emphasizes the difference between the wonder felt and expressed by medieval theologians and philosophers – as a first step to knowledge – and the more negative, exploitative gathering and exhibiting of "wonders" by early modern explorers and their patrons. The Cadog story, whilst apparently conforming to her model, nevertheless nuances it by "allowing" the rustic to exploit his misfortune for financial gain.

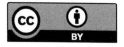

# CHAPTER 8

# Conclusion: Taking the Long View on Medieval Disfigurement

Working on a project that explores the representation of and responses to acquired facial disfigurement in early medieval Europe, I have been struck by the sheer number of instances recorded in medieval evidence. The disruption of the facial features—by far the most visible of sites—resonates with medieval observers; it is threatened as a corporal punishment in legal sources, but penalized if inflicted by anyone other than the king; it features in folkloric tales, often as a warning against transgressive behavior; it is commented upon, often at length, to draw moral lessons. But almost all of this evidence comes from the pens of those observing or imagining facial disfigurement: like many apparently marginal groups in medieval society, the voices of disfigured people themselves are very seldom heard. Yet the patient acceptance of disfigurement or difference is also held up in medieval religious and secular texts as a sign of sanctity or humility before God. The medieval examples offer an opportunity to explore the ambivalence surrounding disfigurement, and try to draw out some questions regarding continuities in the history of people with disfigurements over centuries. Irina Metzler has raised the question as to whether the face-to-face society of the Middle Ages had any concept of disability, and asks whether individuals could have had a "disabled identity."[1] In the present study, the social stigma associated with acquiring a visible facial injury in the early Middle Ages only seems to become an "identity" in legal records of the thirteenth century, when claiming to be a "maimed man"—a status that presumably needed to be permanent—enabled plaintiffs to avoid trial by physical combat. It is certainly the case that the number of examples of recorded

© The Author(s) 2017
P. Skinner, *Living with Disfigurement in Early Medieval Europe*,
DOI 10.1057/978-1-137-54439-1_8

disfigurement increases as we move from the sixth century to the twelfth, and narrative accounts from the latter part of our period do appear to have focused in greater detail on facial appearance than earlier writers. But the exhaustive lists of personal injuries to the head and face contained in early medieval lawcodes suggest that overall levels of concern about facial appearance remained pretty constant in these centuries. The major change—in evidential terms at least—came about with the explosion of medical writings rediscovered in the twelfth century, and a concomitant and well-documented trend toward identification and classification precipitated by Western Europe's engagement (including violence) with the Muslim world.

A substantial proportion of the instances of disfigurement recorded occurs in prescriptive material, and this needs to be acknowledged: the project of recording how people lived with disfigurement relies primarily on actual cases where we know the disfigurement happened. Yet this study has only been able to turn up two or three cases for the entire period where some form of first-person reflection takes place—Wipert, Thietmar, and Walchelin—all three quite late, and all three drawing specific lessons from their different appearance. The first question for further work on disfigurement is thus the nature of the records: at what point will these change from mainly looking *at* people with disfigurements, to a mixture of observations and accounts of the lived experience of looking different? Is the autobiographical account of becoming and being disfigured confined to the most recent century, or are clues to living with disfigurement embedded in earlier letters, diaries and narratives? The early medieval sample privileges reports of deliberate disfigurement over accounts of accidental injury, and focuses almost entirely on when the appearance of male, elite figures, from the lay or clerical sphere, was temporarily or permanently altered. Many lived with their disfigurement afterwards, but it is striking just how many facial injuries were associated with the word "ridicule," and how this specific term persists in sources across our entire period.[2] In a medieval culture that valued honor *and* face, being laughed at, or being the object of not-so-amusing comments, was just as much an injury as physical damage.

What is missing, quite strikingly, is any expression of disgust: here, modern theorists have introduced a concept that is largely absent from the medieval sources. William Ian Miller may relate modern disgust responses to earlier periods, but the "barbarically loathsome" actions of a few were presented with horror expressed at the *actions*, not their results.[3] Authors might express horror and pity, and share with the reader the spectacle of certain acts of mutilation at somewhat greater length than was entirely necessary (my "textual staring"), but they do not describe the aftermath as "disgusting." There was a spectrum associated with the aftermath too: a disfigurement *without* associated impairment and one *with* impairment (of sight, hearing or speech) were classified differently in some of the early laws, and perhaps ridicule shaded into sympathy for the latter category. This distinction has also been made in historiographical practice: only impairment makes it into histories of disability or medical practice, whilst "simple" disfigurement is largely unnoticed and lacks sustained attention from scholars.

Yet, inflicting a deliberate disfigurement was a highly political act, and this study has brought out the significance of mutilation-by-proxy, the attacking of dependents as a means of symbolizing the loss of control or status of the person meant to protect them, be it a king, or a father or—in the specific case of women—a husband. Of course, reports of such attacks still focus our attention on the intended target: the dependents are, often, unfortunate collateral damage (and those mutilated very young were the most damaged of all, facing a lifetime of marginalization). But even the proxies need to be significant in some way—there was no point mutilating a peasant tenant if you wanted to insult the king. One might in fact interpret the threatened mutilation of adulterous women in several lawcodes as a warning to their husbands about the potential shame *they* could suffer at having failed to assert adequate control and protection over their wives, even if this is not explicitly stated in the clauses themselves. Work on medieval violence has picked up on the fact that wives and dependents might be caught up in the downfall of their menfolk or leaders, and toward the twelfth century we certainly see more instances of deliberate mutilations as weapons of humiliation. Whether this is a product of the increase in available written evidence is unclear: the further escalation in the severity of facial violence in the thirteenth century, noted at the start of this study, suggests that this is not simply a matter of the multiplication of texts, but represents a shift away from killing to wounding as a means of settling scores. A question for future research, therefore, might focus on when reports begin of more "ordinary" people with acquired disfigurement (such as some of those documented in the Eyre courts), and explore the reasons for this change.

The stories that disfigurement generated for the early medieval, largely clerical, writers who recorded such incidents seem to fit within something of a predetermined set of parameters drawn from the Bible. And, for many of our writers, the piteous spectacle of those mutilated, or about to be, was an opportunity for others to provide charity, or intervene to plead mercy. It is never stated outright, but disfigurement was, to the elite community we can hear and read about, akin to social death. In some cases the power of a disfigured person's family could shield them from the worst assumptions about their condition, but such protection only lasted as long as they lived; it is interesting that we have a couple of cases of *damnatio memoriae*, whereby later authors, commenting on the same set of circumstances, draw much more robustly negative conclusions about whose fault the disfigurement was (the cases of Young Charles and the Saxon pirate raids of 994 are good examples).

Another issue for historians of disfigurement, therefore, might be how long the framing of disfigurement within religious terms of reference lasted. At what point did the religious framework for understanding disfigurement (act of God, act of wicked people, own fault, disbars further religious or political activity, engenders patience and humility), which is so prominent in the evidence from the early Middle Ages, lessen or disappear, and what replaced it? Although this study ends around 1200 CE, I would hazard a guess that later medieval authors understood and presented disfigurement in very similar ways to those discussed here. Even if more and better skincare remedies (and cover-ups) were being produced, and texts theorizing about surgical repair to the face were being written and circulated by the fifteenth century, the fact remains that faith provided a means of articulating and dealing with the trauma of an acquired disfigurement. Theology Professor Stephen Pattison has recently argued that the Protestant Reformation saw a shift in emphasis from seeing the face of God to hearing and obeying God's word, that is, the opportunity for "face" to play a role in human relations with each other and the divinity diminished sharply, and remains absent today.[4] This hypothesis, convincingly argued, would reward further investigation by historians. Pattison's comments on the isolation, exclusion and shame of those who cannot participate in facial transactions, whether because of disfigurement or neurological conditions impairing facial recognition, resonate loudly with the historical experiences discussed in the present study.

So what about gender? The reality of the early medieval texts is that the vast majority of cases feature, or can be assumed to feature, the disfigurement of men. The minority sample of women is itself interesting in that the *type* or form of the disfigurement they suffer differs from the men: usually specific, inflicted damage to appearance of the face, rather than mutilations of ears or blinding. Males, as we might expect, are also frequently injured in war and at close quarters by swords, clubs and axes. If this did not result in a fatal injury, it left a mark that, I have argued, shamed rather than distinguished the recipient. Rosemary Garland-Thomson has suggested that acquired impairment in adult, white males re-classifies them as among the more socially disadvantaged, who, in the modern American society she was discussing, consist of women and people of color. Depending on the level of disfigurement—and in the medieval spectrum I have explored, this ranges from broken noses and bramble scratches leaving a facial scar on one end, to permanent removal of the eyes or other facial features such as lips, noses or ears on the other—acquired facial disfigurement, too, had the potential to feminize a male victim, particularly if he had been socially active and in the prime of life. The ability to wage war, in particular, was a key feature of elite medieval masculinity (even among some clerics). The dependence inherent in being cared for after disfigurement itself removed a person from their "normal" lives, and whilst they might recover physically, the visible change in their faces clearly provoked interest and inquiry. The rehabilitation of war-wounded men does not feature in the sources, suggesting that this was a process best done in private, and out of sight. It is unlikely to be coincidental that our three first-person accounts are all by clerics, whose masculinity was not compromised in such a devastating way by their condition.

A third question, therefore, centers on the gender imbalance in disfigurement cases. Do women remain in the minority over time, or has disfigurement increasingly become a weapon used only against women? Medieval medical theory, following Aristotelian thought, classified the female body as damaged or lacking anyway. The medieval judicial penalty of castration, threatened and sometimes inflicted upon men, was not available for women, and this may explain why we have instances in medieval law of the female face being a target for punishment and abuse. But what is interesting to me is how reports of female miscreants foreground their sexual morality, even when the deed for which they are being punished might appear to be a whole lot more serious. In fact, medieval authors have a hard time imagining women being violent, and so might equally well ignore evidence of violence against women as trivial compared with the honor games played out between men.

Taking the long view can sometimes be a risky business—medieval specialists might cry "anachronism" when the insights of modern social sciences or cultural studies are applied to medieval texts—or worse still this is "medievalism" and not "medieval studies" (I speak tongue in cheek here; the burgeoning field of medievalism is both intriguing and challenging).

And some of the constraints visible in even this brief report of medieval attitudes toward disfigurement might seem too far distant from modern concerns and priorities to enable a genuine cross-period dialogue that can provide insight both ways. James Partridge, founder and director of the UK charity Changing Faces, stated, in a recent online campaign against an offensive advertisement campaign, that "Changing Faces is determined to challenge any example of prejudicial portrayal because *we are not living in the Middle Ages* [my emphasis]." But medieval attitudes to disfigurement were not so entrenched as to allow me to let his comment go unchallenged. As in modern contexts, reactions were fluid, contingent upon the circumstances of acquisition, and community acceptance of a disfigured face was freighted with similar anxieties about the source of the damage. Another link between the medieval and the modern, I contend, is the fact that disfigurement was and remains a highly-individualized experience: there is a great deal of resistance in contemporary discourse to the idea that facial difference is an undifferentiated, collective experience, and the same appears to be true of medieval cases: the stories are always personal.

There are differences of course. Unlike the medieval past, disfigurement in the present can—provided this is what the patient wants—be mitigated by surgical and cosmetic intervention. And the much wider access to literacy and media means that the voices of people with disfigurements can be heard. But what I would suggest is that we need to take the long view in order to highlight the fact that, whilst the medical ability to address disfigurement has taken enormous strides, and the psychological effects of sudden, acquired disfigurement are now much better understood, reconstructing the history of disfigurement can expose—much as other minority history campaigns have done—the high and low points against which to measure our own, current social attitudes and prejudices.

## Notes

1. Irina Metzler, *Disability in Medieval Europe: Thinking about Physical Impairment during the High Middle Ages* (London: Routledge, 2006), pp. 5–9.
2. *Ibid.*, p. 163, notes the same language in the thirteenth-century miracles of St Elizabeth of Hungary, for example.

3. William Ian Miller, *The Anatomy of Disgust* (Cambridge, MA: Harvard University Press, 1997), 11–22.
4. Stephen Pattison, *Saving Face: Enfacement, Shame, Theology* (Farnham/Burlington, VT: Ashgate, 2013), 2 and 51–75.

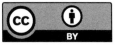

# Appendix 1: Narrative and Archaeological Evidence for Disfigurement

(For disfigurement in legal texts, see below, Appendix 2). NB This list does not claim to be geographically exhaustive: Scandinavia, the Crusader states and the Muslim world, in particular, await their specific studies.

| When | Where | What | Reference |
|---|---|---|---|
| date uncertain | England | sword wound to head bandaged in *Beowulf* | Above, Chap. 7 |
| *Fifth century* | | | |
| [479/80CE] | Byzantium | Illos' missing ear | Theophanes, *Chronographia*, AM5972 |
| [470 s/80s] | Africa/Italy | ears and nose of Theodoric's daughter cut off | Jordanes, *Getica*, XXXVI |
| 5th to 10th C | Low Countries | Healed blade injuries to skull | Panhuysen, "Het scherpe" |
| *Sixth century* | | | |
| early 6th C | Francia | *Pactus Legis Salicae* laws | See Appendix 2 |
| early 6th C | Francia | *Leges Burgundionum* | See Appendix 2 |
| [before 511] | Francia | tonsuring of Chararic and his son | *GT*, II.41 |
| after 533 | Byzantium | *Digest of Justinian* | Above, Chap. 3 |
| [c.555] | Francia | Theodovald cuts off own hair | *GT*, III.18 |
| [c.578] | Francia | hands, feet, ears and nose of Gailen cut off | *GT*, V.18 |
| 580×616 | England, Kent | Laws of King Aethelberht | See Appendix 2 |

© The Author(s) 2017
P. Skinner, *Living with Disfigurement in Early Medieval Europe*,
DOI 10.1057/978-1-137-54439-1

| When | Where | What | Reference |
|---|---|---|---|
| [before 582] | Francia | Count Leudast's mutilated ears, scalping, medical care | GT, V.48, VI.32 |
| before 584 | Francia | condemnation of King Chilperic II as "Nero and Herod of our time" | GT, VI.46 |
| [c.585] | Francia | ears and noses of assassins cut off and let out for "ridicule" | GT, VIII.29, X.18 |
| 585×589 | Francia | death of Duke Rauching: mutilating head | GT, IX.9 |
| 588/9 | Byzantium | Turks get tattoos of cross on forehead to protect from plague | Theophanes, Chronographia, AM6081 |
| [before 596] | Francia | Septimina burnt on face, Droctulf loses ears and is shaven | GT, IX.38 |
| 6th C | England | head injuries, pagan graves | Anderson, "Cranial weapons injuries" |
| 6th C | Francia | rape victim beaten about face | GT, IX.27 |
| 6–8th C | Italy | remains of warriors with head wounds | Rubini and Zaio, "Warriors from the East" |
| 6th–8th C | Germany | healed head wounds in up to 30 skeletons | Mitchell, Medicine, 112 |
| Seventh century | | | |
| c. 600 | England, Kent | Laws of Aethelbehrt | See Appendix 2 |
| early 7th C | Francia | Leges Alamannorum, Pactus | See Appendix 2 |
| before 637 | Ireland | King Congal Cáech disqualified by bee sting in eye | Kelly, Guide, 19 and 239 |
| 608 | Byzantium | blinding mentioned in conspiracy | Theophanes, Chronographia, AM 6101 |
| 625/6 | Byzantium | Emperor Heraclius wounded by spear in face | Theophanes, Chronographia, AM 6118 |
| 640/1 | Byzantium | cutting off Heraklonas' nose, Martina's tongue | Theophanes, Chronographia, AM 6133 |
| 643 | Italy | Edict of King Rothari | See Appendix 2 |
| 654–681 | Spain | Lex Visigothorum | See Appendix 2 |
| [668/9] recte 681 | Byzantium | Tiberius and Heraklius lose noses | Theophanes, Chronographia, AM 6161 |

| When | Where | What | Reference |
|---|---|---|---|
| 694/5 | Byzantium | nose and lips of deposed Emperor Justinian II cut off | Theophanes, *Chronographia*, AM 6187 |
| 697 | Byzantium | nose-cutting of another imperial candidate (Leontios) | Theophanes, *Chronographia*, AM 6190 |
| 7th C | E Francia | *Lex Ribvaria* | See Appendix 2 |
| 7th C? | Ireland | eye put out by holly sprig, shame | *The Wooing of Étaín*, in *Early Irish Myths and Sagas* |
| 7th C? | Ireland | bestial facial features | *The Destruction of Da Derga's Hostel*, in *ibid.* |
| 7th C? | Ireland | women who loved Cú Chulaind put out one eye in his likeness | *Death of Aife's Only Son*, in *ibid.* |
| 7th C? | Ireland | Éogan's eye put out by a spear | *Tale of Macc Da Thó's Pig*, in *ibid.* |
| late 7th C? | Ireland | Book of Aicill | See Appendix 2 |
| 7th–8th C | Ireland | *Bretha Déin Chécht* | See Appendix 2 |
| *Eighth century* | | | |
| early 8th C | Ireland | *Bretha Nemed Toísech* | See Appendix 2 |
| early 8th C | Ireland | *Bretha Crólige* | See Appendix 2 |
| [705] | Byzantium | restoration of Justinian II with prosthetic gold nose and ears | Paul the Deacon, *History of the Lombards*, VI.31; Agnellus of Ravenna, c. 137 |
| [705–798] | Byzantium | blindings reported by Theophanes, including that of Constantine by Empress Irene | Theophanes, *Chronographia*, AM 6198, 6205, 6210, 6211, 6235, 6257, 6263, 6284, 6285, 6289, 6291 |
| 726 | Byzantium | *Ecloga* | See Appendix 2 |
| 726–750 | Italy | *Leges Langobardorum* | See Appendix 2 |
| 730–750 | Byzantium | George Limnaiotes, nose slit; Paul of Kaioumas, nose cut off | *Dumbarton Oaks Hagiography Database* |
| 731 | Francia | *Leges Alamannorum, Lex* | See Appendix 2 |
| 740 s | E Francia | *Lex Baiwariorum* | See Appendix 2 |
| 751 | Francia | Childeric III's hair cut | Einhard, *Vita*, I.1 |

| When | Where | What | Reference |
|------|-------|------|-----------|
| before 764/5 | Byzantium | torture and mutilation of holy men: cut off noses, eyes gouged out, hands cut off, ears cut off, whipped, hair shaved, beards soaked in pitch and burnt | *Vie d'Étienne le jeune*, c. 56 |
| 775×820 | Byzantium | Theodore and Theophanes 'Graptoi' | *Byzantine Defenders*, ed. Talbot, 204 |
| before 794 | Francia | cruelty of Queen Fastrada causes blindings | Einhard, *Vita*, III.20 |
| late 8th C | Francia | *Lex Salica* | See Appendix 2 |
| 799 | Italy | attempted deposition and facial mutilation of Pope Leo III | Einhard, *Vita*, III.28; Notker, *Gesta*, I.26 |
| [late 8th C] | Francia/ Byzantium | envoys to Byzantium breach protocol, threatened with blinding | Notker, *Gesta*, II.6 |
| late 8th/early 9th C | Francia | *Lex Salica Karolina* | See Appendix 2 |
| *Ninth century* | | | |
| early 9th C | Frisia | *Lex Frisionum* | See Appendix 2 |
| after 801 | Francia | *admonitio* on correct marriage | Add. ad Pippini et Karoli M. Capitularia, no. 121, *MGH Cap. Reg. Franc.*, I |
| 803/4 | Byzantium | Blinding of "Bardarios" | Theophanes, *Chronographia*, AM 6296 |
| 805 | Francia | capitulary of Thionville | See Appendix 2 |
| 810/11 | Byzantium | Khan Krum's mutilation of Christians including cutting off ears | Theophanes, *Chronographia*, AM 6303 |
| 817 | Francia | Louis the Pious—wound to back of ear | *Annales Regni Francorum* |
| [before 840] | Francia | Louis the Pious hires justiciar to mete out retaliative punishment | Notker, *Gesta*, II.21 |
| 866 | Italy | Pope Nicholas I condemns confessions extracted by beating around the head | *MGH Epp. Karol. Aevi*, IV, 595 |
| 870 | Francia | Louis the German—treatment of rotting flesh | *Annales Bertiniani* |

| When | Where | What | Reference |
|------|-------|------|-----------|
| 870 s | England | Ebba of Coldingham and her nuns self-mutilate faces | Pulsiano, "Blessed bodies" |
| 864 | Francia | Young Charles, son of Charles the Bald, slashed across face with a sword, survives two years | *Annales Bertiniani*, Ado of Vienne, Regino of Prum |
| 877 | S Italy | Sergius, *magister militum* of Naples, blinded and exiled | Erchempert, *Historia*, c. 39 |
| 880 s | Francia | highlighting of red hair | Notker, *Gesta*, I.18 |
| 886×912 | Byzantium | *Novels* of Leo VI | See Appendix 2 |
| 9th C | Switzerland (St Gall) | remedies for wounds to face | Jörimann, *Frühmittelalterliche Rezeptarien* |

*Tenth century*

| When | Where | What | Reference |
|------|-------|------|-----------|
| 899×924 | England | Helmstan's scratched face | Fonthill Letter |
| [after 925] | England | attempt to blind King Athelstan | Wm of Malmesbury, *Gesta Regum*, II.137 |
| early 10th C | England | cure for "blisters on a man's *neb*" | Ps-Apuleius, in *Leechbooks*, ed. Cockayne, I, 87 |
| early 10th C | England | remedy for broken head | Bald's *Leechbook* I, I.1, and III.33, ed. Cockayne, II, 19–26, 327 |
| early 10th C | England | remedy for blotches on face | Bald's *Leechbook* I, I.8, 32, 33, ed. Cockayne, II, 53, 77–81 |
| early 10th C | England | surgery for hare lip | Bald's *Leechbook* I.13, ed. Cockayne, II, 59 |
| 929 | France | the medic Deroldus becomes bishop of Amiens | *Annals* of Flodoard of Reims |
| [before 944] | Normandy | Riulf blinded in prison | Wm of Malmesbury, *Gesta Regum*, II.145 |
| 950×1120 | England | Peri-mortem injuries to head and face | Patrick, "Approaches" |
| 954 | France | Louis IV suffers from "elephantiasis" | *Annals* of Flodoard of Reims |
| 959×975 | England | laws of Edgar | See Appendix 2 |
| [960 s/970 s] | S. Italy | blinding of Greeks in Calabria by Otto II's men | *Thietmar*, II.15 |
| 960×1100 | England | surgery on head injury? | Mays, "A possible case" |
| [965] | Italy | Pope John XIII slapped around the face | *MGH, SS*, III, 719 |

| When | Where | What | Reference |
|------|-------|------|-----------|
| [before 972] | Germany | Bishop Michael of Regensburg missing ear | *Thietmar*, II.27 |
| late 10th C | England | Matthew's eyes "gouged out with a sword" | Above, Chap. 4, n.12 |
| [990×995] | Germany | blinding of a man of Bishop Bernward of Wurzburg | *Thietmar*, IV.21 |
| [993] | England | Aethelred blinds Aelfric's son | Wm of Malmesbury, *Gesta Regum*, II.165 |
| [994] | Germany | pirates cut off noses, hands and feet of Saxon hostages | Adam of Bremen, II.xxxi (29), *Thietmar* IV.23–25 |
| 998 | Italy | cut off hands and ears, and blinding of deposed pope John XVI by Otto III | *Rodulf Glaber*, tr. France, I.12; John the Deacon, *MGH SS*, VII |
| [mid 10th C] | Germany/N Italy | Henry of Bavaria orders blinding of bishop of Salzburg | *Thietmar*, II.40 |
| 10th C | Wales | Laws of Hywel Dda | See Appendix 2 |
| 10th C | Germany | Bamberg recipe collection | Jörimann, *Frühmittelalterliche Rezeptarien* |
| before 1003 | France | Gerbert of Aurillac's letters include comments on medicine | *Letters of Gerbert*, tr. Lattin |
| undated | England | Anglo-Saxon child with hare lip | Crawford, *Childhood*, 95 |
| undated | England | Anglo-Saxon child with fibrous dysplasia of jawbone | Craig and Craig, "Diagnosis" |

*Eleventh century*

| When | Where | What | Reference |
|------|-------|------|-----------|
| 1000 | Germany | Otto III restores face of dead Charlemagne with gold nose tip | *MGH, SS rer. Germ.*, XXI |
| 1006 | England | blinding of Wulfheah and Ufegeat | *Anglo-Saxon Chronicle* |
| c.1009 | Russia | Wipert's account of being blinded | *MGH SS*, IV, 569 |
| 1014 | England | Cnut mutilates ears, noses and hands of Anglo-Saxon hostages | *Anglo-Saxon Chronicle* |
| before 1018 | Germany | Thietmar's nephew performs a retaliative blinding | *Thietmar*, IV.21 |
| before 1018 | Germany | Thietmar's reflection on his own facial deformity | *Thietmar*, IV.75 |

| When | Where | What | Reference |
|------|-------|------|-----------|
| before 1018 | Bohemia | blinding of Boleslav III (d.1037) | Thietmar, V.30 |
| before 1018 | eastern Germany | Liutici cut hair to make peace | Thietmar, VI.25 |
| before 1018 | Germany | bad teeth—inability to chew | Thietmar, VI.64 |
| before 1018 | Germany | outer/"inner" sight | Thietmar, VII.55 and 67 |
| before 1018 | Germany | shaving and flogging of six men | Thietmar, VIII.22 |
| 1020 × 1023 | England | Laws of Cnut | See Appendix 2 |
| 1028 × 1050 | Byzantium | Empress Zoe blinds indiscriminately | Psellos, Chronographia, VI.157 |
| before 1030 | France | Fulbert of Chartres' medical allusions | Letters and Poems of Fulbert |
| [1030s] | Italy/ Byzantium | Theodwin shaved of beard and hair | Amatus, II.13 |
| 1031 | Germany | Ebbo's letter with medical terminology | MGH Briefe in der deutsche Kaiserzeit III |
| 1036 | England | blinding of Alfred son of Aethelred, lives in monastery | Anglo-Saxon Chronicle; Wm of Malemesbury, Gesta Regum, II.188 |
| 1036 | England | blinding of Alfred goes wrong—knife goes too far | Wm of Poitiers, Gesta Guillelmi, I.4 |
| 1041 | Bulgaria | nose cut off and blinding of usurper Dolianus | Michael Psellos, Chronographia, IV. 49 |
| 1042 | Byzantium | Empress Zoe's hair cut | Psellos, Chronographia, V.23 |
| 1042 | Byzantium | blinding of Emperor Michael V and the nobilissimus Constantine | Psellos, Chronographia, V.40–50 |
| 1043 | Byzantium | John Orphanotrophos blinded | Michael Psellos, Chronographia, V.14 |
| [c.1045] | France | William Talvas blinds and castrates William of Giroie | Orderic, III.ii.15 |
| 1050–14th C | Norway | trauma injuries, St Mary's church Oslo | Brødholt, "Skeletal trauma" |
| 1050s? | Byzantium | Basil Sclerus blinded; Tornikios and Vatatzes condemned to blinding | Michael Psellos, Chronographia, VI.15; VI.123 |
| 1052 × 1077 | S Italy | Gisulf II of Salerno gouging out eyes of prisoners | Amatus, VIII.2, 3, 11 |
| before 1060 | France | incompetence of medic treating Henry I of France | Orderic, III.ii.79 |

| When | Where | What | Reference |
|------|-------|------|-----------|
| [1066] | England | King Harold "survives" arrow wound in eye at Hastings | Gerald of Wales, *Journey*, II.11 |
| 1066 | Italy | blinding, cutting of nose and lips of Arioald | Andrea da Strumi, *Passione* |
| [c.1070] | S Italy | Robert Guiscard extracts teeth of, and blinds, William "Mascabeles" | Anna Komnena, *Alexiad*, I.11 |
| before 1072 | Italy | facial punishment of Ardericus | Letters of Peter Damian, no. 85 |
| [1074] | Byzantium | fake blinding of Roussel | Anna Komnena, *Alexiad*, I.4 |
| 1075/6 | Normandy | Blinding of Bretons who had opposed William | *Anglo-Saxon Chronicle* |
| before 1081 | Byzantium | blinding of Basilacius | Anna Komnena, *Alexiad*, I.9 |
| [1082/3] | Byzantium | cruelty of Robert Guiscard and Normans | Anna Komnena, *Alexiad*, V.5 |
| 1086 | England | blinding for poachers of king's deer | *Anglo-Saxon Chronicle* |
| 1091 | France | Walchelin the priest's scarred face | *Orderic*, VIII.17 |
| before 1093 | Germany | St Ulrich of Zell injures own eye with a stick | *Vita S. Udalrici* |
| c.1094 | Byzantium | blinding and rehabilitation of Nicephorus Diogenes | Anna Komnena, *Alexiad*, IX.9 |
| 1095 | England | William of Eu | *Anglo-Saxon Chronicle* |
| late 11th C | France | Robert of Courcy loses right eye in battle | *Orderic*, X.7 |
| late 11th/ early 12th C | France | Alais of Soissons has a cleric blinded and his tongue cut out | Guibert of Nogent, III.16, in *Self and Society*, ed. Benton |
| late 11th/ early 12th C | Normandy | Ralph the "Ill-Tonsured" active | *Orderic*, III.ii.69–70 |
| 11th/12th C | Wales | shaming of the beard in *Mabinogion* | Multiple examples: see above, Chap. 2, note 55 |
|  | Wales | removal of beard/whiskers in *Mabinogion* | Above, Chap. 2, note 57 |

*Twelfth century*

| When | Where | What | Reference |
|------|-------|------|-----------|
| 1106/7 | Byzantium | Anemas brothers shaved completely, threatened with blinding; shaving of traitor Gregory | Anna Komnena, *Alexiad*, XII.6; XII.8 |

| When | Where | What | Reference |
|------|-------|------|-----------|
| 1106×1112 | Normandy | Bishop Gaudry's "African man" carries out blinding | Guibert of Nogent, III.7, in *Self and Society*, ed. Benton |
| [before 1111] | S Italy/ Byzantium | Bohemond threatens blindings | Anna Komnena, *Alexiad*, XI.10 |
| [before 1112] | Normandy | Gérard of Quierzy one-eyed | Guibert of Nogent, III.5, in *Self and Society*, ed. Benton |
| 1112 | Normandy | murder and mutilation of Bishop Gaudry | Guibert of Nogent, III.8–9, in *Self and Society*, ed. Benton |
| [before 1116] | France | mutilations of eyes | Guibert of Nogent, III.3, in *Self and Society*, ed. Benton |
| c.1116 | Turkey | blinding of Malik-Shah | Anna Komnena, *Alexiad*, XV.6 |
| 1117 | England | Wm Giffard, bishop of Winchester saves a child who was to be deprived of [his?] eyes for committing theft | *English Lawsuits from William I to Richard I*, vol. 1, no 210, ed. van Caenegem |
| c.1119 | Normandy | blinding of Ralph of Harenc's son; blinding and nose-cutting of Eustace of Breteuil's daughters | *Orderic*, XII.10 |
| 1124 | England | six thieves blinded and castrated | *Anglo-Saxon Chronicle* |
| 1124 | Normandy | Henry I orders blinding of Luke of La Barre | *Orderic*, XII.39 |
| before 1125 | France | "blemished exterior a matter for sorrow" | Guibert of Nogent, I.2, in *Self and Society*, ed. Benton |
| before 1125 | France | "blindness" to inner self | Guibert of Nogent, I.19, in *Self and Society*, ed. Benton |
| before 1125 | France | hideous face a sign of evil | Guibert of Nogent, III.8, in *Self and Society*, ed. Benton |
| 1126 | Germany | mutilation of eyes, nose, lips, cheeks and ears of Heldolf | *Chronicon Montis Sereni*, ed. Ehrenfeuchter |
| before 1142 | Normandy | medical allusions | *Orderic*, VIII.26 |
| c.1147 | Flanders | William permanently scarred on head by sword at Avesnes | *MGH SS*, XIV |
| before 1158 | Netherlands | Oda of Brabant disfigures herself | *AASS*, XI, 20 April |

| *When* | *Where* | *What* | *Reference* |
|--------|---------|--------|-------------|
| 1162/4 | England | Thomas Becket rejects corporal punishment but a cleric accused of theft judged by secular court, TB caused him to be branded (*cauteriari*) to placate king—on face? | *English Lawsuits, vol. 2,* no 416, ed. van Caenegem |
| [1165] | | Heretics vanquished by ordeal and after their faces were branded (*facie cauteriata*) expelled from the kingdom | *English Lawsuits, vol. 2,* no 426, ed. van Caenegem, citing Ralph de Diceto, I, 318. |
| 1166 | S Italy | *Ecloga ad Procheiron Mutata* | See Appendix 2 |
| after 1170 | England | Thomas Becket postumously restores Ailward of Westoning's eyes | *English Lawsuits, vol. 2,* no 471, ed. Van Caenegem |
| 1177 | England | St William of York restores the eyes of two victims of injustice | *English Lawsuits, vol. 2,* nos 504 and 505, ed. van Caenegem |
| after 1179 | Kingdom of Jerusalem | battlefield injuries, Vadum Iacob castle | Mitchell *et al.*, "Weapon injuries" |
| [before 1191] | Wales | blinding by saint | Gerald of Wales, *Journey,* I.1 |
| [before 1191] | France | blinded prisoner learns way around | Gerald of Wales, *Journey,* I.11 |
| [before 1191] | Wales | legitimacy proven by inherited scar | Gerald of Wales, *Journey,* II.7 |
| [before 1191] | Wales | Iorwerth "Fat-Nose" | Gerald of Wales, *Journey,* II.8 |
| [before 1191] | Orkneys | Hugh of Shrewsbury hit by arrow in eye | Gerald of Wales, *Journey,* II.7 |
| 1191 | S Italy | Richard of Acerra's cheeks pierced by arrow | *Liber ad Honorem Augusti,* XV |
| c.1194 | Wales | Welsh people take great care of their teeth, shave their beards and cut hair short | Gerald of Wales, *Description of Wales,* I.11 |
| 12th C | S Italy | cosmetics improve an ugly woman | *De Ornatu Mulierum,* ed. Green |
| late 12th C | France | tale of daughters born with noseless faces | Marie de France, *Bisclavret* |
| late 12th/ early 13th C | France | blinding, pulling out beard whiskers, cutting off ears | *Raoul de Cambrai,* ed. Kay |

| When | Where | What | Reference |
|------|-------|------|-----------|
| *Thirteenth century* | | | |
| 1201 | England (Cornwall) | John de Bosco accuses Odo de Hay of wounding him *"in capite ita quod ossa de capite suo extrahuntur unde maimatus est."* | Thirteenth-century English material without reference here is discussed above, Chap. 3 |
| 1201 | | Edith of St Teath wounded in the head so that 16 bones were extracted | |
| 1201 | | Serlo of Inniscaven gravely wounded so that three bones were extracted from his head | |
| 1201 | | Edmer of Penburthen wounded in the head so that 28 bones were extracted | |
| 1201 | | Anger of Penhale wounded so that four bones taken from his head | |
| 1201 | | Warin of Bodwannick wounded in the head so that bones were extracted, and in the nose | |
| 1201 | | Peter Burill accuses Anketill de Wingoli of giving him four wounds to his head | |
| 1202 | England (Essex) | William de la Dune and his wife Joscea accuse Michael Trenchard of wounding them on the head with a staff | *Pleas before the King of his Justices 1198–1202, vol. 2,* nos 384–386, ed. Stenton, 89–90. |
| 1202 | | William of Brienon: knife wound in the jaw | |
| 1202 | England (Lincs) | Astin of Wispington accused Simon of Edlington of putting out his eye. | |
| 1203 | England (Shropshire) | Alice Crithecreche condemned to blinding | Discussed above, Chap. 5 |
| 1208 | England (York) | Reiner of Garton accuses Hugh reeve of Ellerker of inflicting a *plagam in capite* | *Pleas vol. 2,* no 3445, ed. Stenton, 103. |
| after 1217 | England (Worcester) | Thomas of Elderfield's eyes restored by St Wulfstan | Wheatley, *Stumbling Blocks,* 175–179 |

| When | Where | What | Reference |
| --- | --- | --- | --- |
| 1218 | England (Yorkshire) | A plea dismissed by the justices because the victim (whose case was brought by his son) had neither died nor lost his sight | |
| 1231 | S Italy | *Liber Augustalis* | See Appendix 2 |
| 1245 | Italy | Genoese archers' eyes and hands mutilated | *MGH, SS*, XVIII |
| 1248 | England (Berkshire) | Robert of Denmead wounded in the head with a fork [*furca*] and a hatchet | |
| 1250 | Cyprus | Assizes | See Appendix 2 |
| 1256 | England (Shropshire) | spear strike below the eye, fatal eight days later | |
| 1256 | | Walter of Wottenhull's claim that Thomas of Willaston had hit him on the head with a stick was dismissed | |
| 1256 | | Simon of Preen claimed he had been injured in the back and head with a sword | |
| 1259 | Italy | Ezzelino da Romano mutilates the people of Friuli | *MGH, SS* XIX, 136 |
| 1267 | Italy | Theoderic of Bologna's *Surgery* | ed. Campbell and Cotton |
| 13th C | England | remains of male with cranial trauma, St Mary Spital | Powers, "Cranial trauma" |
| 13th C | Southern France | Multiple Albigensian crusade mutilations | Above, Chap. 4 |
| c.1251 | Germany | Berchtold bishop of Passau blinds and mutilates ears of one of his clergy | *MGH SS*, XXV |
| 13th C | Italy | Aldevrandus's deformed head | Salimbene, *MGH SS*, XXXII |
| late 13th C | France/Italy | remedies for "trivial" facial conditions | Demaitre, "Skin and the city" |
| before 1270 | Hungary | St Margaret of Hungary fails to get permission to mutilate her face | *AASS*, III, 28 January |
| before 1297 | Italy | St Margaret of Cortona fails to get permission to mutilate her face | *AASS*, VI, 22 February |

# Appendix 2: Disfigurement in Early Medieval Lawcodes

| Text | Place/date | Injury | Reference |
|---|---|---|---|
| *Pactus Legis Salicae*, ed. Eckhardt | Francia, early 6th C | pulling beard/hair | III.104 |
| | | wounding, blood falls to ground | XVII.3 |
| | | head wound exposing brain | XVII.4 |
| | | head wound removing three bones | XVII.5 |
| | | wound, cannot be staunched | XVII.7 |
| | | cutting hair (boy, girl) | XXIV.2–3 |
| | | removing eye | XXIX.1 |
| | | cutting off nose | XXIX.1 |
| | | injuring front teeth | XXIX.1 |
| | | cut out tongue | XXIX.1 |
| | | cutting off ear | XXIX.3 |
| | | knocking out tooth | XXIX.5 |
| *Leges Burgundionum*, ed. de Salis | Francia, early 6th C | pulling hair (man) | V.4–5 |
| | | facial wound (triple penalty as not concealed by clothes) | XI.2 |
| | | knocking out teeth (noble, freeman, inferior, slave) | XXVI.1–5 |
| | | cutting hair of woman in own house; she is not to retaliate | XXXIII.1–5, XCII.1–6 |

© The Author(s) 2017
P. Skinner, *Living with Disfigurement in Early Medieval Europe*,
DOI 10.1057/978-1-137-54439-1

| Text | Place/date | Injury | Reference |
|------|-----------|--------|-----------|
| Laws of Aethelberht of Kent, ed. Oliver | England, 560×616 | pulling hair | c.33 |
| | | exposing bone | c.34 |
| | | cutting bone | c.35 |
| | | breaking scalp | c.36 |
| | | breaking scalp and skull | c.36.1 |
| | | making deaf | c. 38 |
| | | cut off ear | c.39 |
| | | pierce ear | c.40 |
| | | gash ear | c.41 |
| | | gouge out eye | c.42 |
| | | damage (*weorðeþ*) eye or mouth | c.43 |
| | | pierce the nose | c.44 |
| | | pierce one cheek/side[1] (*hleore*) | c.44.1 |
| | | pierce both cheeks/sides | c.44.2 |
| | | gash nose | c.45 |
| | | shatter jaw bone | c.47 |
| | | damage to teeth (front, incisors, canines, rest) | cc.48–48.3 |
| | | damage speech | c. 49 |
| | | slight or serious disfigurement *Æt þam lærestan wlitewamme And æt þam maran* | cc.60, 60.1 |
| | | hit in nose, levels of wound visibility | cc.61–61.4 |
| | | removal of servant's eye or foot | c. 80 |
| *Leges Alamannorum, Pactus*, ed. Eckhardt | Francia, early 7th C | injury to head revealing brain | Pactus I.1 |
| | | broken skull, bones that sound extracted | Pactus I.4 |
| | | fractured skull | Pactus I.5 |
| | | injure eye, pupil remains | Pactus V.1 |
| | | take out eye | Pactus V.2 |
| | | injure ear | Pactus VI.1 |
| | | remove ear, deafness | Pactus VI.2 |
| | | way-blocking | Pactus XVIII.1 |
| | | cutting woman's hair | Pactus XVIII.7 |

| Text | Place/date | Injury | Reference |
|------|-----------|--------|-----------|
| *Leges Langobardorum*, ed. Bluhme, Rothari's Edict | Italy, 643 | way-blocking a woman or girl | c. 26 |
| | | way-blocking a man, no physical injury | c.27 |
| | | beaten up freeman | c. 41 |
| | | hitting with fist or slapping | c. 44 |
| | | head injury, skin broken, covered by hair | c. 46 |
| | | head injury, bone extracted makes sound | c. 47 |
| | | take out eye | c. 48 |
| | | cut off nose | c. 49 |
| | | cut off lip, teeth appear | c. 50 |
| | | damage to teeth | cc. 51–2 |
| | | cut off ear | c. 53 |
| | | injury to face | c. 54 |
| | | nose and ear wounds healing to a scar | cc. 55–6 |
| | | head injury to slave or semi-free | c. 78 |
| | | head injury to slave or semi-free, bone broken, medic attends | c. 79 |
| | | injury to face, slave or semi-free | c. 80 |
| | | take out eye, slave or semi-free | c. 81 |
| | | cut off nose, slave or semi-free, doctor | c. 82 |
| | | cut off ear, slave or semi-free, doctor | c. 83 |
| | | cut off lip, slave or semi-free, doctor | c. 84 |
| | | damage teeth, slave or semi-free, front or back | cc. 85–6 |
| | | head injury, field slave, broken skin | c. 103 |
| | | face injury, field slave | c. 104 |
| | | take out eye, field slave | c. 105 |
| | | cut off nose, field slave | c. 106 |
| | | cut off, ear, field slave | c. 107 |
| | | cut off lip, field slave | c. 108 |
| | | damage to teeth, field slave, front or back | c. 109 |
| | | who does the injury finds the doctor | c. 128 |

| Text | Place/date | Injury | Reference |
|------|-----------|--------|-----------|
| | | no need to marry blind or leprous bride | c. 180 |
| | | disfiguring horses | c. 341 |
| | | removing eye of one-eyed man | c. 377 |
| | | violence of women *inhonestum* | c. 378 |
| | | pulling beard or hair of man | c. 383 |
| *Lex Ribvaria*, ed. Beyerle and Buchner | E Francia, 7th C | hitting someone, blood falls to ground | II |
| | | ear injury, causing hearing loss or not | V.1 |
| | | nose injury, affecting mucus or not | V.2 |
| | | taking out eye; injury to eye blinding | V.3 |
| | | injuring eye, ear or nose of slave | XXVII |
| | | touching woman | XLIII |
| *Lex Visigothorum*, ed. K. Zeumer | Spain, 654–681 | prostitute scalped (*decalvata*) | III.4.17 |
| | | injury to head, to skin, to bone, broken bone | VI.4.1 |
| | | scalping (*decalvare*), "shameful injuries" to face (*turpibus maculis*). Retaliation to slapping and punching forbidden | VI.4.3 |
| | | injury or removal of nose so that the *pars turpata* shows, lips and ears | VI.4.3 |
| | | on medical practice, including removal of cataracts | XI.1.1–8 |
| | | Jewish women carrying out circumcisions to lose noses | XII.3.4 |
| *Book of Aicill* | Ireland, late 7th C? | injuries in female fights not actionable | Kelly, *Guide*, 79 |
| *Eighth century Bretha Déin Chécht* | Ireland, 7th–8th C | degree of blemish | c. 10, in Kelly, *Guide*, 131 |
| | | degrees of facial wound to lords and apprentices | c. 13, in Kelly, *Guide*, 8 |
| | | compensation to victim of facial injury for every public assembly attended | c. 31, in Kelly, *Guide*, 132 |
| | | six classes of tooth injury | c. 34, in Kelly, *Guide*, 132 |
| *Bretha Nemed Toísech* | Ireland, early 8th C | competent physician heals without blemish | Kelly, *Guide*, 57 |

| Text | Place/date | Injury | Reference |
|------|-----------|--------|-----------|
| *Bretha Crólige* | Ireland, early 8th C | victim examined by doctor, assailant pays for lasting blemish | Kelly, *Guide*, 129 |
| *Leges Langobardorum* ed. Bluhme, Liutprand | Italy, 726 | shaving/scalping and branding of forehead and face of recidivist thief | c. 80 |
| *Ecloga*, ed. Freshfield | Byzantium, 726 | removal of perjurer's tongue | XVII.2 |
| | | blinding of thief from a sanctuary | XVII.5 |
| | | cutting-off or slitting of the nose for sexual offences | XVII.23–27, 30–34 |
| *Leges Alamannorum, Lex*, ed. Eckhardt | Francia, 731 | obstructing woman and uncovering hair | Leges ALVI/ BLVIII |
| | | shed blood that reaches the ground | *Leges* ALVII.2/ BLIX.2 |
| | | fractured skull | *ibid.* 3 |
| | | bone extracted from head makes sound | *ibid.* 4 |
| | | doctor loses bone | *ibid.* 5 |
| | | doctor touching brain | *ibid.* 6 |
| | | brain swells, doctor uses "silk" | *ibid.* 7 |
| | | remove ear, not deaf | *Leges* ALVII.8/ BLX.1 |
| | | remove ear deeply, deafens | ALVII.9/ BLX.2 |
| | | cut off half ear | ALVII.10/ BLX.3 |
| | | injure upper eyelid, eye cannot close | ALVII.11/ BLXI.1 |
| | | injure lower eyelid, cannot hold tears | ALVII.12/ BLXI.2 |
| | | injure eye, sight "as if through glass" | ALVII.13/ BLXI.3 |
| | | injure eye, blinding | ALVII.14/ BLXI.4 |
| | | pierce nose | ALVII.15/ BLXII.1 |
| | | remove top of nose, cannot hold mucus | ALVII.16/ BLXII.2 |
| | | remove whole nose | ALVII.17/ BLXII.3 |
| | | injure upper lip, teeth visible | ALVII.18/ BLXIII.1 |
| | | injure lower lip, cannot hold saliva | ALVII.19/ BLXIII.2 |

| Text | Place/date | Injury | Reference |
|------|------------|--------|-----------|
| | | knock out both top front teeth | ALVII.20/ BLXIII.3 |
| | | knock out one top front tooth | ALVII.21/ BLXIII.4 |
| | | knock out "marczan" tooth | ALVII.22/ BLXIII.5 |
| | | knock out other tooth | ALVII.23/ BLXIII.6 |
| | | knock out bottom front teeth | ALVII.24/ BLXIII.7 |
| | | knock out one bottom front tooth | ALVII.25/ BLXIII.8 |
| | | cut out tongue, separate penalties for loss of speech or remaining able to be understood | ALVII.26/ BLXIV.1 |
| | | other facial injury not covered by hair or beard | ALVII.27/ BLXIV.2 |
| | | tonsuring another against their will | ALVII.28/ BLXV.1 |
| | | shaving beard of another | ALVII.29/ BLXV.2 |
| | | all penalties for injury double for women | ALIX.2/ BLXVII.2 |
| *Leges Langobardorum*, ed. Bluhme, Liutprand | Italy, 731 | women involved in violence | c. 123 |
| | 731 | injuring woman relieving herself | c. 125 |
| | 733 | stealing clothes of woman bathing | c. 135 |
| *Lex Baiwariorum*, ed. Liber | E Francia, 740 s | drawing blood | IV.2, V.2, VI.2 |
| | | wound cannot be staunched, broken scalp or fractured skull | IV.4, VI.3 |
| | | Injury, bone extracted | IV.5, V.4, VI.4 |
| | | head injury exposing brain (freeman, freedman, slave) | IV.6, V.5, VI.5 |
| | | take out eye | IV.9, V.6, VI.6 |
| | | pierce nose | IV.13, VI.8 |
| | | pierce ear | IV.14 |
| | | damage lower lip, cannot contain saliva, or lower eyelid, cannot contain tears | IV.15 |
| | | knock out front and other teeth | IV.16, VI.10 |

| Text | Place/date | Injury | Reference |
|------|-----------|--------|-----------|
| | | damage lips of slave | VI.9 |
| | | remove ear of slave | VI.11 |
| *Leges* | Italy, 750 | shaving | c.4 |
| *Langobardorum*, ed. | | | |
| Bluhme, Aistulf | | | |
| *Lex Salica*, ed. | late 8th C | skull injury, bone removed | XXII.3 |
| Eckhardt | | | |
| | | injury drawing blood | XXIII.2 |
| | | cutting hair of boy or girl | D, XXXV.1–2 |
| | | removing eye | D, XLVIII.10 |
| | | injuring nose or ear | D, XLVIII.11 |
| | | cutting tongue cannot speak | D, XLVIII.12 |
| | | knocking out tooth | D, XLVIII.13 |
| | | way-blocking man or woman | D, L.1–2 |
| *Lex Salica Karolina*, | late 8th | causing injury, blood falls to | XV.2 |
| ed. Eckhardt | –early 9th C | ground | |
| | | head injury, 3 bones removed | XV.3 |
| | | head injury, 3 bones and brain | XV.4 |
| | | visible | |
| | | wound cannot be staunched | XV.6 |
| | | take out eye, cut off ear or nose | XVI.1 |
| | | take out eye | XVI.13 |
| | | cut off nose | XVI.14 |
| | | cut off ear | XVI.15 |
| | | cut out tongue, cannot speak | XVI.16 |
| | | knock out tooth | XVI.17 |
| | | touching a woman | XXII.1–4 |
| | | cutting hair of boy or girl | XXXIII.2–3 |
| | | way-blocking man or woman | XXXVIII.1–2 |
| *Ninth century* | | | |
| *Lex Frisionum*, ed. | Frisia, early | head injury, loss of hearing | XXII.1 |
| Richthofen | 9th C | | |
| | | head injury, mute but hearing | XXII.2 |
| | | injury, blood shed | XXII.3 |
| | | head injury exposing skull | XXII.5 |
| | | head injury, broken bone | XXII.6 |
| | | sword blow to head touching | XXII.7 |
| | | brain membrane | |
| | | sword blow to head breaking | XXII.8 |
| | | membrane | |
| | | cut off ear | XXII.9 |
| | | cut off nose | XXII.10 |
| | | cut forehead upper wrinkle | XXII.11 |
| | | cut forehead lower wrinkle | XXII.12 |

| Text | Place/date | Injury | Reference |
|------|------------|--------|-----------|
| | | cut forehead wrinkle closest to eyes | XXII.13 |
| | | damaging eyebrows | XXII.14 |
| | | wound eyelid | XXII.15 |
| | | pierce nose | XXII.16 |
| | | cut off mustache | XXII.17 |
| | | cut lower jaw | XXII.18 |
| | | damage to front/canine/back tooth | XXII.19–21 |
| | | cut through collarbone | XXII.22 |
| | | injure eye causing blindness | XXII.45 |
| | | take out whole eye | XXII.46 |
| | | pulling beard or hair | XXII.65 |
| | | bone comes out of wound; makes sound | XXII.71–4 |
| | | pierce both jaws and tongue with arrow | XXII.85 |
| | | hit head making deaf and mute | *Add.Sap.* III.8 |
| | | cut off ear | *Add.Sap.* III.9 |
| | | cut off nose | *Add.Sap.* III.10 |
| | | pierce one side of the nose | *Add.Sap.* III.11 |
| | | pierce nose septum | *Add.Sap.* III.12 |
| | | pierce nose with arrow three holes | *Add.Sap.* III.13 |
| | | pierce jaw | *Add.Sap.* III.14 |
| | | cut eyebrows | *Add.Sap.* III.15 |
| | | facial injury visible at 12 feet | *Add.Sap.* III.16 |
| | | cut off mustache | *Add.Sap.* III.17 |
| | | hit eye and mouth causing bruise | *Add.Sap.* III.18 |
| | | cut off eyelid | *Add.Sap.* III.19 |
| | | cut through three wrinkles of forehead | *Add.Sap.* III.20 |
| | | cut through one wrinkle of forehead | *Add.Sap.* III.21 |
| | | head injury sensitivity to head and cold | *Add.Sap.* III.22 |
| | | head injury breaking skull | *Add.Sap.* III.23 |
| | | head injury bone extracted | *Add.Sap.* III.24 |
| | | lodging sword in bone | *Add.Sap.* III.25 |
| | | exposing bone | *Add.Sap.* III.26 |
| | | leaving sunken scar | *Add.Sap.* III.34 |
| | | knock out canine tooth | *Add.Sap.* III.37 |
| | | knock out back tooth | *Add.Sap.* III.38 |

| Text | Place/date | Injury | Reference |
|---|---|---|---|
| | | pull/pull out hair | *Add.Sap.* III.39–40 |
| | | knock out eye | *Add.Sap.* III.47 |
| | | knock out pupil of eye | *Add.Sap.* III.48 |
| | | injure eye | *Add.Sap.* III.59 |
| | | pierce nose | *Add.Sap.* III.63 |
| | | pierce "wall" bone in head—cheek? | *Add.Sap.* III.64 |
| | | pierce lower jaw | *Add.Sap.* III.65 |
| | | cut off tongue | *Add.Sap.* III.74 |
| Capitulary of Thionville | Francia, 805 | conspirators to cut each others' noses off | *MGH Capit. reg. Franc.* I, no 44 |
| *Novels* of Leo VI, ed. Noailles and Dain | Byzantium, 886×912 | removal of nose of both parties in adultery | Novel 32 |
| | | armed accomplices of rapist to lose noses and be shaved to the skin | Novel 35 |
| | | penalty for taking out eye or complete blinding is removal of one eye and a fine | Novel 92 |
| *Tenth century* Laws of Hywel Dda² | Wales, c.950 | physician of court to charge for attending to head wounds cut to brain; details of his practice | Book of Blegywryd, tr. Richards, 41; LLyfr Iorwerth, tr. Jenkins, 24–25 |
| | | cut off ear, cut tongue | Book of Blegywryd, tr. Richards, 63; LLyfr Iorwerth, tr. Jenkins, 196 |
| | | cut off ear wound closes causing deafness | LLyfr Iorwerth, tr. Jenkins, 196 |
| | | knocking front tooth = conspicuous scar | Book of Blegywryd, tr. Richards, 64; Cyfnerth, tr. Jenkins, 196 |

| Text | Place/date | Injury | Reference |
|------|-----------|--------|-----------|
| | | injury to back tooth; injury to canine tooth | Book of Blegywryd, tr. Richards, 64; LLyfr Iorwerth, tr. Jenkins, 196 |
| | | head injury so brain visible (one of the "dangerous wounds") | Book of Blegywryd, tr. Richards, 64; LLyfr Iorwerth, tr. Jenkins, 197 |
| | | on medical assistance and payment | Book of Blegywryd, tr. Richards, 64; LLyfr Iorwerth, tr. Jenkins, 197 |
| | | bones removed from skull, make sound | Book of Blegywryd, tr. Richards, 64; LLyfr Iorwerth, tr. Jenkins, 197 |
| | | pulling, pulling out or cutting hair | Book of Blegywryd, tr. Richards, 64; LLyfr Iorwerth, tr. Jenkins, 198 |
| | | disinheriting of blemished heir, cannot serve king | Book of Blegywryd, tr. Richards, 78 |
| | | attacking someone's stallion; detailed | Book of Blegywryd, tr. Richards, 89; Damweiniautr. Jenkins, 172–3 |
| | | blind or speech impaired cannot be judges | Book of Blegywryd, tr. Richards, 99; *Triads*, tr. Roberts, 201 |
| | | blood spilt from head to ground | Book of Blegywryd, tr. Richards, 109; LLyfr Iorwerth, tr. Jenkins, 197 |
| | | woman wishing blemish on man's beard | LLyfr Iorwerth, tr. Jenkins, 52 |

| Text | Place/date | Injury | Reference |
|------|-----------|--------|-----------|
| | | accidental burning | Damweiniautr. Jenkins, 171 |
| | | conspicuous scars include to face | LLyfr Iorwerth, tr. Jenkins, 197 |
| | | injury to eyelid and eyelashes | Cyfnerth, tr. Jenkins, 198 |
| | | hitting woman permitted but not to head | LLyfr Iorwerth, tr. Jenkins, 53 |
| | | kiss, grope, have sex with woman | *Triads*, tr. Roberts, 105 |
| 959×975 | England | law of Edgar, prescribing blinding, removal of ears, slitting of the nose, scalping and amputation of hands and feet for a convicted thief | Wormald, *Making*, 125–6 |
| *Eleventh century* | | | |
| II Cnut, tr. Whitelock | England, 1020×3 | blinding, cutting off ears, nose and upper lip or scalp of recidivist offender | 30.5 |
| | | branding convicted slave | 32 |
| | | cut off nose and ears of adulterous woman | 53 |
| *Twelfth century* | | | |
| Ecloga ad Procheiron Mutata, ed. Freshfield | S Italy, 1166 | thief blinded for third offence | XX[XVIII].4 |
| | | beating on the head | XX[XVIII].31 |
| | | blinding | XX[XVIII].32 |
| | | splitting nose (interpersonal violence) | XX[XVIII].33 |
| | | knocking out teeth | XX[XVIII}.34 |
| | | injuring neighbor's beard so as to disfigure him[3] | XX[XVIII].38 |
| | | nose-slitting for sexual offences | XX[XIX] |
| | | shaving and slitting noses of those abetting abduction of woman; if abduction unarmed, abettors shaved | XXII[XXVII].2 |

| Text | Place/date | Injury | Reference |
|---|---|---|---|
| | | slit nose of married woman having sex with slave | XXIII[XXXI].1 |
| | | priest with nosebleed not to officiate, but can if only teeth are bleeding | XXXI[XXII].23 |
| | | freeman injured during building maintenance can claim for loss of earnings but not disfigurement/injury | XXXIV.30 |
| *Thirteenth century* | | | |
| *Liber Augustalis*, tr. Powell | S Italy, 1231 | one-eyed person duelling | I.40 [40] |
| | | physicians examined and licenced | III.44–45 [1, 23] |
| | | nose-slitting of adulterous woman | III.54 [52] |
| | | pimps and madams punished as adulterers | III.59, 84 [61] |
| | | mothers who prostitute their daughters have noses slit | III.80 [57], 85 [62] |
| | | cut out tongue of blasphemers | III.91 [68] |
| *Assizes of Cyprus*, tr. Coureas | Cyprus, c.1250 | on doctors treating skull injuries | I.225 |
| | | slave summoning master to court to lose tongue | I.16 |
| | | challenging judgment of court and having no money to pay fine—lose half tongue | I.253 |
| | | thief branded (location unspecified) | I.281–2 |

## NOTES

1. Miller, Eye for an Eye, 114, translates 'cheek', but Oliver's edition, renumbering the clauses, suggests that the nose is being referred to still.
2. Traditionally ascribed to Hywel, but surviving in mss of the late twelfth and early thirteeth centuries
3. See above, Chap. 1, note 42, regarding the problems translating this clause

# Bibliography

## Primary Sources

### England/Wales/Ireland/Scotland

Aethelberht of Kent, *Laws*, ed. L. Oliver http://www.earlyenglishlaws.ac.uk/laws/texts/abt/

*Ancrene Wisse: a Corrected Edition of the Text in Cambridge, Corpus Christi College MS 402, with variants from other Manuscripts*, ed. Bella Millett, drawing on E. J. Dobson with notes by Richard Dance (Oxford: Oxford University Press for the Early English Texts Society, 2005).

*Ancrene Wisse: Guide for Anchoresses*, tr. Hugh White (London: Penguin, 1993).

*The Anglo-Saxon Chronicle*, tr. G. S. Garmonsway (London: Everyman, 1953).

*The Anglo-Saxon Chronicle: a revised translation*, ed. Dorothy Whitelock (London: Eyre and Spottiswoode, 1961).

Charles-Edwards, T. M., *The Welsh Laws* (Cardiff: University of Wales Press, 1989).

*The Earliest Welsh Poetry*, tr. Joseph P. Clancy (London: Macmillan, 1970).

*Early Irish Myths and Sagas*, tr. with notes by Jeffrey Gantz (London: Penguin, 1981).

*English and Norse Documents relating to the Reign of Ethelred the Unready*, tr. M. Ashdown (Cambridge: Cambridge University Press, 1930).

*English Historical Documents*, I, tr. D. Whitelock (2nd edition, London: Routledge, 1979).

*English Lawsuits from William I to Richard I*, 2 vols, ed. R. C. Van Caenegem (Selden Society Publications 106 and 107, London: The Selden Society, 1990–1991).

© The Author(s) 2017

P. Skinner, *Living with Disfigurement in Early Medieval Europe*,
DOI 10.1057/978-1-137-54439-1

Gerald of Wales, *The Journey Through Wales/The Description of Wales*, tr. L. Thorpe (London: Penguin, 1978).

*Gesta Guillelmi of William of Poitiers*, ed. and trans. R. H. C. Davis and M. Chibnall (Oxford: Clarendon Press, 1998).

Kelly, Fergus, *A Guide to Early Irish Law* (Dublin: Institute for Advanced Studies, 1988).

*Klaeber's Beowulf, 4th Edition*, ed. R. D. Fulk, Robert E. Bjork and John D. Niles (Toronto: Toronto University Press, 2008).

*The Laws of Hywel Dda (The Book of Blegywryd)*, tr. M. Richards (Liverpool: Liverpool University Press, 1954).

*The Laws of Hywel Dda: Law Texts from Medieval Wales*, tr. Dafydd Jenkins (Llandysul, Gomer Press, 1986).

*Leechdoms, Wortcunning and Starcraft of Early England*, ed. O. Cockayne, 3 vols (London, Longmans Green, 1864–1866).

*The Legal Triads of Medieval Wales*, ed. Sara Elin Roberts (Cardiff: University of Wales Press, 2007).

*The Life of St Cadog/Vita Sancti Cadoci*, c.36, in *Vitae Sanctorum Britanniae et Geneaologiae*, ed. A. W. Wade-Evans (Cardiff: University of Wales Press, 1944), 24–141.

*The Mabinogion*, tr. Gwyn Jones and Thomas Jones (London: Everyman, 1949).

*Pleas before the King or his Justices*, 4 vols ed. D. M. Stenton (Selden Society Publications, 67–8, 83–4, London: Bernard Quaritch, 1948–1967).

*Rogeri de Wendover, Chronica*, ed. H. Coxe (London: Sumptis Societatis, 1842).

*The Roll and Writ File of the Berkshire Eyre of 1248*, ed. M. T. Clanchy (Selden Society Publications, 90, London: The Selden Society, 1973).

*The Roll of the Shropshire Eyre of 1256*, ed. A. Harding (Selden Society Publications, 96, London: The Selden Society, 1980).

*Rolls of the Justices in Eyre...for Gloucestershire, Warwickshire and Staffordshire, 1221, 1222*, ed. D. M. Stenton (Selden Society Publications, 59, London: Bernard Quaritch, 1940).

*Rolls of the Justices in Eyre...for Yorkshire in 3 Henry III (1218–1219)*, ed. D. M. Stenton (Selden Society Publications, 56, London: Bernard Quaritch, 1937).

*Select Pleas of the Crown, Volume I: AD 1200–1225*, ed. F. W. Maitland (Selden Society Publications, 1, London: Bernard Quaritch, 1888).

William of Malmesbury, *Gesta Regum Anglorum/The History of the English Kings*, ed. R. A. B. Mynors, R. M. Thomson and M. Winterbottom, 2 vols, I (Oxford: Clarendon Press, 1998).

## FRANCE/GERMANY/LOW COUNTRIES

[*Magistri*] *Adam Bremensis Gesta Hammaburgensis Ecclesiae Pontificum*, 3rd ed., ed. Bernhard Schmeidler, *MGH SS rer. Germ.*, II (Hannover and Leipzig: Hahn, 1917).

Adam of Bremen, *History of the Archbishops of Hamburg-Bremen*, tr. Francis J. Tschan with introduction by Timothy Reuter (New York: Columbia University Press, 2002).

Ex Adonis Archiepiscopi Viennensis Chronico, ed. I. de Arx, *MGH SS* II (Hannover: Hahn, 1829).

*Annales Bertiniani*, ed. G. Waitz, *MGH SS rer. Germ.*, V (Hannover: Hahn, 1883).

*Annales Cameracenses*, *MGH SS*, XVI, ed. G. H. Pertz (Hannover: Hahn, 1859).

*The Annals of Flodoard of Reims, 919–966*, tr. Steven Fanning and Bernard Bachrach (Toronto: Toronto University Press, 2011).

*The Annals of Fulda: Ninth-Century Histories vol II*, tr. Timothy Reuter (Manchester: Manchester University Press, 1992).

*The Annals of St Bertin: Ninth-Century Histories vol I*, tr. Janet L. Nelson (Manchester: Manchester University Press, 1991).

*Bernardi Cremifanensis Historiae*, *MGH SS*, XXV, ed. G. H. Pertz (Hannover: Hahn, 1880).

*The Book of St Foy*, tr. Pamela Sheingorn (Philadelphia: Pennsylvania University Press, 1995).

*Carolingian Chronicles: Royal Frankish Annals and Nithard's Histories*, tr. B. W. Scholz (Ann Arbor: University of Michigan Press, 1970).

*Chronicon Laetiense*, ed. I. Heller, *MGH SS*, XIV, ed. G. H. Pertz (Hannover: Hahn, 1883).

*Chronicon Montis Sereni*, ed. E. Ehrenfeuchter, *MGH SS* XXIII, ed. G. Waitz (Hannover: Hahn, 1874).

*Chronicon Novaliciense*, ed. G. H. Pertz, *MGH SS rer. Germ.*, XXI (Hannover: Hahn, 1846).

*The Ecclesiastical History of Orderic Vitalis*, ed. M. Chibnall, 6 vols (Oxford: Clarendon Press, 1969–1980).

Einhard and Notker the Stammerer, *Two Lives of Charlemagne*, tr. L. Thorpe (London: Penguin, 1969).

*Einhardi Vita Karoli Magni*, ed. O. Holder-Egger, *MGH SS rerum. Germ.* XXV (Hannover: Hahn, 1911).

*Frühmittelalterliche Rezeptarien* (= *Beiträge zur Geschichte der Medizin, Heft 1*), ed. J. Jörimann (Leipzig and Zurich: Orell Füssli, 1925).

*Gesta Guillelmi of William of Poitiers*, ed. and trans. R. H. C. Davis and M. Chibnall (Oxford: Clarendon Press, 1998).

*The Gesta Normannorum Ducum of William of Jumièges, Orderic Vitalis and Robert of Torigni*, ed. E. M. C. van Houts, 2 vols (Oxford: Clarendon Press, 1992).

*Gregorii Episcopi Turoniensis Libri Historiarum X*, ed. B. Krusch and W. Levison, *MGH SS Rer Merov.*, I (Hannover: Hahn, 1951).

Gregory of Tours, *History of the Franks*, tr. Lewis Thorpe (London: Penguin, 1974).

*The History of the Albigensian Crusade: Peter of Les-Vaux-de-Cernay's Historia Albigensis,* tr. W. A. Sibly and M. D. Sibly (Woodbridge: Boydell, 1998).

*The Letters and Poems of Fulbert of Chartres,* ed. and tr. F. Behrends (Oxford: Clarendon Press, 1976).

*Leges Alamannorum,* ed. K. A. Eckhardt, *MGH LL nat. Germ.,* V.1 (Hannover: Hahn, 1966).

*Leges Burgundionum,* ed. L. R. de Salis, *MGH LL nat. Germ.,* II.1 (Hannover: Hahn, 1892).

*Lex Baiwariorum,* ed. E. Liber, *MGH LL. Nat. Germ.,* V.2 (Hannover: Hahn, 1926).

*Lex Frisionum,* ed. K. de Richthofen, *MGH LL,* III, ed. G. Pertz (Hannover: Hahn, 1863).

*Lex Ribvaria,* ed. F. Beyerle and R. Buchner, *MGH LL nat. Germ.,* III.2 (Hannover: Hahn, 1954).

*Lex Salica* and *Lex Salica Karolina,* ed. K. Eckhardt, *MGH LL nat. Germ.,* IV.2 (Hannover: Hahn, 1959).

*Lupi Abbatis Ferrariensis Epistolae,* in *MGH Epp. Merovingici et Karolini Aevi,* IV (Berlin: Weidmann, 1925).

*MGH Capitularia Regum Francorum I,* ed. A. Boretius (Hannover: Hahn, 1883).

*MGH Die Briefe in der deutschen Kaiserzeit III: die ältere Wormser Briefsammlung,* ed. W. Bulst (Weimar: Böhlau, 1949).

*MGH* Epistolae Merovingici et Karolingici Aevi, IV (Berlin: Weidmann, 1925).

Notker, *Gesta Karoli, MGH SS rer. Ger. n.s.,* XII, ed. H. Haefele (Berlin: Weidmann, 1959).

Orderic Vitalis, *Ecclesiastical History,* ed. Marjorie Chibnall, 6 vols, (Oxford: Oxford University Press, 1969–80).

*Ottonian Germany: the* Chronicon *of Thietmar of Merseburg,* tr. David A. Warner (Manchester: Manchester University Press, 2001).

*Pactus Legis Alamannorum,* ed. K. A. Eckhardt, *MGH LL nat. Germ., V.1* (Hannover: Hahn, 1966).

*Pactus Legis Salicae,* ed. K. Eckhardt, in *MGH Leges Nat. Germ.,* IV.1 (Hannover: Hahn, 1962).

*Raoul de Cambrai,* ed. and tr. Sarah Kay (Oxford: Clarendon Press, 1992).

*Reginonis Abbatis Prumiensis Chronicon,* ed. F. Kurze, *MGH SS rer. Germ.,* L (Hannover: Hahn, 1890).

*Rodulfi Glabri Historiarum Libri Quinque/Rodulfus Glaber The Five Books of the Histories,* ed. and tr. John France (Oxford: Clarendon Press, 1989).

*Self and Society in Medieval France: The Memoirs of Abbot Guibert of Nogent,* ed. and tr. John Benton (New York: Harper and Row, 1970).

*Thietmar Mersebergensis Episcopi Chronica,* ed. Robert Holtzmann, *MGH SSRG* n.s. IX (Berlin: Weidmann, 1935).

*Vita S. Adalberti Episcopi, MGH SS* IV, ed. G. H. Pertz (Hannover: Hahn, 1841).

*Vita S. Udalrici Prioris Cellensis, MGH SS*, XII, ed. G. H. Pertz (Hannover: Hahn, 1856).

*Vita Ven. Oda Praemonstratensis, AASS.*, XI, 20 April.

*Walteri Vita Karoli Comitis Flandriae*, in *MGH SS*, XII, ed. G. H. Pertz (Hannover: Hahn, 1856).

## ITALY

*Agnelli Liber Pontificalis Ecclesiae Ravennatis*, ed. O. Holder-Egger, *MGH SSRLI*, ed. G. Waitz (Hannover: Hahn, 1878).

Amatus of Montecassino, *The History of the Normans*, tr. Prescott N. Dunbar with introduction by G. A. Loud (Woodbridge: Boydell, 2004).

*Andrea da Strumi, Arioaldo: passione del santo martire milanese*, tr. M. Navoni (Milan: Jaca Book, 1994).

*Bartholomaei Scribae Annales, MGH SS*, XVIII, ed. G. H. Pertz (Hannover: Hahn, 1863).

*De B. Margarita Poenit. Tertii Ord. S. Francisci, Cortonae in Etruria, Vita a Confessore Scripta et Aliis, AASS* VI, February 22.

*Benedicti S. Andreae Monachi Chronicon, MGH SS* III, ed. G. H. Pertz (Hannover: Hahn, 1839).

*Chronica Fratris Salimbene Ordinis Minorum. Liber de Praelatio*, ed. O. Holder-Egger, *MGH SS*, XXXII, ed. G. H. Pertz (Hannover: Hahn, 1913).

*Die Chronik des Saba Malaspina*, ed. W. Koller and A. Nitschke (Hannover: Hahn, 1999).

*Erchemperti Historia Langobardorum Beneventanorum, MGH SSRLI*, ed. G. Waitz (Hannover: Hahn, 1878).

*Iohannis Diaconi Chronicon Venetum et Gradense, MGH SS* VII, ed. G. H. Pertz (Hannover: Hahn, 1846).

*Leges Langobardorum*, ed. F. Bluhme, *MGH LL*, IV, ed. G. H. Pertz (Hannover: Hahn, 1868).

*The Letters of Gerbert with his Papal Privileges as Sylvester II*, trans. Harriett Pratt Lattin (New York: Columbia University Press, 1961).

*The Letters of Peter Damian 61–90*, tr. Owen J. Blum (Washington DC: Catholic University of America Press, 1998).

*Liber ad Honorem Augusti di Pietro da Eboli*, ed. G. B. Siragusa (Rome: Istituto Storico Italiano, 1906).

*The Liber Augustalis or Constitutions of Melfi promulgated by the Emperor Frederick II for the Kingdom of Sicily in 1231*, tr. J. M. Powell (Syracuse, NY: Syracuse University Press, 1971).

*The Lombard Laws*, tr. K. F. Drew (Philadelphia: Pennsylvania University Press, 1973).

*MGH Die Briefe in der deutschen Kaiserzeit, IV.2: Die Briefe des Petrus Damiani II*, ed. K. Reindel (Munich: MGH, 1988).

*MGH Epp. Saeculi XIII e Regestis Pontificum Romanorum Selectae*, ed. C. Rodenberg, III (Berlin: Weidmann, 1894).

*Pauli Historia Langobardorum*, ed. L. Bethmann and G. Waitz, *MGH SSRLI*, ed. G. Waitz (Hannover, Hahn, 1878).

*I Placiti del "Regnum Italiae,"* ed. C. Manaresi (Rome: Tipografia del Senato, 1955, 1957 and 1960).

*Rolandini Patavini Chronica*, ed. P. Jaffé, *MGH SS*, XIX, ed. G. H. Pertz (Hannover: Hahn, 1866).

*The Surgery of Theoderic, c. AD1267*, tr. E. Campbell and J. Cotton (New York: Appleton-Century-Crofts, 1955).

*The Theodosian Code and Novels, and the Sirmondian Constitutions*, ed. and tr. C. Pharr (New Jersey: The Lawbook Exchange, 2001).

*The Trotula: a Medieval Compendium of Women's Medicine*, ed. Monica H. Green (Philadelphia: University of Pennsylvania Press, 2001).

## Iberia/North Africa

Jordanes, *Getica*, tr. C. C. Mierow (Princeton: Princeton University Press, 1915).

*Leges Visigothorum*, in *MGH LL. Nat. Germ.* I, ed. K. Zeumer (Hannover and Leipzig: Hahn, 1902).

## Byzantium, the Balkans and Eastern Europe

Anna Comnène, *Alexiade*, ed. and tr. Bernard Leib, 3 vols (Paris: Les Belles Lettres, 1967).

Anna Komnena, *Alexiad*, tr. E. R. A. Sewter (London: Penguin, 1969).

*B. Margaritae Hungariae Virginis*, *AASS* III, 28 January.

*Byzantine Defenders of Images: Eight Saints' Lives in English Translation*, tr. A.-M. Talbot (Washington: Dumbarton Oaks, 1998).

*The Chronicle of Theophanes Confessor: Byzantine and Near Eastern History AD284–813*, tr. Cyril Mango and R. Scott with the assistance of G. Greatrex (Oxford: Clarendon Press, 1997).

*The Digest of Justinian*, tr. and ed. A. Watson, 2 vols (Philadelphia: University of Pennsylvania Press, 1985).

*Dumbarton Oaks Hagiography Database* at http://www.doaks.org/research/byzantine/resources/hagiography-database, [Accessed 9 June 2014].

*Fourteen Byzantine Rulers: the* Chronographia *of Michael Psellos*, tr. E. R. A. Sewter (London: Penguin, 1979).

*A Manual of Later Roman Law: the Ecloga ad Procheiron Mutata*, tr. E. H. Freshfield (Cambridge: Cambridge University Press, 1927).

*A Manual of Roman Law: The Ecloga published by the Emperors Leo III and Constantine V of Isauria at Constantinople, 726,* tr. E. H. Freshfield (Cambridge, Cambridge University Press, 1926).

Macrides, R., "Justice under Manuel I Komnenos: Four Novels on court business and murder," *Fontes Minores,* 6 (1984): 99–204, reprinted in *ead., Kinship and Justice in Byzantium, 11th-15th Centuries* (Aldershot: Variorum, 1999), Essay IX.

Michele Psello, *Imperatori di Bisanzio (Cronografia),* ed. and tr. Salvatore Impellizari, Ugo Criscuolo and Siliva Ronchey, 2 vols (Milan: Fondazione Lorenzo Valla/Mondadori, 1984).

[Pope Nicholas I's letter to the Bulgarians, 866], *MGH Epp Karol. Aevi* IV (Berlin: Weidmann, 1925).

*Les Novelles de Léon VI Le Sage,* ed. and tr. P. Noailles and A. Dain (Paris: Les Belles Lettres, 1944).

*Ο ΠΡΟΧΕΙΡΟC ΝΟΜΟC: Imperatorum Basilii, Constantini et Leonis Prochiron,* ed. C. E. Zachariae v. Lingenthal (Heidelberg: Mohr, 1837).

*Theophanis Chronographia,* ed. C. de Boor, 2 vols (Hildesheim: Georg Olms, 1963).

*La vie d'Étienne le Jeune par Étienne le Diacre.* ed. and tr. M.-F. Auzépy (Ashgate: Variorum, 1997).

## EASTERN MEDITERRANEAN

*The Assizes of the Lusignan Kingdom of Cyprus,* tr. Nicholas Coureas (Nicosia: Cyprus Research Centre, 2002).

*The Chronicle of Ibn al-Athir for the Crusading Period from al-Kamil fi'l-Ta'rikh Part 3: the Years 589–629,* tr. D. S. Richards (Aldershot: Ashgate, 2008).

[Polemon] *Seeing the Face, Seeing the Soul: Polemon's Physiognomy from Classical Antiquity to Medieval Islam,* ed. Simon Swain (Oxford: Oxford University Press, 2007).

## SECONDARY WORKS

Abulafia, Anna Sapir, "Theology and the commercial revolution: Guibert of Nogent, St Anselm and the Jews of northern France," in *Church and City, 1000–1500: Essays in Honour of Christopher Brooke,* ed. D. Abulafia, M. Franklin and M. Rubin (Cambridge: Cambridge University Press, 1992), 23–40.

Agamben, Giorgio, "The face", in *id., Means without End: Notes on Politics,* tr. V. Binetti and C. Casarino (Minneapolis: Minnesota University Press, 2000) [originally published as *Mezzi senza fine* (NP: Bollati Boringhieri, 1996)].

Agamben, Giorgio, Homo Sacer: *Sovereign Power and Bare Life*, tr. D. Heller-Roazen (Stanford: Stanford University Press, 1998) [originally published as Homo Sacer: *il potere sovrano e la nuda vita* (Torino: Einaudi, 1995)].

Aird, W., *Robert Curthose Duke of Normandy, c. 1050–1134* (Woodbridge: Boydell, 2008).

Althoff, Gerd, *Otto III* (University Park: Pennsylvania State Press, 2003).

Amundsen, Darryl, *Medicine, Society and Faith in the Ancient and Medieval Worlds* (Baltimore: Johns Hopkins University Press, 1996).

Anderson, T., "Cranial weapon injuries from Anglo-Saxon Dover," *International Journal of Osteoarchaeology*, 6.1 (1998): 10–14.

*Anger's Past: The Social Uses of an Emotion in the Middle Ages*, ed. B. H. Rosenwein (Ithaca and London: Cornell University Press, 1998).

Ariès, Philippe, *L'Enfant et la vie familiale sous l'Ancien Régime* (Paris: Plon, 1960) [Translated into English by Robert Baldick as *Centuries of Childhood: A Social History of Family Life* (New York: Vintage, 1962)].

Bachrach, Bernard S., *Early Carolingian Warfare: Prelude to Empire* (Philadelphia: Pennsylvania University Press, 2001).

Baker, Naomi, *Plain Ugly: the Unattractive Body in Early Modern Culture* (Manchester: Manchester University Press, 2010)

Baker, Peter, *Honour, Exchange and Violence in Beowulf* (Woodbridge: Boydell, 2013).

Balzaretti, Ross, "'These are things men do, not women': the social regulation of female violence in Langobard Italy," in *Violence and Society in the Medieval West*, ed. G. Halsall (Woodbridge: Boydell, 1998), 175–192.

Banham, Debby, "A millennium in medicine? New medical texts and ideas in England in the eleventh century," in *Anglo-Saxons: Studies presented to Cyril Roy Hart*, ed. Simon Keynes and Alfred P. Smyth (Dublin: Four Courts Press, 2006), 230–242.

Baraz, D., *Medieval Cruelty: Changing Perceptions from Late Antiquity to the Early Modern Period* (Ithaca, NY: Cornell University Press, 2003).

Barnes, Colin, *"Cabbage Syndrome": the Social Construction of Dependence* (London/New York/Philadelphia: The Falmer Press, 1990).

Bartlett, Robert, "Symbolic meanings of hair in the middle ages," *Transactions of the Royal Historical Society*, 6th series, 4 (1994): 43–60.

Bashour, M., "History and current concepts in the analysis of facial attractiveness," *Plastic and Reconstructive Surgery*, 118 (2006): 741–756.

Bates, David, "Anger, emotion and a biography of William the Conqueror," in *Gender and Historiography: Studies in the Earlier Middle Ages in Honour of Pauline Stafford*, ed. J. L. Nelson, S. Reynolds and S. M. Johns (London: Institute of Historical Research, 2012), 21–33.

*The Battle of Maldon, AD991*, ed. D. Scragg (Oxford: Basil Blackwell in association with the Manchester Centre for Anglo-Saxon Studies, 1991).

Bennett, Judith, *History Matters: Patriarchy and the Challenge of Feminism* (Philadelphia: University of Pennsylvania Press, 2006).

Berger, John, *Ways of Seeing* (London: Penguin, 1972, repr. 2008).

Biernoff, Suzannah, "The rhetoric of disfigurement in First World War Britain," *Social History of Medicine*, 24.3 (2011): 666–685.

Bildhauer, Bettina, *Medieval Blood* (Cardiff: University of Wales Press, 2006).

Bishop. Edward, *McIndoe's Army: the Story of the Guinea Pig Club and its Indomitable Members* (London: Grub Street, 2004).

Bloch, Marc, *Feudal Society* (French first edition 1939, English translation London: Routledge, 1961).

*Bodies of Knowledge: Cultural Interpretations of Illness and Medicine in Medieval Europe*, ed. Sally Crawford and Christina Lee (BAR International Series 2170/ Studies in Early Medicine 1, Oxford: Archaeopress, 2010).

Boeckl, Christine M., *Images of Leprosy: Disease, Religion and Politics in European Art* (Kirksville, Missouri: Truman State University Press, 2011).

Boswell, John, *The Kindness of Strangers: the Abandonment of Children in Western Europe from Late Antiquity to the Renaissance* (Chicago: Chicago University Press, 1988).

*Boundaries of the Law: Geography, Gender and Jurisdiction in Medieval and Early Modern Europe*, ed. A. Musson (Aldershot: Ashgate, 2005).

Bourdieu, Pierre, *Outline of a Theory of Practice* (Cambridge, 1977).

Bradbury, Jim, *The Medieval Archer* (Woodbridge: Boydell, 1985).

Bragg, Lois, "Disfigurement, disability and dis-integration in *Sturlinga Saga*," *alvíssmál*, 4 (1994 [1995]): 15–32.

Braidotti, Rosi, *Patterns of Dissonance: A Study of Women in Contemporary Philosophy* (Cambridge: Polity Press, 1991).

Brenner, Elma, "Recent perspectives on leprosy in medieval western Europe," *History Compass*, 8.5 (2010): 388–406.

Brenner, Elma, *Leprosy and Charity in Medieval Rouen* (Woodbridge: Boydell, 2015).

Brødholt, E. T., and P. Holck, "Skeletal trauma in the burials from the royal church of St Mary in medieval Oslo," *International Journal of Osteoarchaeology*, 22.2 (2012): 201–218.

Brubaker, Leslie, and John Haldon, *Byzantium in the Iconoclast Era c.680–850: a History* (Cambridge: Cambridge University Press, 2011).

Bruce, Vicky, and Andy Young, *Face Perception* (London and NY: Psychology Press, 2012).

Buc, Philippe, *The Dangers of Ritual: Between Early Medieval Texts and Social Scientific Theory* (Princeton: Princeton University Press, 2002).

Burgwinkle, William, *Sodomy, Masculinity and Law in Medieval Literature: France and England, 1050–1230* (Cambridge: Cambridge University Press, 2004).

Burt, Ronald S., *Brokerage and Closure: an Introduction to Social Capital* (Oxford: Oxford University Press, 2005).

Butler, Sara, *The Language of Abuse: Marital Violence in Later Medieval England* (Leiden and Boston: Brill, 2007).

Bynum, Caroline Walker, "Why all the fuss about the body? A medievalist's perspective," *Critical Enquiry*, 22 (1995): 1–33.

Bynum, Caroline Walker, *The Resurrection of the Body* (New York: Columbia University Press, 1995).

Bynum, Caroline Walker, "Wonder," *American Historical Review*, 102 (1997): 1–17.

Cameron, M. L., "Bald's Leechbook: its sources and their use in compilation," *Anglo-Saxon England*, 12 (1983): 153–182.

Cameron, M. L., "Bald's Leechbook and cultural interactions in Anglo-Saxon England," *Anglo-Saxon England*, 19 (1990): 5–12.

Cameron, M. L., *Anglo-Saxon Medicine* (Cambridge: Cambridge University Press, 1993).

Camporesi, Piero, *The Incorruptible Flesh: Body Mutation and Mortification in Religion and Folklore*, tr. T. Croft-Murray and H. Elsom (Cambridge: Cambridge University Press, 1988) [originally published as *La carne impassibile* (Milan: Il Saggiatore, 1983)].

Carrel, Helen, "The ideology of punishment in late medieval English towns," *Social History* 34 (2009): 301–320.

Cassidy-Welch, Megan, "Images of blood in the *Historia Albigensis* of Peter des Vaux-de-Cernay," *Journal of Religious History*, 35 (2011): 478–491.

*Castration and Culture in the Middle Ages*, ed. Larissa Tracy (Cambridge: D. S. Brewer, 2013).

Caviness, M., *Visualizing Women in the Middle Ages* (Philadelphia: University of Pennsylvania Press, 2001).

Charles-Edwards, Thomas, "Honour and status in some Irish and Welsh prose tales," *Eriu*, 29 (1978): 123–141.

Classen, Albrecht, *Violence in Medieval Courtly Literature: a Casebook* (New York: Garland, 2004).

Cock, Emily, "'Lead[ing] 'em by the nose into publick shame and derision': Gaspare Tagliacozzi, Alexander Read and the lost history of plastic surgery," *Social History of Medicine*, 28.1 (2015): 1–21.

*Codierungen von Emotionen im Mittelalter/Emotions and Sensibilities in the Middle Ages*, ed. Stephen C. Jaeger and Ingrid Kasten (Berlin: De Gruyter, 2003).

Collins, Randall, "Three faces of cruelty: towards a comparative sociology of violence," *Theory and Society*, 1 (1974): 415–440.

Connor, Carolyn L., *Women of Byzantium* (New Haven: Yale University Press, 2004).

Cowell, Andrew, "Violence, history and the Old French epic of revolt," in *Violence and the Writing of History in the Medieval Francophone World*, ed. Noah D. Guynn and Zrinka Stahuljak (Cambridge: D. S. Brewer, 2013), 19–34.

Craig, E., and G. Craig, "The diagnosis and context of a facial deformity from an Anglo-Saxon cemetery at Spofforth, North Yorkshire," *International Journal of Osteoarchaeology*, 23 (2013): 621–9.

Crawford, Sally, *Childhood in Anglo-Saxon England* (Stroud: Sutton, 1999).

*Cuckolds, Clerics and Countrymen: Medieval French Fabliaux*, ed. and tr. John DuVal and Raymond Eichmann (Fayetteville: University of Arkansas Press, 1982).

Cule, John, "The court mediciner and medicine in the laws of Wales," *Journal of the History of Medicine and Allied Sciences*, 21 (1966): 213–266.

D'Aronco, Maria A., "How 'English' is Anglo-Saxon medicine: the Latin sources for Anglo-Saxon medical texts," in *Britannia Latina: Latin in the Culture of Great Britain from the Middle Ages to the Twentieth Century*, ed. Charles Burnett and Nicholas Mann (London: Warburg Institute, 2005), 27–41.

D'Aronco, Maria A., "The transmission of medical knowledge in Anglo-Saxon England: the voices of manuscripts," in *Form and Content of Instruction in Anglo-Saxon England in the Light of Contemporary Manuscript Evidence, Papers presented at the International Conference, Udine, 6–8 April 2006*, ed. by Patrizia Lendinara, Loredana Lazzari, and Maria A. D'Aronco, (Fédération Internationale des Instituts d'Études Médiévales, Textes et Études du Moyen Âge, 39, Turnhout: Brepols, 2007), 35–58.

d'Cruze, Shani, and Louise A. Jackson, *Women, Crime and Justice in England since 1660* (London: Palgrave Macmillan, 2009).

Dale, Thomas E. A., *Relics, Prayer and Politics in Medieval Venetia: Romanesque Painting in the Crypt of Aquileia Cathedral* (Princeton: Princeton University Press, 1997)

*The Dark Side of Childhood in Late Antiquity and the Middle Ages*, ed. Katariina Mustakallio and Christian Laes (Oxford: Oxbow, 2011).

Darling, Linda, "Mirrors for princes in Europe and the Middle East: a case of historiographical incommensurability", in *East Meets West in the Middle Ages and Early Modern Times: Transcultural Experiences in the Premodern World*, ed. A. Classen (Berlin: DeGruyter, 2013), 223–242.

Das, Sukla, *Crime and Punishment in Ancient India (c. AD 300 to AD 1100)* (New Delhi, Abhinar Publications, 1977).

*The Dating of Beowulf: a Reassessment*, ed. Leonard Neidorf (Woodbridge: Boydell, 2014).

Davies, R. R., "The status of women and the practice of marriage in late-medieval Wales," in *The Welsh Law of Women: Studies presented to Professor Daniel A. Binchy on his 80th Birthday*, ed. Dafydd Jenkins and Morfydd Owen (Cardiff: University of Wales Press, 1980), 93–114.

Davies, Wendy, *Small Worlds: The Village Community in Early Medieval Brittany* (Berkeley: University of California Press, 1988).

de Certeau, M., "Outils pour écrire le corps," *Traverses*, 14/15 (1979): 3–14.

de Jong, Mayke, *In Samuel's Image: Childhood Oblation in the Early Medieval West* (Leiden: Brill, 1996).

de Vriendt, S., "Doven in de middeleeuwen: drie vragen aan mediëvisten," in *Een School spierinkjes: Kleine opstellen over Middelnederlandse artes-literatuur*, ed. W.P. Gerritsen, Annelies van Gijsen and Orlanda S.H. Lee (Middeleeuwse studies en bronnen, 26, Hilversum: Verloren, 1991), 168–171.

Delaporte, François, *Anatomy of the Passions*, tr. S. Emanuel (Stanford: Stanford University Press, 2008) [originally published as *Anatomie des passions* (Paris: PUF, 2003)].

Demaitre, Luke, *Leprosy in Premodern Medicine* (Baltimore: Johns Hopkins University Press, 2007).

Demaitre, Luke, "Skin and the city: cosmetic medicine as an urban concern," in *Between Text and Patient: The Medical Enterprise in Medieval and Early Modern Europe*, ed. Florence Eliza Glaze and Brian K. Nance (Florence: SISMEL-Edizioni del Galluzzo, 2011), pp. 97–120.

Demaitre, Luke, *Medieval Medicine: the Art of Healing from Head to Toe* (Santa Barbara: Praeger, 2013).

*Difference and Identity in Francia and Medieval France*, ed. Meredith Cohen and Justine Firnhaber-Baker (Farnham and Burlington: Ashgate, 2010).

*The Dilemma of Difference: a Multidisciplinary View of Stigma*, ed. Stephen C. Ainlay, Gaylene Becker and Lerita M. Coleman (New York and London: Plenum Press, 1986).

*Disability in the Middle Ages: Reconsiderations and Reverberations*, ed. Joshua Eyler (Aldershot: Ashgate, 2010).

*Disembodied Heads in Medieval and Early Modern Culture*, ed. C. G. Santing, B. Baert and A. Traninger (Leiden: Brill, 2013).

Dockray-Miller, Mary, *Motherhood and Mothering in Anglo-Saxon England* (New York: Palgrave, 2000).

Douglas, Mary, *Purity and Danger: an Analysis of Concepts of Pollution and Taboo* (2nd edition, London: Routledge, 2002).

Dutton, Paul Edward, and Herbert Kessler, *The Poetry and Paintings of the First Bible of Charles the Bald* (Ann Arbor: University of Michigan Press, 1997).

Dutton, Paul Edward, *Charlemagne's Mustache and Other Cultural Clusters of a Dark Age* (London/New York: Palgrave Macmillan, 2004).

Dutton, Paul Edward, "Keeping secrets in a dark age," in *Rhetoric and the Discourses of Power in Court Culture: China, Europe and Japan*, ed. D. R. Knechtges and E. Vance (Seattle: University of Washington Press, 2005), 169–198.

*Ear, Nose and Throat in Culture*, ed. W. Pirsig and J. Willemot (Ostend: G. Schmidt, 2001).

Earley, P. Christopher, *Face, Harmony and Social Structure: An Analysis of Organizational Behavior across Cultures* (Oxford and New York: Oxford University Press, 1997).

*Early Medieval Studies in Memory of Patrick Wormald*, ed. Stephen Baxter, Catherine Karkov, Janet Nelson and David Pelteret (Aldershot: Ashgate, 2009).

Easton, Martha, "Pain, torture and death in the Huntingdon Library *Legenda aurea*," in *Gender and Holiness: Men, Women and Saints in Late Medieval Europe*, ed. Sam Riches and Sarah Salih (London: Routledge, 2005), 49–64.

Eco, Umberto, *On Beauty: the History of a Western Idea*, tr. A. McEwan (London: Secker and Warburg, 2004).

Eco, Umberto, *On Ugliness* (London: Harvill Secker, 2007).

Elias, Norbert, *The Civilizing Process vol 1: The History of Manners, vol 2: State Formation and Civilization* (German first edition 1939, English translation Oxford: Blackwell, 1969 and 1982).

Erdal, Y. S., and Ö. D. Erdal, "A review of trepanations in Anatolia with new cases," *International Journal of Osteoarchaeology*, 21.5 (2011): 505–534.

Evans, G. R., *Law and Theology in the Middle Ages* (London and New York: Routledge, 2002).

*Fama: the Politics of Talk and Reputation in Medieval Europe*, ed. Thelma Fenster and Daniel Lord Smail (Ithaca, NY: Cornell University Press, 2003).

Farmer, Sharon, *Surviving Poverty in Medieval Paris* (Ithaca, NY: Cornell University Press, 2002).

Favazza, Armando R., *Bodies under Siege: Self-mutilation and Body Modification in Culture and Psychiatry* (2nd ed., Baltimore: Johns Hopkins University Press, 1996).

*The Final Argument: the imprint of violence on society in medieval and early modern Europe*, ed. Donald J. Kagay and L. J. Andrew Villalon (Woodbridge: Boydell, 1998).

*Fleshly Things and Spiritual Matters: Studies on the Medieval Body in Honour of Margaret Bridges*, ed. Nicole Nyffenegger and Katrin Rupp (Newcastle: Cambridge Scholars Press, 2011).

Flint, Valerie J., "The early medieval *medicus*, the saint - and the enchanter," *Social History of Medicine* 2.2 (1989): 127–145.

Flood, John, *Representations of Eve in Antiquity and the English Middle Ages* (New York: Routledge, 2011).

Fornaciari, A., and V. Giuffra, "Surgery in the early middle ages: evidence of cauterisation from Pisa," *Surgery*, 151 (2012): 351–2.

Foucault, Michel, *Discipline and Punish: the Birth of the Prison*, tr. A. Sheridan (New York: Allen Lane, 1977 [originally published in French Paris: Gallimard,1975]).

Foucault, Michel, *Care of the Self: the History of Sexuality vol. 3*, tr. R. Hurley (London: Penguin, 1990).

Foyster, Elizabeth, *Manhood in Early Modern England: Honour, Sex and Marriage* (London: Longman, 1999, repr. Oxford: Routledge, 2014).

*Framing Medieval Bodies*, ed. Sarah Kay and Miri Rubin (Manchester: Manchester University Press, 1994).

Freedman, Paul, "Atrocities and the execution of peasant rebel leaders in late medieval and early modern Europe," *Medievalia et Humanistica*, n.s. 31 (2005): 101–113.

Frembgen, J. Wasim, "Honour, shame and bodily mutilation: cutting off the nose among tribal societies in Pakistan," *Journal of the Royal Asiatic Society*, 16 (3), (2006): 243–60.

Garland, Lynda, *Byzantine Empresses: Women and Power in Byzantium, AD527–1204* (London: Routledge, 1999).

Garland-Thomson, Rosemarie, "From wonder to error: a genealogy of freak discourse in modernity," in *Freakery: Cultural Spectacles of the Extraordinary Body*, ed. R. Garland Thomson (New York: New York University Press, 1996), 1–19.

Garland-Thomson, Rosemarie, *Staring: How We Look* (Oxford: Oxford University Press, 2009).

Geller, Jay, *On Freud's Jewish Body: Mitigating Circumcisions* (New York: Fordham University Press, 2007).

Geltner, Guy, "Medieval prisons: between myth and reality, hell and purgatory," *History Compass*, 4 (2006): 1–14.

Geltner, Guy, *The Medieval Prison: a Social History* (Princeton: Princeton University Press, 2008).

Geltner, Guy, *Flogging Others: Corporal Punishment and Cultural Identity from Antiquity to the Present* (Amsterdam: AUP, 2014).

Geremek, Bronislaw, *The Margins of Society in Late Medieval Paris* (Cambridge: Cambridge University Press, 1987).

Gillingham, John, "Killing and mutilating political enemies in the British Isles from the late 12th to the early 14th century: a comparative study," in *Britain and Ireland 900–1300: Insular Responses to Medieval European Change*, ed. B. Smith (Cambridge: Cambridge University Press, 1999), 114–134.

Gilman, Sander, *Making the Body Beautiful: a Cultural History of Aesthetic Surgery* (Princeton/Oxford: Princeton University Press, 1999).

Girón-Negrón, Luis M., "How the go-between cut her nose: two Ibero-medieval translations of a *Kalilah wa Dimnah* story," in *Under the Influence: Questioning the Comparative in Medieval Castile*, ed. Leyla Rouhi and Cynthia Robinson (Leiden: Brill, 2005), 231–259.

Glaze, Florence Eliza, "Gariopontus and the Salernitans: textual traditions in the eleventh and twelfth centuries," in *"La Collectio Salernitana" di Salvatore de Renzi*, ed. D. Jacquart and A. Paravicini Bagliani (Florence: SISMEL-Edizioni del Galluzzo, 2009), 149–90.

Gluckmann, Max, "The peace in the feud," *Past and Present*, 8 (1955): 1–14.

Goffart, W., *The Narrators of Barbarian History* (Princeton: Princeton University Press, 1988).

Goffman, Erving, *Stigma: Notes on the Management of Spoiled Identity* (Englewood Cliffs, NJ: Prentice-Hall/London: Penguin, 1963).

Gonthier, Nicole, *Le châtiment du crime au Moyen Âge (XIIe-XVIe siècles)* (Rennes: Presses universitaires de Rennes, 1998).

Goodich, Michael, *Other Middle Ages: Witnesses at the Margins of Medieval Society* (Philadelphia: University of Pennsylvania Press, 1998).

Goudsblom, Johan, "Public health and the civilizing process," *Milbank Quarterly*, 64.2 (1986): 161–188.

Grabar and Carl Nordenfalk, *Early Medieval Painting* (Paris: Skira, 1957).

Grabes, Herbert, *The Mutable Glass: Mirror-Imagery in Titles and Texts of the Middle Ages and English Renaissance* (Cambridge: Cambridge University Press, 1982).

Green, Monica, "Bodily essences: bodies as categories of difference," in *A Cultural History of the Human Body in the Medieval Age*, ed. Linda Kalof (London: Bloomsbury, 2010), 149–172.

Gretsch, Mechthild, "The language of the 'Fonthill letter'," *Anglo-Saxon England*, 23 (1994): 57–102.

Griffiths, Fiona, *The Garden of Delights: Reform and Renaissance for Women in the Twelfth Century* (Philadelphia: University of Pennsylvania Press, 2006).

Grig, Lucy, "Torture and truth in late antique martyrology," *Early Medieval Europe*, 11.4 (2002): 321–336.

Groebner, Valentin, "Losing face, saving face: noses and honour in the late medieval town," *History Workshop Journal*, 40 (1995): 1–15.

Groebner, Valentin, *Defaced: the Visual Culture of Violence in the Later Middle Ages* (New York: Zone Books, 2004).

Groebner, *Who Are You? Identification, Deception and Surveillance in Early Modern Europe* (New York: Zone Books, 2007).

Hallaq, Wael B., *An Introduction to Islamic Law* (Cambridge, Cambridge University Press, 2009).

Halsall, Guy, "Playing by whose rules? A further look at Viking atrocity in the ninth century," *Medieval History*, 2.2 (1992): 3–12.

Halsall, Guy, *Warfare and Society in the Barbarian West, 450–900* (London: Routledge, 2003).

Hanawalt, Barbara, *Growing up in Medieval London: The Experience of Childhood in History* (New York and Oxford: Oxford University Press, 1995).

Head, Constance, *Justinian II of Byzantium* (Madison: University of Wisconsin Press, 1972).

Herrin, Judith, "Blinding in Byzantium," in *Polypleuros nous: Miscellanea für Peter Schreiner zu seinem 60 Geburtstag* (München: Saur, 2000): 56–68.

*Histoire de la Vergogne [History of Shame]*, Rives Méditerranéennes, 31 (2008).

*History-Writing and Violence in the Medieval Mediterranean*, ed. A. Liuzzo-Scorpo and J. Wood, *Al-Masāq: Journal of the Medieval Mediterranean*, 27 (2015).

Hodgson, Geoffrey, "Dermatology and history in Wales (Cymru)," *British Journal of Dermatology*, 90 (1974): 699–712.

Holck, P., "Two 'medical' cases from medieval Oslo," *International Journal of Osteoarchaeology*, 12.3 (2002): 166–172.

Hollis, Stephanie, "The social milieu of Bald's Leechbook," *AVISTA Forum Journal*, 14 (2004): 11–16.

*Honour and Shame: the Values of Mediterranean Society*, ed. J. Peristiany (Chicago: Chicago University Press, 1966).

Horden, Peregrine, "The year 1000: medical practice at the end of the first millennium," *Social History of Medicine*, 13 (2000): 201–219.

Horden, Peregrine, "Religion as medicine: music in hospitals," in *Religion and Medicine in the Middle Ages*, ed. Peter Biller and Joseph Ziegler (York: University of York, 2001), 135–153.

Horden, Peregrine, "The earliest hospitals in Byzantium, western Europe and Islam," *Journal of Interdisciplinary History*, 35 (2005): 361–389.

Horden, Peregrine, *Hospitals and Healing from Antiquity to the Later Middle Ages* (Aldershot: Variorum, 2008).

Horden, Peregrine, "Medieval medicine," in *The Oxford Handbook of the History of Medicine*, ed. M. Jackson (Oxford: Oxford University Press, 2011), 41–59.

Horden, Peregrine, "What's wrong with early medieval medicine?" *Social History of Medicine*, 24.1 (2011): 5–25.

Horton, Richard, "Offline: the moribund body of medical history," *The Lancet*, vol 384, issue 9940 (2014): 292.

*Hostage-Taking and Hostage Situations: the Medieval Precursors of a Modern Phenomenon*, ed. Matthew Bennett and Katherine Weikert (Abingdon: Routledge, forthcoming).

Hudson, John, "Violence, theft and the making of the English Common Law," in *Crime and Punishment in the Middle Ages: Papers presented at the 10th annual medieval workshop, University of Victoria, British Columbia, 8 February 1997*, ed. T. Haskett (Victoria, BC: Humanities Centre of the University of Victoria, 1998), 19–35.

Huizinga, Johan, *Waning of the Middle Ages* (Dutch first edition 1919, English translation published London: Edward Arnold, 1924).

*Icon and Word: the Power of Images in Byzantium*, ed. Antony Eastwood and Liz James (Aldershot: Ashgate, 2003).

Insley, Charles, "Rhetoric and ritual in late Anglo-Saxon charters," in *Medieval Legal Process: Physical, Spoken and Written Performance in the Middle Ages*, ed. Marco Mostert and Paul Barnwell (Turnhout: Brepols, 2011), 109–121.

Jacquart, Danielle, and Claude Thomasset, *Sexualité et savoir médical au moyen âge* (Paris: PUF, 1985).

Johns, Susan, *Noblewomen, Aristocracy and Power in the Twelfth-Century Anglo-Norman Realm* (Manchester: Manchester University Press, 2003).

Johnson, Lizabeth, "Attitudes towards spousal violence in medieval Wales," *Welsh History Review*, 24 (2009): 81–115.

Jones, E. E., A. Farina, A. Hastorf, H. Markus, D. Miller and R. A. Scott, *Social Stigma: the Psychology of Marked Relationships* (New York: Freeman, 1984).

Kaeuper, Richard, *Chivalry and Violence in Medieval Europe* (Oxford: Oxford University Press, 2001).

Kaldellis, Anthony, *The Argument of Psellos's* Chronographia (Leiden: Brill, 1999).

Karras, Ruth Mazo, *Sexuality in Medieval Europe: Doing unto Others* (New York: Routledge, 2005).

Kershaw, Paul, *Peaceful Kings: Peace, Power and the Early Medieval Imagination* (Oxford: Oxford University Press, 2011).

Kessler, Herbert, *Seeing Medieval Art* (New York: Broadview, 2004).

Kosto, Adam J., *Hostages in the Middle Ages* (Oxford: Oxford University Press, 2012).

Koziol, Geoffrey, "Review article - The dangers of polemic: is ritual still an interesting topic of historical study?", *Early Medieval Europe*, 11 (2002): 367–388.

Kristeva, Julia, *Powers of Horror: an Essay on Abjection*, tr. L. S. Roudiez (New York: Columbia University Press, 1982) [originally published as *Pouvoirs de l'horreur* (Paris: Seuil, 1980)].

Landi, Antonio, Maria C. Facchini, Antonio Saracino and Giuseppe Caserta, "Historical aspects," in *Reconstructive Surgery in Hand Mutilation*, ed. Guy Foucher (London: Martin Dunitz, 1997), 3–12.

*The Languages of Gift in the Early Middle Ages*, ed. Wendy Davies and Paul Fouracre (Cambridge: Cambridge University Press, 2014).

Larrington, Carolyne, "The psychology of emotion and the study of the medieval period," *Early Medieval Europe*, 10 (2001): 251–6.

*Law and Society in Byzantium: Ninth-Twelfth Centuries*, ed. Angeliki Laiou and Dieter Simon (Washington: Dumbarton Oaks, 1994).

*Law, Laity and Solidarities: Essays in Honour of Susan Reynolds*, ed. Pauline Stafford, Janet Nelson and Jane Martindale (Manchester: Manchester University Press, 2001).

Le Goff, Jacques, "Merchant's time and church's time in the middle ages," in *id., Time, Work and Culture in the Middle Ages*, tr. A. Goldhammer (Chicago, Chicago University Press, 1980), 29–42.

Le Goff, Jacques, *Medieval Civilization, 400–1500*, tr. J. Barrow (Oxford: Blackwell, 1988).

Leung, Angela K., and Dov Cohen, "Within- and between-culture variation: individual differences and the cultural logics of honor, face and dignity culture," *Journal of Personality and Social Psychology*, 100.3 (2011): 507–526.

Leyser, Conrad, "Long-haired kings and short-haired nuns: writing on the body in Caesarius of Arles," *Studia Patristica*, 24 (1993): 143–150.

Leyser, Conrad, "Masculinity in flux: nocturnal emission and the limits of celibacy in the early middle ages," in *Masculinity in Medieval Europe*, ed. D. M. Hadley (London: Longman, 1998), 103–119.

Maleon, Bogdan-Petrou, "La role de la mutilation dans la lutte politique a Byzance," in *Le corps et ses hypostases en Europe et dans la société roumaine du*

*Moyen Âge à l'époque contemporaine*, ed. Constanţa Vintilă- Ghiţulescu et Alexandru-Florin Platon (Bucharest: New Europe College, 2010), 125–146.

Maleon, Bogdan-Petrou, "The impossible return: about the status of deposed and mutilated emperors," *Medieval and Early Modern Studies for Central and Eastern Europe*, 3 (2011): 31–49.

Manchester, Keith, "Medieval leprosy: the disease and its management," in *Medicine in Early Medieval England: Four Papers*, ed. Marilyn Deegan and D. G. Scragg (Manchester: Centre for Anglo-Saxon Studies, 1987), 27–32.

Marlin, John, "The Investiture Contest and the rise of Herod plays in the twelfth century," *Early Drama, Art and Music Review*, 23 (2000): 1–18.

Marshall, Claire, "The politics of self-mutilation: forms of female devotion in the late middle ages," in *The Body in Late Medieval and Early Modern Culture*, ed. Darryl Grantley and Nina Taunton (Aldershot: Ashgate, 2000), 11–22.

Martinez Pizarro, Joaquín, *Writing Ravenna: The* Liber Pontificalis *of Andrea Agnellus* (Ann Arbor: University of Michigan Press, 1995).

Matter, E. Ann, "Theories of the passions and the ecstasies of late medieval religious women," *Essays in Medieval Studies*, 18 (2001): 1–16.

Mauss, Marcel, *The Gift: the Form and Reason for Exchange in Archaic Societies* (London: Cohen and West, 1954).

Mays, S. A., "A possible case of surgical treatment of cranial blunt force injury from medieval England," *International Journal of Osteoarchaeology*, 16.2 (2006): 95–103.

McCall, Andrew, *The Medieval Underworld* (Stroud: Sutton, 2004).

McCormick, Michael, *Eternal Victory: Triumphal Rulership in Late Antiquity, Byzantium and the Early Medieval West* (Cambridge: Cambridge University Press, 1986).

McGlynn, Sean, *By Sword and Fire: Cruelty and Atrocity in Medieval Warfare* (London: Weidenfeld and Nicolson, 2008).

McIlvenny, Paul, "The disabled male body 'writes/draws back': graphic fictions of masculinity in the autobiographical comic *The Spiral Cage*," in *Revealing Male Bodies*, ed. Nancy Tuana, William Cowling, Maurice Harrington, Greg Johnson and Terrance MacMullan (Bloomington/Indianapolis: Indiana University Press, 2002), 100–124.

McKinley, J., "A probable trepanation from an early Anglo-Saxon cemetery at Oxborough, Norfolk," *International Journal of Osteoarchaeology*, 2.4 (1992): 333–335.

McVaugh, Michael, "Surface meanings: the identification of apostemes in medieval surgery," in *Medical Latin from the Late Middle Ages to the 18th Century: Proceedings of the ESF Exploratory Workshop in the Humanities organized under the supervision of Albert Derolez, Brussels, 3–4 September 1999*, ed. W. Bracke and H. Deumans (Brussels: ESF, 2000), 13–29.

McVaugh, Michael, *The Rational Surgery of the Middle Ages* (Firenze, SISMEL-Edizioni del Galluzzo, 2006).

Meaney, Audrey, "Variant versions of Old English medical remedies and the compilation of Bald's Leechbook," *Anglo-Saxon England*, 13 (1984): 235–268.

*Medicine across Cultures*, ed. H. Selin and H. Shapiro (Berlin: Springer, 2003).

*Medicine and the Law in the Middle Ages*, ed. Wendy Turner and Sara Butler (Leiden: Brill, 2014).

*Medieval Mothering*, ed. J. Carmi Parsons and Bonnie Wheeler (New York: Garland, 1996).

Mellinkoff, Ruth, *The Mark of Cain: An Art Quantum* (Berkeley: University of California Press, 1981).

Mellinkoff, Ruth, *Outcasts: Signs of Otherness in Northern European Art of the Late Middle Ages*, 2 vols (Berkeley: California University Press, 1993).

Merback, Mitchell, *The Thief, the Cross and the Wheel: Pain and the Spectacle of Punishment in Medieval and Renaissance Europe* (London: Reaktion Books, 1999).

Metzler, Irina, *Disability in Medieval Europe: Thinking about Physical Impairment during the High Middle Ages* (London/New York: Routledge, 2006).

Metzler, Irina, *A Social History of Disability in the Middle Ages: Cultural Considerations of Physical Impairment* (London/New York: Routledge, 2013).

Miller, Andrew G., "'Tails' of masculinity: knights, clerics and the mutilation of horses in medieval England," *Speculum* 88 (2013): 958–995.

Miller, Sarah Alison, *Medieval Monstrosity and the Female Body* (London: Routledge, 2010).

Miller, Timothy, *The Birth of the Hospital in the Byzantine Empire* (Baltimore: Johns Hopkins University Press, 1985).

Miller, Timothy S., and John W. Nesbitt, *Walking Corpses: Leprosy in Byzantium and the Medieval West* (Ithaca, NY: Cornell University Press, 2014).

Miller, William Ian, *Bloodtaking and Peacemaking: Feud, Law and Society in Saga Iceland* (Chicago: Chicago University Press, 1990).

Miller, William Ian, *The Anatomy of Disgust* (Cambridge, MA: Harvard University Press, 1997).

Miller, William Ian, *Humiliation and Other Essays on Honor, Social Discomfort and Violence* (Ithaca/London: Cornell University Press, 1998).

Miller, William Ian, *Eye for an Eye* (Cambridge: Cambridge University Press, 2006).

Mirrer, Louise, "The 'unfaithful wife' in medieval Spanish literature and law," in *Medieval Crime and Social Control*, ed. Barbara Hanawalt and David Wallace (Minneapolis: University of Minnesota Press, 1999), 143–155.

Mitchell, Piers D., *Medicine in the Crusades: Warfare, Wounds and the Medieval Surgeon* (Cambridge: Cambridge University Press, 2004).

Mitchell, Piers D., "The torture of military captives in the crusades to the medieval Middle East," in *Noble Ideals and Bloody Realities: Warfare in the Middle Ages*, ed. N. Christie and M. Yazigi (Leiden: Brill, 2006), 97–118.

Mitchell, Piers D., "Trauma in the crusader period city of Caesarea: a major port in the medieval eastern Mediterranean," *International Journal of Osteoarchaeology*, 16.6 (2006): 493–505.

Mitchell, Piers D., Y. Nagar and R. Ellenbaum, "Weapon injuries in the 12th century crusader garrison of Vadum Iacob castle, Galilee," *International Journal of Osteoarchaeology*, 16.2 (2006): 145–155.

*Monks and Nuns, Saints and Outcasts*, ed. Lester K. Little, Sharon H. Farmer and Barbara H. Rosenwein (Ithaca, NY: Cornell University Press, 2000).

Moore, Alison M., "History, memory and trauma in photography of the *tondues*: visuality of the Vichy past through the silent image of women," *Gender and History*, 17 (2005), 657–681.

Moore, R. I., *The Formation of a Persecuting Society* (Oxford: Blackwell, 1987, 2nd ed., 2007).

Morris, Colin, *The Discovery of the Individual, 1050–1200* (New York and London: Harper and Row, 1972).

Moss, Candida, "Heavenly healing: eschatological cleansing and the resurrection of the dead in the holy church," *Journal of the American Academy of Religion*, 79 (2011): 991–1017.

*Motherhood, Religion and Society in Medieval Europe*, ed. Conrad Leyser and Lesley Smith (Farnham: Ashgate, 2011).

Mounsey, Chris, "Variability: beyond sameness and difference," in *The Idea of Disability in the 18th Century*, ed. Chris Mounsey (Plymouth: Bucknell University Press, 2014), 1–30.

Mulvey, Laura, *Visual and Other Pleasures: Theories of Representation and Difference* (Bloomington: Indiana University Press, 1989).

*Music as Medicine: the History of Music Therapy since Antiquity*, ed. Peregrine Horden (Aldershot: Ashgate, 2000).

Musson, A., "Crossing boundaries: attitudes to rape in late medieval England," in *Boundaries of the Law: Geography, Gender and Jurisdiction in Medieval and Early Modern Europe*, ed. A. Musson (Aldershot: Ashgate, 2005), 84–101.

Nash, Tina, *Out of the Darkness* (London: Simon and Schuster, 2012).

*Negotiating the Gift: Premodern Figurations of Exchange*, ed. A. Giladi, V. Groebner and B. Jussen (Göttingen: Vandenhoeck and Ruprecht, 2003).

Neuman, A. A., *The Jews in Spain*, I (Philadelphia: JPS, 1942).

*Noble Ideals and Bloody Realities: Warfare in the Middle Ages*, ed. N. Christie and M. Yazigi (Leiden: Brill, 2006).

Nokes, Richard Scott, "The several compilers of Bald's Leechbook," *Anglo-Saxon England*, 33 (2004): 51–76.

Olivelle, Patrick, "Penance and punishment: marking the body in criminal law and social ideology of ancient India," *Journal of Hindu Studies*, 4 (2011): 23–41.

Oliver, Lisi, "Sick maintenance in Anglo-Saxon law," *Journal of English and Germanic Philology*, 107.3 (2008): 303–326.

Oliver, Lisi, "Protecting the body in early medieval law," in *Peace and Protection in the Middle Ages*, ed. T. B. Lambert and D. Rollason (Durham: Centre for Medieval and Renaissance Studies, 2009), 60–77.

Oliver, Lisi, *The Body Legal in Barbarian Law* (Toronto: Toronto University Press, 2011).

Orme, Nicholas, *Medieval Children* (Yale: Yale University Press, 2003).

Ortner, D. J., "Human skeletal paleopathology," *International Journal of Paleopathology*, 1 (2011): 4–11.

Osborn Taylor, Henry, *The Medieval Mind: A History of the Development of Thought and Emotion in the Middle Ages*, 2 vols (London: Macmillan, 1911; repr. Cambridge, MA: Harvard University Press, 1959 and 1962).

Owens, L. S., "Craniofacial trauma in the prehispanic Canary Islands," *International Journal of Osteoarchaeology*, 17.5 (2007): 465–478.

*The Oxford Handbook of Women and Gender*, ed. Judith Bennett and Ruth Mazo Karras (Oxford: Oxford University Press, 2013).

Panhuysen, Raphael G. A. M., "Het scherp van de snede: sporen van geweld in vroegmiddeleeuws Maastricht," *Archeologie in Limburg*, 92 (2002): 2–7.

Parker, S. J., "Skulls, symbols and surgery: a review of the evidence for trepanation in Anglo-Saxon England and a consideration of the motives behind the practice," in *Superstition and Popular Magic in Anglo-Saxon England*, ed. D. Scragg (Manchester: Manchester Centre for Anglo-Saxon Studies, 1989), 73–84.

Partridge, James, *Changing Faces: the Challenge of Facial Disfigurement* (London: Penguin, 1990).

Patlagean, Evelyne, "Byzance et le blason pénal du corps," in *Du châtiment dans la cité: supplices corporels et peine de mort dans le monde antique: Table ronde, (Rome, 9–11 novembre 1982)* (Rome: École française de Rome, 1984), 405–427.

Patrick, P., "Approaches to violent death: a case study from early medieval Cambridge," *International Journal of Osteoarchaeology*, 16.4 (2006): 347–354.

Pattison, Stephen, *Saving Face: Enfacement, Shame, Theology* (Aldershot: Ashgate, 2013).

Pendergast, Mark, *Mirror Mirror: A History of the Human Love Affair with Reflection* (New York: Basic Books, 2003).

Phillips, Susan E., *Transforming Talk: the Problem with Gossip in Late Medieval England* (University Park: Penn State University Press, 2007).

Pilsworth, Clare, "Medicine and hagiography in Italy, 800–1000," *Social History of Medicine*, 13.2 (2000): 253–264.

Pilsworth, Clare, "'Can you just sign this for me John?': Doctors, charters and occupational identity in early medieval northern and central Italy," *Early Medieval Europe*, 17 (2009): 363–388.

Pilsworth, Clare, *Healthcare in Early Medieval Northern Italy: More to Life than Leeches* (Turnhout: Brepols, 2014).

Piper, Katie, *Beautiful* (London: Ebury Press, 2011).

Poggi, G., *Durkheim* (Oxford: Oxford University Press, 2000).

Polanichka, Dana, and Alex Cilley, "The very personal history of Nithard: family and honour in the Carolingian world," *Early Medieval Europe*, 22 (2014): 171–200.

*Politiques des émotions au Moyen Âge*, ed. Damian Boquet and Piroska Nagy (Florence: SISMEL-Edizioni del Galluzzo, 2010).

Pollock, F., and F. W. Maitland, *The History of English Law before the Time of Edward I*, 2 vols (Cambridge: Cambridge University Press, 1895).

Pormann Peter E., and Emilie Savage-Smith, *Medieval Islamic Medicine* (Edinburgh: Edinburgh University Press, 2010).

Porter, Martin, "A persistent fisnomical consciousness, c.400BC-c.1470CE," in *id., Windows of the Soul: The Art of Physiognomy in European Culture, 1470–1780* (Oxford: Oxford University Press, 2005).

Pouchelle, M.-C., *The Body and Surgery in the Middle Ages*, tr. R. Morris (Oxford, Polity Press, 1990).

Power, Eileen, *Medieval Women* (Cambridge: Cambridge University Press, 1975).

Powers, N., "Cranial trauma and treatment: a case study from the medieval cemetery of St Mary Spital, London," *International Journal of Osteoarchaeology*, 15 (2005): 1–14.

*Practical Medicine from Salerno to the Black Death*, ed. Luis Garcia-Ballester, Roger French, Jon Arrizabalaga and Andrew Cunningham (Cambridge: Cambridge University Press, 1994).

Prag, J., and R. Neave, *Making Faces: Using Forensic and Archaeological Evidence* (London, British Museum Press, 1997).

*Le prince au miroir de la littérature politique de l'Antiquité aux Lumières*, ed. F. Lachaud and L. Scordia (Rouen: Publications des universités de Rouen et du Havre, 2007).

*Property and Power in the Early Middle Ages*, ed. Wendy Davies and Paul Fouracre (Cambridge: Cambridge University Press, 1995).

Pugh, Tison, and Angela Jane Weisl, *Medievalisms: Making the Past in the Present* (Abingdon: Routledge, 2013).

Pulsiano, Philip, "Blessed bodies: the *vitae* of Anglo-Saxon female saints," *Parergon* 16.2 (1999): 1–42.

Rawcliffe, Carole, *Leprosy in Medieval England* (Woodbridge: Boydell, 2006).

Reisberg, D., and S. Habakuk, "A history of facial and ocular prosthetics," *Advances in Ophthalmic Plastic Reconstructive Surgery*, 8 (1990): 11–24.

*Religion and the Body*, ed. Sarah Coakley (Cambridge: Cambridge University Press, 1997).

Reynolds, Susan, "Early medieval law in India and Europe: a plea for comparison," *Medieval History Journal*, 16 (2013): 1–20.

Richards, Mary P., "I-II Cnut: Wulfstan's *Summa?*", in *English Law before Magna Carta*, ed. Stefan Jurasinski, Lisi Oliver and Andrew Rabin (Leiden: Brill, 2010), 137–156.

Richards, Peter, *The Medieval Leper and his Northern Heirs* (Cambridge: Brewer, 1977).

Richardson, Kristina L., *Difference and Disability in the Medieval Islamic World: Blighted Bodies* (Edinburgh: Edinburgh University Press, 2012).

Risse, Guenter P., *Mending Bodies, Saving Souls: a History of Hospitals* (Oxford: Oxford University Press, 1999).

Roberts, Charlotte, and Keith Manchester, *The Archaeology of Disease*, 3rd ed. (Stroud: Sutton, 2005).

Roffey, Simon, and Katie Tucker, "A contextual study of the medieval hospital and cemetery of St Mary Magdalen, Winchester, England," *International Journal of Paleopathology*, 2.4 (2012): 170–180.

Rosenwein, Barbara H., "Writing without fear about early medieval emotions," *Early Medieval Europe*, 10 (2001): 229–234.

Rosenwein, Barbara H., "Worrying about emotions in history," *American Historical Review*, 107 (2002): 821–845.

Rosenwein, Barbara H., "Identity and emotions in the early middle ages," in *Die Suche nach den Ursprüngen: Von der Bedeutung des frühen Mittelalters*, ed. Walter Pohl (Vienna: VÖAW, 2004), 129–137.

Rosenwein, Barbara H., "Histoire de l'émotion: méthodes et approches," *Cahiers de civilisation médiévale*, 49.193 (2006): 33–48.

Rosenwein, Barbara H., *Emotional Communities in the Early Middle Ages* (Ithaca, NY: Cornell University Press, 2006).

Roth, Norman, *Jews, Visigoths and Muslims in Medieval Spain: Cooperation and Conflict* (Leiden: Brill, 1994).

Rubin, Stanley, *Medieval English Medicine* (London: David & Charles, 1974).

Rubin, "The Anglo-Saxon physician," in *Medicine in Early Medieval England: Four Papers*, ed. Marilyn Deegan and D. G. Scragg (Manchester: Centre for Anglo-Saxon Studies, 1987), 7–15.

Rubini, M., and P. Zaio, "Warriors from the East: skeletal evidence of warfare from a Lombard-Avar cemetery in central Italy (Campochiaro, Molise, 6th-8th century AD)," *Journal of Archaeological Science*, 38 (2011): 1551–1559.

Runciman, Steven, "The Empress Irene the Athenian," in *Medieval Women*, ed. Baker, 101–118.

Sanborn, L., "Anglo-Saxon medical practices and the *Peri Didaxeon*," *Revue de l'Université d'Ottawa*, 55 (1985): 7–13.

Sauerländer, Willibald, "The fate of the face in medieval art," in *Set in Stone: the Face in Medieval Sculpture*, ed. C. T. Little (New York: Metropolitan Museum, 2006), 3–17.

Segal, Einat, "Sculpted images from the eastern gallery of the St-Trophime cloister in Arles and the Cathar heresy," in *Difference and Identity in Francia and Medieval France*, ed. Meredith Cohen and Justine Firnhaber-Baker (Farnham and Burlington: Ashgate, 2010), 67–69.

*Set in Stone: the Face in Medieval Sculpture*, ed. C. T. Little (New York: Metropolitan Museum of Art, 2006).

*The Settlement of Disputes in Early Medieval Europe*, ed. Wendy Davies and Paul Fouracre (Cambridge: Cambridge University Press, 1986).

*Shame between Punishment and Penance: the Social Uses of Shame in the Middle Ages and Early Modern Times*, ed. Bénédicte Sère and Jörg Wettlaufer (Florence: SISMEL-Edizioni del Galluzzo, 2013).

Shanmugarajah, K., S. Gaind, A. Clarke and P. E. M. Butler, "The role of disgust emotions in the observer response to facial disfigurement," *Body Image*, 9 (2012): 455–461.

Shaw, W., "Folklore surrounding facial deformity and the origins of facial prejudice," *British Journal of Plastic Surgery* 34 (1981): 237–246.

Sheehan, Sarah, "Losing face: Heroic discourse and inscription in flesh in *Scéla Mucce Meic Dathó*," in *The Ends of the Body: Identity and Community in Medieval Culture*, ed. Suzanne Conklin Akbari and Jill Ross (Toronto: Toronto University Press, 2013), 132–152.

Shoham, S., *The Mark of Cain: the Stigma Theory of Crime and Social Deviation* (Jerusalem: Israel University Press, 1970).

Shoham-Steiner, Ephraim, "Poverty and disability: a medieval Jewish perspective," in *The Sign Languages of Poverty*, ed. Gerhard Jaritz (Vienna: VÖAW, 2007), 75–94.

Shoham-Steiner, Ephraim, *On the Margins of a Minority: Leprosy, Madness and Disability among the Jews of Medieval Europe* (Detroit: Wayne State University Press, 2014).

Singer, Julie, *Blindness and Therapy in Late Medieval French and Italian Poetry* (Woodbridge: Boydell and Brewer, 2011).

Skey, Miriam Anne, "The iconography of Herod in the Fleury Playbook and in the visual arts," in *The Fleury Playbook: Essays and Studies*, ed. C. Clifford Flanigan, Thomas P. Campbell and Clifford Davidson (Kalamazoo: Medieval Institute, 1985), 120–143.

Skinner, Patricia, *Health and Medicine in Early Medieval Southern Italy* (Leiden: Brill, 1997).

Skinner, Patricia, "'The light of my eyes': medieval motherhood in the Mediterranean", *Women's History Review*, 6.3 (1997): 391–410.

Skinner, "A cure for a sinner: sickness and healthcare in medieval southern Italy," in *The Community, the Family and the Saint: Patterns of Power in Early Medieval Europe*, ed. J. Hill and M. Swann (Leeds/Turnhout: Brepols, 1998), 297–309.

Skinner, Patricia, "'And her name was?' Gender and naming in medieval southern Italy," *Medieval Prosopography*, 20 (1999): 23–49.

Skinner, Patricia, "The gendered nose and its lack: 'medieval' nose-cutting and its modern manifestations", *Journal of Women's History*, 26.1 (2014): 45–67.

Skinner, Patricia, "Marking the face, curing the soul? Reading the disfigurement of women in the later middle ages," in *Medicine, Religion and Gender in Medieval Culture*, ed. Naoë Kukita Yoshikawa (Woodbridge: Boydell, 2015), 287–318.

Skinner, Patricia, "Visible prowess? Reading men's head and face wounds in early medieval Europe to 1000CE," in *Wounds and Wound Repair in Medieval Culture*, ed. Larissa Tracy and Kelly de Vries (Leiden: Brill, forthcoming).

Skoda, Hannah, *Medieval Violence: Physical Brutality in Northern France, 1270–1330* (Oxford: Oxford University Press, 2013).

Smail, Daniel Lord, "Violence and predation in later medieval Mediterranean Europe," *Comparative Studies in Society and History*, 54.1 (2012): 7–34.

Sontag, Susan, *Regarding the Pain of Others* (New York: Picador, 2003).

Sperati, G., "Amputation of the nose through history," *Acta Otorhinolaryngologica Italica*, 29 (2009): 44–50.

Stafford, Pauline, "Sons and mothers: family politics in the Middle Ages," in *Medieval Women: Essays presented to Professor Rosalind M. T. Hill*, ed. Derek Baker (Oxford: Blackwell, 1978), 79–100.

Stafford, Pauline, *Gender, Family and the Legitimation of Power* (Aldershot: Ashgate, 2006).

*Stigma: the Experience of Disability*, ed. Paul Hunt (London: Geoffrey Chapman, 1966).

Stone, Rachel, "Kings are different: Carolingian mirrors for princes and lay morality," in *Le prince au miroir de la littérature politique de l'Antiquité aux Lumières*, ed. F. Lachaud and L. Scordia (Rouen: Publications des universités de Rouen et du Havre, 2007), 69–86.

*The Stranger in Medieval Society*, ed. F. R. P. Akehurst and Stephanie Cain Van d'Elden (Minneapolis: Minnesota University Press, 1997).

*Le sujet des émotions au Moyen Âge*, ed. Damian Boquet and Piroska Nagy (Paris: Editions Beauchesne, 2009).

*Symposium on Byzantine Medicine: Dumbarton Oaks Papers* 38, ed. John Scarborough (Washington: Dumbarton Oaks Research Library, 1985).

Tajfel, Henri, "Intergroup relations, social myths and social justice in social psychology", in *The Social Dimension*, ed. H. Tajfel, II (Cambridge: Cambridge University Press, 1984).

Tibbetts Schulenberg, Jane, *Forgetful of their Sex: Female Sanctity and Society c.500–1100* (Chicago: Chicago University Press, 1998).

*The Treatment of Disabled Persons in Medieval Europe*, ed. Wendy Turner and Tory Vandeventer Pearman (Lampeter: Edwin Mellen, 2010).

Treharne, Elaine, *Living through Conquest: the Politics of Early English* (Oxford: Oxford University Press, 2012).

Upson-Saia, Kristi, "Resurrecting deformity: Augustine on wounded and scarred bodies in the heavenly realm", in *Disability in Judaism, Christianity, and Islam: Sacred Texts, Historical Traditions, and Social Analysis*, ed. Darla Schumm and Michael Stoltzfus (New York: Palgrave Macmillan, 2011), 93–122.

van Eickels, Klaus, "Gendered violence: castration and blinding as punishment for treason in Normandy and Anglo-Norman England," *Gender and History*, 16.3 (2004): 588–602.

van Krieken, Robert, "Violence, self-discipline and modernity: beyond the 'civilizing process'," *Sociological Review*, 37.2 (1989): 193–218.

Vandeventer Pearman, Tory, *Women and Disability in Medieval Literature* (New York: Palgrave Macmillan, 2011).

*Violence and Society in the Early Medieval West*, ed. Guy Halsall (Woodbridge: Boydell, 2002).

*Violence and the Writing of History in the Medieval Francophone World*, ed. Noah D. Guynn and Zrinka Stahuljak (Cambridge: D. S. Brewer, 2013).

*Violence in Medieval Society*, ed. R. W. Kaeuper (Woodbridge: Boydell, 2000).

*Violences souveraines au Moyen Âge*, ed. F. Feronda *et al.* (Paris: PUF, 2010).

Vives, E., and D. Campilo, "Hipertrofia de un cornete nasal en una mujer procente del cementerio medieval de Sant Marçal en Avinyó (Barcelona)," in *XXVII Congreso internacional de historia de la medicina, 31 agosto-6 septiembre 1980: actas* (Barcelona, Acadèmia de Ciències Mèdiques de Catalunya I Balears, 1981), 669–670.

Waldron, Tony, *Palaeopathology* (Cambridge: Cambridge University Press, 2008).

Wallace-Hadrill, J. M., *The Long-Haired Kings and other Studies on Frankish History* (New York: Barnes and Noble, 1962).

Watkin, T. G., *The Legal History of Wales* (Cardiff: University of Wales Press, 2007).

Watts, Richard J., *Politeness* (Cambridge: Cambridge University Press, 2003).

*Weapons and Warfare in Anglo-Saxon England*, ed. Sonia Chadwick Hawkes (Oxford: Oxford Committee for Archaeology, 1989).

Weston, Simon, *Going Back: Return to the Falklands* (London: Penguin, 1992).

Wheatley, Edward, *Stumbling Blocks before the Blind: Medieval Constructions of a Disability* (Ann Arbor: University of Michigan Press, 2010).

*Why the Middle Ages Matter: Medieval Light on Modern Injustice*, ed. C. Chazelle, S. Doubleday, F. Lifschitz and A. Remensnyder (New York: Routledge, 2012)

Wickham, Chris, "Gossip and resistance among the medieval peasantry," *Past and Present*, 160 (1998): 3–24.

Wickham, Chris, *Courts and Conflict in Twelfth-Century Tuscany* (Oxford: Oxford University Press, 2003).

Wilson, Dudley, *Signs and Portents: Monstrous Birth from the Middle Ages to the Enlightenment* (London and New York: Routledge, 1993).

Wilson, Stephen, *The Means of Naming: a Social History* (London: UCL Press, 1998).

*Women in the Middle East: Perceptions, Realities and Struggles for Liberation*, ed. H. Afshar (Basingstoke: Macmillan, 1993).

*Women Writers of the Middle Ages: a Critical Study of Texts from Perpetua to Marguerite Porete*, ed. Peter Dronke (Cambridge: Cambridge University Press, 1984).

Wormald, Patrick, *Legal Culture in the Early Medieval West: Law as Text, Image and Experience* (London: Hambledon, 1999).

Wormald, Patrick, *The Making of English Law: King Alfred to the Twelfth Century*, vol 1 (Oxford: Blackwell, 1999).

*Wounds and Wound Repair in Medieval Culture*, ed. Kelly DeVries and Larissa Tracy (Leiden: Brill, 2015).

*Wounds in the Middle Ages*, ed. Anne Kirkham and Cordelia Warr (Aldershot: Ashgate, 2014).

*The Year 1000: Medical Practice at the End of the First Millennium*, ed. Peregrine Horden and Emilie Savage-Smith, *Social History of Medicine*, 13.2 (2000).

Yuval-Davis, N., *Gender and Nation* (London: Sage, 1997).

Zemon Davies, Natalie, *The Return of Martin Guerre* (Cambridge, MA: Harvard University Press, 1984).

Zemon Davies, Natalie, "Remaking impostors: from Martin Guerre to Sommersby," *Hayes Robinson Lecture Series*, 1 (Egham: Royal Holloway University of London, 1997).

# INDEX

---

Note: Page numbers followed by "n" denote notes.

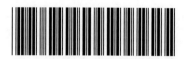